EVOLUTION
of
HOMOEOPATHIC REPERTORIES
and
REPERTORISATION

EVOLUTION
of
HOMOEOPATHIC REPERTORIES
and
REPERTORISATION

Dr. Jugal Kishore

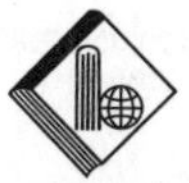

B. Jain Publishers (P) Ltd.
An ISO 9001 : 2000 Certified Company
USA—EUROPE—INDIA

EVOLUTION OF HOMOEOPATHIC REPERTORIES AND REPERTORISATION

First Edition : 1998
Revised Edition: 2004
3rd Impression: 2009

Published by Kuldeep Jain for
B. JAIN PUBLISHERS (P) LTD.
An ISO 9001 : 2000 Certified Company
1921/10, Chuna Mandi, Paharganj, New Delhi 110 055 (INDIA)
Tel.: 91-11-2358 0800, 2358 1100, 2358 1300, 2358 3100
Fax: 91-11-2358 0471 • Email: info@bjain.com
Website: www.bjainbooks.com

Printed in India by
J.J. Offset Printers

ISBN: 978-81-319-0804-4

CONTENTS

INTRODUCTION

During my early adventures in the discoveries of the role of homoeopathic medicine in sickness, I became excited by the work done by the early pioneers in the field of Repertory making. Boenninghausen's Therapeutic Book was my first love in this area, and now I remember with nostalgia and a little surprise also, how a number of good cases were cured with the help of this little book. Gradually, I got introduced to quite a number of other workers, especially Kent and Boger, and that led me to discover how the concept and philosophy of indexing out vast Materia Medica changed from one author to another. Unless we understand the basis of structure behind the Repertories, we cannot do justice to the study of any single Repertory. There was a kind of evolution taking place all the time, and this has to be understood properly by the students of homoeopathy.

This excitement, coupled with the practical experience in the clinics, made me look every where for the sources of Repertory making. Later on, I was able to develop an Integrated Card Repertory, which was in a way, a precursor of the present Computerised Repertories. I have tried in the book, to give some information about the birth, growth and development of the repertories in general, and I have also given various requirements for utilizing different Repertories, their advantages and disadvantages. A number of repertorial case records, by different clinicians and myself, have been given.

In my work, I have been blessed with the devotion and dedicated assistance of my young colleagues, in the area of research in Homoeopathic literature, who worked hard, and enabled me to finalize this book. It was specially Dr. Rashmi Pasricha who managed to get the relevant material properly organized and processed it through the computer. Without her professional commitment, I could not have finished this work.

I hope that both the practitioners and the students of Homoeopathic medicine will find this material worthy of their time spent on reading it.

November 30, 1997 Dr. Jugal Kishore

THE AUTHOR

Dr. Jugal Kishore graduated from the former Christian College, Lahore (Punjab University) securing the highest aggregate marks. He won merit scholarships all through in school and college. He graduated in Homoeopathic Medicine securing first position in merit from faculty of Homoeopathic Medicine, Bengal and later he was awarded MD (Homoeopathic Medicine) by Homoeopathic Medical Council of West Bengal. He was conferred Honorary Fellowship by the Homoeopathic Federation, Pakistan as well as by the Homoeopathic Association of Ceylon. Ever since then, he has been in private practice. His vast experience of several decades to the service of mankind, has placed him in the list of few most eminent Homoeopathic physicians and consultants of the world.

Throughout his professional career, Dr. Jugal Kishore has served numerous top professional positions such as Honorary Physician to the President of India for four terms; President of Central Council of Homoeopathy; Honorary Advisor in Homoeopathy to the Government of India from 1972 to 1979; President of All India Homoeopathic Association of India for two terms; Chief National Executive of International Homoeopathic Medical Organization; Honorary Founder Director of Nehru Homoeopathic Medical College, New Delhi; Special invitee of The International Research Council; President of the Asian Homoeopathic Medical League; Chairman Sharda Boiron Laboratories Pvt. Ltd. in collaboration with France; Professor Emeritus of Rajasthan University to guide MD students; Consultant in the field of training and evaluation by Northampton University etc. The list is so long that it may require a special booklet. Presently also, he is Visiting Professor and Honorary Consultant Nehru homoeopathic Medical College, New Delhi; Chairman Emeritus of Sharda Boiron Lab. Pvt. Ltd.; President of the Governing Body of Central Council of Research in Homoeopathy, Govt. of India and Executive Committee of Central Council of Research in Homoeopathy, Govt. of India.

Dr. Jugal Kishore is author of world's largest Card Repertory, a punch-card system for analysing indicated remedy in chronic and difficult cases. He has contributed many outstanding articles in the National and International Periodicals of repute. Young medical doctors are trained in the clinic of Dr. Jugal Kishore with the very idea of sharing his vast and unlimited experience to the new generation for serving the humanity in future.

Dr. Jugal Kishore has made original contribution on the provings and actual application of Saraca Indica, Sulphurous acid, Cynadon dac, Abroma augusta, M & B 693 and Tylophora indica.

He has travelled intensively and extensively in India and all over the world for professional purposes since he has always looked at the problems of millions of suffering mankind from the humanitarian angle to service selflessly.

THE BOOK

This book details the history of the birth, growth and development of Homoeopathic Repertories. It started during Hahnemann's time, as the Homoeopathic pioneers needed some sort of Index for the symptoms of the Homoeopathic remedies. The growth of the Materia Medica compelled them to such ready reference and indices.

For the students of Homoeopathic Medicine, the author indicates the importance of knowing the background and the genius behind the work done by different workers. He has enumerated different Repertories, and how, apart from working as mere indices, they could be utilised as philosophic and scientific guides for proper case taking, evaluation of symptoms and different ways of analysis of the indicated remedies.

The author was stimulated and excited by the efforts and achievements of these pioneers and tried to pass on, at least, some part of its to the students, teachers and readers.

Hahnemann's principles, as laid down in the Organon, and his philosophical guidance has been dove-tailed in the relevant portion of the different chapters of the book.

This kind of the book is needed badly by the profession, teachers and students, especially, for the post-graduate students of Homoeopathic Repertory.

Chapter One

THE REPERTORIES IN GENERAL

Introduction:

A homoeopathic physician, who is keenly interested in doing the best for his patient in the given circumstances has a very difficult task regarding the choice of remedies unlike the 'allopathic' colleagues. There may be different pathways for helping a patient but, the ideal, the most scientific and 'most' curative is the practice of classical homoeopathy, but this kind of practice requires a deep and extensive study of homoeopathic Materia Medica, accumulation of experience or learning at the feet of more experienced practicing teachers or 'gurus', development of perceptive qualities of mind and heart and possible spiritual bent of mind.

Luckily, one of the great instruments at his disposal for sifting through the maze of symptoms of such a large number of remedies in the Materia Medica is the 'Homoeopathic Repertory'. Unfortunately, the homoeopathic repertory suffers from handicaps because of inherent difficulties in their structuring. There are scores of repertories, big and small, but none is perfect or can be complete, although we have to depend on them all the same, with all their limitations.To use these instruments effectively, their structure, historical and evolutionary developments have to be thoroughly studied in depth, before we can utilize them properly. They, too, will always remain the servant and not the master. Card repertories and now Computers are again a second fine of servants, and have to be utilized very carefully, as they can mislead one, if the right structuring of the software is not done or the right kind of inquiry inputs are not made.

Even then it is the Materia Medica ultimately, coupled with clinical experience which is the last court of appeal for judgement making.

The Repertory-making is a never-ending activity. It requires to be nourished time and again and that is when we have to lay the right foundation for correct parameters for data collection and indexing. This applies to both written books or any other kind of storage or activating of such a data in Computers.

What is a Repertory?

The word Repertory has originated from the Latin word 'REPERTORIUM' which means 'an inventory; a table or a compendium, where the contents are so arranged that they are easy to find'. It is a store house for finding something; a veritable treasury. It is essentially a classified index for a mass of knowledge; in short, a dictionary or an index. Hence, basically, the Homoeopathic Repertory is an index to the huge mass of symptoms of various drugs of the Homoeopathic Materia Medica.

It adds nothing, changes nothing, but serves merely as a guide to the mass, lets us say the labyrinth of the Materia Medica. In a Repertory, we have separation by analysis for the purpose of classification and ready reference; in Materia Medica, a combination by synthesis to enable us to study drug effects in their grand unity and relationship. All of us repertorise when we prescribe a drug. Most of us use only our own mental repertory, which is naturally limited because of our limited capacity to remember all the details. In Repertory we can have an arrangement whereby we do the regional and symptomatic classification and indexing of the remedies of our Materia

Medica.

The indexing of such varieties of signs, symptoms and expressions, encompassing the man as a whole, both in his mental and physical expressions of sickness, whether artificially produced or in its natural form, is a task of very great difficulty. This is why we find different authors or compilers producing different repertories with different modes of indexing. Two different authors may not mean the same thing by even a common expression like 'Pain'.

Need for a Repertory

The introduction and development of the Homoeopathic Materia Medica by Hahnemann was a unique phenomenon in the history of medicine. No system of medicine had discovered and put down in ink such minute details about medicines and their characteristics. All these facts were mostly noted from experiments on healthy human beings. As the volume of the Homoeopathic Materia Medica expanded and remedies multiplied, it became a problem to apply this knowledge according to the directions laid down by Hahnemann. In his own time, Hahnemann, too, became conscious about the need for suitable indices to the growing 'Materia Medica'. As early as 1805 in his famous 'Fragmenta de viribus medica mentorum positivis' published in Latin, the first part contained symptoms which were observed in the provers and the second part formed the index, or the repertory. It is, thus seen that Hahnemann was the first Repertorian or father of Homoeopathic Repertory.

As the inscription on the first page indicates that Hahnemann had referred to Repertories in his directions for treatment of chronic diseases. Here were Hahnemann and his disciples, who knew their remedies better and most intimately because they had experimented on their own bodies and had suffered. They could not forget the exact impressions. During Hahnemann's time, he and his disciples had proved about 100 remedies. In spite of the smaller number of drugs and their close intimacy with the details of symptoms, Hahnemann and his band of workers started to bend their genius to the making of Repertories. In comparison with the small number of remedies at that time, it is estimated that by 1921, we had 1600 remedies listed in our Materia Medica, out of which 1300 were tested on human body. In 1955 the number had gone to about 2000, out of which 1500 have been tested on human beings. Imagine somebody trying to select a remedy from the ten volumes of Allen's Encyclopaedia. This is well nigh an impossible task. To quote Dr. P. Schmidt, "How many homoeopaths know these by their symptoms, even by their names; many of them are absolutely unknown. How many know the symptoms of 'Linaria Vulgaris' - repeated fainting fits and the frequent need to urinate at night; and of 'Macuna Urens', that plant from Venezuela, which causes such burning and is always associated with haemorrhoids? No one can know everything, and that is why, in all honesty, one must admit that no conscientious homoeopathic doctor can practice homoeopathy in a serious and really scientific way without a Repertory". Repertories had to be made to serve as a ready index to the vast structure of homoeopathic symptomatology. This is why, men like Boenninghausen applied their mind to the discovery of better methods of selecting the similimum. To meet the challenge of the exploding Materia Medica, the Homoeopathic Repertory was born.

Difficulties in making a Repertory

Our Materia Medica, which is built up not only on the data from human 'provings' but also on clinical findings and confirmations of action of the remedies, is itself a very complex entity because of the complexity of human beings themselves. To classify and tabulate mental symptoms is one of the most complicated task. Different people conceive or understand differently the different words or symptoms expressing the mental or emotional feelings or complaints. That is why, a number of authors have given numerous cross-references in the chapters concerned with mental symptoms or Mind.

Even in the area of different pains and sensations, one cannot be very sure of what the prover has exactly meant by a kind of pain.

Our task would have been much easier, if we had only to deal with objective signs and symptoms, but the subjective symptoms of provers and hence, of patients have a great value. Then there is the difficulty of placing and indexing of associated symptoms (concomitants).

Apart from these things, there are a very large number of drugs or remedies which have to be indexed. There are some remedies which have much larger data than others with the result that remedies like Sulphur, Belladonna, Bryonia, Calc carb, Sepia etc. have been over-indexed. Hence, in repertorisation of clinical cases, some of these polycrests elbow out other important but lesser proved drugs. The indicated remedy may be one of the latter.

Sometimes Repertory makers placed very similar or same symptoms in different places because the provers or proving masters had given different expressions. Let us take the case of a pre-maturely looking old patient. One has not only to see in 'Generalities' - old age, premature, but also see under 'Face' - expression, old looking.

No repertory can serve fully and accurately an index to the Materia Medica. It is well-nigh an impossibility. For example, patients talk of 'coldness and numbness of the heels' or complain of 'pain in left groin extending to left thigh, a raging pain as if an injection bursting through a fine blood-vessel' or a complex symptom, 'pain, during menses, located in the forehead, aggravated by stooping, and extending to occiput, with sweating of forehead' etc. One can imagine the difficulties of indexing such symptoms.We have to break up these symptoms and place or index them in suitable areas of functions etc.

It required many men of genius to solve the problems

of indexing the symptoms of our Materia Medica. It was and is still a very tricky problem. They had each a different solution or way of solving it. The best and the perfect has yet to be discovered.

Very often, the authors themselves had to give cross-references or pointers for seeing other similar rubrics. Boger, in his Repertory, has given a very large number of cross-references in his chapter on Mind.

Kent has often mentioned 'see other rubrics'. For example, under 'Mind - Fear, men of', he has referred to see also 'Fear, people of ' (page 46). Similarly 'Mind, childish behaviour' (page 11), see also 'Mind, foolish behaviour' (page 48); Fear (See Anxiety). Very often we find that one becomes anxious from fear. These two emotions are so closely intermingled. Similarly 'Hurry' and 'Impatience' have to be carefully analysed. An impatient person may be driven to hurry. In normal activities he may not be hurried.

Kent has refered us to 'Malicious' and 'Misanthropy' when he has taken up the rubric of 'Hatred'. There are numerous such examples. This proves, beyond any doubt, the difficulties of indexing mental symptoms in our Repertories. A student of Repertory has to, therefore, go deeply into the mental picture of the patient and make an adequate search for the right rubric.

Because of these difficulties, different authors of different Repertories naturally started making Repertories in different ways, which again created confusion amongst the students and practitioners. The controversies between followers of Boenninghausen and Kentian Repertories continue even to this day. In those days, our old masters did not possibly have the opportunity or facilities to sit together and work out common standard i.e. commonly accepted format and structure of our Repertory.

Even today, there is a need for having an international

forum for malting an integrated Repertory and review the guidelines laid down for indexing the newer provings. Even before this is done, this forum could be used also for verifying the authenticity of the 'Provings' material.

It is, therefore, very important to understand deeply the evolution and development of the Homoeopathic Repertory and the philosophy behind the construction of each Repertory. A Repertory is only as good as a knowledge of structural arrangement and understanding of the author's directions for use.

There are, however, homoeopathic prescribers who spurn the use of Repertories. For them it is a closed chapter. They consider it a waste of their time even to open these books. Dr. Neatby of England, admitted in one of the professional meetings that he had found no use for his Kent's Repertory and had to dispose it off to a second-hand bookseller. Dr. Boger once remarked that there were homoeopathic doctors who never had anything to do with the Repertory and had never opened one in their life time. They were sleepers and must be waked up. They must remember that Repertories like husbands are a necessary evil. It is not possible to do without them, unless they develop their brains to a giant size.

Skill in the use of a Repertory is some hundred of times more valuable than the most prodigious feats in the memorizing of symptoms. It is singularly easy for the practitioners, who depend much upon memory, to fall into oft-travelled ruts, which grow deeper, with each easy, thoughtless, habitual process of his mind.

For example, 'Worse from motion' infallibly calls up Bryonia as 'better from motion' does Rhustox, because we have grooves in our mind that make these phrases lead us to the remedies named. Yes, in certain circumstances Bryonia, though worse from beginning to move like Rhustox, is better by movement later on. Many other remedies that are worse from motion, and many others that are better, therefore, should be given a chance to prove their appropriateness, and it is by the use of a Repertory that they can be given due weight and proper consideration.

It is the curse of memorized keynotes that they strongly converge the mind towards ruts and routine prescribing causing a few of the polycrests to occupy an unduly prominent place in our armamentarium.

The use of Repertories and their study frees the mind from bondage of fixed ideas about symptoms and the tyranny of a few important remedies.

Dr. J.B.S. King wrote in 1909 in his editorial in the Medical Advance, the urgent need for improving the educational systems in the Homoeopathic Medical Colleges in America, especially with regard to the teaching of Materia Medica. We in India too, had followed similar modes and curriculae of teaching in our early Medical Colleges. In the following words, he has emphasized the imperative need for study of Repertories.

"It is a remark of Benjamin Franklin, that because he had a very good memory in his youth, he had learned to depend upon it to such an extent, that when his faculties became impaired with age, he was unable to supplement them successfully by using memoranda, never having formed that excellent habit in his early days.

Homoeopathic students with retentive memories, who study Materia Medica on the memorising method, fostered by the prevalent inadequate system of teaching, are not unlikely to find themselves in the position complained of by Franklin.

By the aid of 'Keynote' or 'characteristics', ten or twelve striking symptoms of each of a dozen polycrests and 3 or four symptoms of twenty less important ones are memorised On this slender basis, the student plumes himself on his knowledge, gets a standing of 100 and smilingly receives the congratulations of his friends. This is not an over-estimate of the amount of Materia Medica learnt, nor an under-estimate of high esteem in which he holds himself. Hundreds of graduates of Homoeopathic colleges have gone forth and still go forth this way

Memory is the meanest of the faculties required in this study; it should be only a servant, yet by the usual methods of teaching, it is exalted to the first rank.

How to find the one remedy (out of at least three or four hundred), that is needed to cure a given case, is the most important information that can possibly be given to the prospective prescriber. This cannot be done by any man's memory, but only from the skillful use of our records. Indispensable to the successful prosecution of this search, is the use of a Repertory, that is of a book in which remedies are collected according to the state of the body."

I have intentionally emphasised the points raised by Dr. J.B.S. King, because in our Institutions in India, we have been following what was happening in American Homoeopathic Colleges. It is still being followed in some of our colleges here.

But recently the pendulum has swung to the other side with the result that the students, especially in Europe, depend only on Repertory and fail to grasp the finer nuances, which have been handed down to us by experienced authors of Materia Medica. They try to learn Materia Medica from the rubrics of the Repertory.

In actual practice, there are two kinds of cases that come to every physician. One is the case that may be prescribed for, with certainty of success on the symptoms that are styled characteristic and peculiar. In some cases, however, the Repertory is necessary where drug picture is not clearly marked or there is absence of the dependable characteristic symptoms.

In every case , one does not go through the elaborate process of repertorising 10 or 15 rubrics as in some of the cases, the cardinal or deciding symptom can unlock the mysteries of the indicated remedy. That is why, very careful case-taking and then proper evaluation of the symptoms is a must before consulting the Repertories or Materia Medica. It seems paradoxical to the beginner to be told that proper case taking and evaluation of the symptoms requires a fairly deep knowledge of Homoeopathic Repertories, Materia Medica and of course, Homoeopathic philosophy.

The following is the case cited by a colleague of ours, Dr. Usmani, which will illustrate my point. Of course, many such examples can be cited, especially when a train of complaints or symptoms have followed a particular causation like a sudden grief, fright, or a severe infection.

"This is the case of chronic bronchial catarrh (wheezy chest) which defied all treatment. A barely one year old had frequent attacks of bronchitis which was often accompanied by diarrhoea. Slightest exposure to cold or ingestion of cold food or drinks would bring on the attack. She had tardy dentition and started standing or walking rather late. All sorts of medicines were prescribed like Ant-tart, Ipecac, Calc-carb, Lycopodium, Sulphur, Belladonna, Spongia and Bacillinum. There was only temporary relief. One day the mother casually remarked that it was a problem to get the child to bed, that she was unusually lively and active before going to sleep. She would cry if you made her lie down by force. She would get up and start playing by herself. Now there are two remedies that have the symptom - 'Excitement before going to sleep' i.e. Psorinum and Nat-mur. The latter was prescribed, which restored the child to perfect health in an astonishly short time."

The functions and uses of Repertory

The Repertory has two functions:-

(i) The primary, as a simple and straight-forward index to the Materia Medica (which itself is a very complex and difficult function because of the complexity of our Materia Medica).

(ii) Secondary (but of prime importance to the Homoeopathic practitioner), as a distinct system for the purpose of helping him in the elimination of the non-indicated drugs.

These two functions are closely related and are two different stages of the evolutionary development of the Homoeopathic Repertory.

The Repertory, whatever be its structure or its approach, aims at simplifying the work of the seeker after the similimum. It helps us in the comparison of the character and intensity of the symptoms in the patient to the symptoms in the Materia Medica.It brings out the different competing remedies into a bolder relief and helps us in the short-cuts to the Materia Medica.

The related remedies which might follow or replace the first prescription are also brought into focus.

Materia Medica contains the symptoms of remedies, whereas the Repertory as an index relates the remedies to the symptoms. Here the relationship is mutually complimentary.

Sometimes the use of the Repertory, as merely an index of the Materia Medica, is required in search for the indicated remedy. Here it is tantamount to use of Key-note symptoms or rare, strange and peculiar symptoms, which are usually familiar to the good students of Homoeopathic Materia Medica. Here the beginner or the novice may spend much more time in trying to take all the symptoms and running through the Repertory. Of course, proper evaluation and then taking such decisions requires a lot of study and experience. Here the

Repertory's primary function as an index to our Materia Medica is illustrated

Let me cite Late **Dr. P. Sankaran's** cases illustrating this point. But one may remember that complicated cases, without clearly marked key-note type of symptoms, have to be run through proper Repertorial analysis and thumbing of a few pages of Repertory will not help.

Here Hahnemann has warned us, that it is ultimately the totality of the case which is the final determinant of the remedy which covers the patient in his entirety as far as possible as it covers also his 'miasmatic' tendencies and background. If the so called peculiar symptom does not lead us to such a remedy, the result will be only palliative and will remove one or a few symptoms and not cure the patient.

1. "One of my patients came to me with several symptoms all looking like Lachesis. Lachesis, however, failed to give satisfaction. Then she gave me a good symptom that she invariably developed palpitation after bath. It did not depend upon the exertion of the bath nor on whether hot or cold water was used but upon the bath itself. When I referred to Kent's Repertory, again it came to my rescue. Under the rubric 'Palpitation, bathing agg.'(P874), only one drug was found- Am-carb(Am-carb is very similar to lachesis; it is incidentally an antidote to snake poison). This drug was found to cover the other symptoms of the patient also and it completely cured her of her whole disorder, including an eczema."

2. "About three years back, I was called to see a young married lady suffering from retention of urine. Some five weeks earlier, she had developed fever which had been treated with Chloromycetin. The temperature had dropped to normal but on the same day she had developed retention of urine. Not being relieved by any medicine, she had to be catheterised four times a day. It was thought that the retention would gradually

disapper but it did not. So a neurologist was consulted who found nothing abnormal and thought it must be due to shock. She was discharged from the hospital without any specific treatment being suggested and so she had to continue to catheterise herself four times a day till I saw her.

Since there was the possibility of a fright having caused the condition, I gave her Opium in potency with no good result. Thereupon, I consulted Dr.S.R.Phatak who diagnosed it as hysterical. On looking into Kent's Repertory, under the rubric 'Bladder, retention of urine, in hysteria', we found only one drug and that too in bold type- Zinc. So she was given Zinc-met 200. With the second dose of Zinc-met, she had a copious flow of urine without resorting to the catheter. Since then she has neither required the catheter nor any dose of any medicine."

3. "A young girl of 20 consulted me for a peculiar and embarassing disorder. She had itching of the nose, which, at first, came on every time she started eating but which later on appeared even at the sight of food. So bad was the disorder that she had not been able to eat anything for nearly a month. She had to liquefy her food and drink it up. She had consulted several skin specialists but they could not relieve her. They had actually directed her to a psychiatrist. When she applied to me for medicine, I doubted if such a symptom could be found even in homoeopathy. But when I referred to Kent's Repertory, to my surprise, I found the rubric 'Itching of the nose while eating' - Jatropa and Lachesis. Between the two, I preferred Lachesis, because she was loquacious, and one dose of this relieved her completely."

Dr.P Schmidt has described a case about a physician of Chicago. He had an array of symptoms, but among those there was one, that was very curious. Every time he went to pass a stool, his nose would run. Dr. Schmidt opened the Repertory and found at once the only remedy given under the rubric 'Nose, coryza, stool, during'(p328) was Thuja. Further questioning of the patient disclosed that he had a history of Gonorrhoea and warts and Thuja eliminated the whole symptom-complex.

In acute conditions, there is usually presence of well marked characteristic symptoms, which any student of Homoeopathic Materia Medica would be able to utilize and prescribe the medicine, either by his memory of Materia Medica or by thumbing one or two pages of the Repertory. I once had one patient suffering from acute viral fever

Mrs. C had fever with chill for the last three days, possibly of the viral origin. There was afternoon temperature. There was no thirst practically although temperature rose to 101.5 degree F. The whole of the left side of the body was aching. There was irritation in the throat. Pulsatilla 200 was given on the indications- One sided complaints, Pain left sided and Thirstless during fever. Next day, there was no fever and the patient was very much better in every way. Although thirstlessness in fever is characteristic of Pulsatilla, but there are many other remedies having this symptom. Other accompanying symptoms led us unerringly to the correct similimum.

The study and use of Repertories makes our Materia Medica more interesting. Actually the repertory stimulates the study of the Materia Medica. In the annals of Homoeopathy, we have found that those who were keen students of Repertory, were also masters of Materia Medica . Actually the Repertory is **Materia Medica made available at our finger-tips.** It leads one up to that something in Materia Medica, which one seeks in the most expeditious manner possible. Dr. J.T. Kent, who compiled one of the greatest Repertories of all times, was also a great exponent of our Materia Medica. His lectures on it are a great monument. Dr. Tyler, who was an expert in the use of Repertories, was in the habit of studying one drug daily from the Materica Medica. Such examples are easy to find.

To suggest remedics for a case, the Repertory is better than a Consulting Physician, because it contains more information, which is better classified, more exact, and easier to follow. Then it never forgets anything, has no favourite remedies but mentions with equal promptness the most obscure ones and the polycrests, when they have any bearing upon a case.

The Repertory helps, also, to be more objective and keep our prejudices in abeyance regarding our tendency to prescribing on one or two characteristic symptoms. It, very often, leads us to a remedy or remedies, one could hardly have imagined or thought of in a particular case. Those, who do not use Repertories, tend to develop some favourite remedies, but repertorial studies help us in shaking off these shackles. They open out possibilities, which would have been a closed book to us.

The Repertory helps us in evaluating properly the case and the individual symptoms. It makes us more particular about the accuracy of the anamnesis and subsequent classification of symptoms. It helps us, indirectly, in separating the symptoms of the patient from those of illness, pathognomic and also non-pathognomic ones.

It helps us in the art of interrogation and the framing of intelligent questions. Without its knowledge, even the case taking can often be an ineffective affair. Dr. P. Schmidt once said that it teaches us humility and the constant need to crush and utterly nullify all our prejudices. He said, "Repertory is not just an index but an extremely useful instrument to know and handle. It is a wonderful thing, a positive brain whose prodigious riches, one must know how to use".It is a frequent companion and helper. Regular repertorial work is a refresher course in Materia Medica. Repertory does not restrict the Materia Medica, it makes it, on the other hand, more available.

Limitations of Repertory

In spite of all that could be said in praise of Repertories, they cannot decide the remedy for us. The beginners expect too much from the Repertory. Any cut and dried plan for figuring out a remedy with mathematical precision is foredoomed to failure. There are too many imperfections in our knowledge of the Materia Medica, case-taking, evaluation of symptoms and construction of Repertories. The Repertory can never be a magic key to the remedy or a push-button for our solutions. This will apply equally to the computerisation of Repertory.

There is no question of mathematical equations between the symptoms of a patient and those in the Materia Medica from a study of Repertories. The Repertories are only meant for guiding us to the group of likely remedies in the Materia Medica. The trouble arises when we abuse the secondary function of the repertory and let it usurp the functions of the Materia Medica. This attempt places repertory in an untrue light; has led many to expect something of it, which it cannot do properly and thus obscuring the proper function. The final decision should always be with the Materia Medica and original provings. The sole function of the Repertory is to point out where in the Materia Medica the evidence is most likely to be found out. Now and then, a correct prescription is made, with the help of a Repertory alone; hence the misconception that it can perform the latter function unaided by Materia Medica. It is condemned wrongly for failure where it should not be expected to succeed.

Repertory is a peculiar index and although its function is like that of the piano, yet like the latter, a decent and considerable attainment can be obtained only by practice. Some tend to blame the instrument. In a way, Repertory is a fairly faithful instrument; it gives you back what you put into it, nothing more, nothing less. If you put the wrong things in, you get the wrong things out. The Repertory, how-so-ever complete, cannot select the remedy for us. At its best, it should point out a few remedies having resemblance to the case before us as Boenninghausen said, " lead the way into a field of related remedies".

It is the province of the Repertory to suggest, that of the Materia Medica to decide. In my view, one of the chief merits of the Repertory, though it is a limitation, consists in its not being too positive, but revealing more than one possible remedies for a case, always inviting reference to the Materia Medica, and in giving opportunity for the exercise of good judgement, which must always be the dominant factor in making a difficult prescription.

The best Repertory

What is the best Repertory? Kent once answered, "The best is that which one makes oneself". It is, indeed, a profound statement. Unless we are conversant intimately with the philosophy and structure of a Repertory, we cannot utilise it properly. To understand the Repertories, an evaluation of their historical development is very essential.

Historical development of the Repertory

Many compilations resulted as various minds approached the problem academically. Profound study and comparisons ultimated in what we today know as Repertories. A Repertory is only as good as one's efficient knowledge of its structural arrangement and understanding of the author's directions for its use. No body can understand any Repertory, unless we study the historical development of the concept of Repertory and the gradual progression of the various Repertories, discovering the thinking behind this concept, which inspired those who drew them up, and also to see how they did it.

The earlient Repertory, as mentioned already, was born as early as 1805, when Hahnemann published in Latin his famous "Fragmenta de viribus medicamentorum positivis". The first part contained symptoms observed and the second part formed the index or Repertory.

Contrary to general impressions, it must be recorded that Hahnemann was the first to make a Repertory and that he did have a repertory to use in his daily practice. He had four volumes of this reference book consisting of 4239 pages, with slits to hold little square papers, of which he had cut off the corners, so as to slip them into the slits, and be able to change them at need. In 1829, Hahnemann wrote to his friend Rummel, "How useful will be a good alphabetical Repertory once it is completed". In about 1829, he assigned a young doctor, Ernst Ferdinand Ruckert to arrange a Repertory of the remedies. This was to form the last volume of the Chronic Diseases. Ruckert worked on it from 1829 to 1830 and his work was constantly checked and consulted on the bedside by Hahnemann, but this attempt was not successful and has remained limited to a manuscript form, housed now in Hael's Museum in Robert Bosch Hospital, Stuttgart, West Germany.

It is said that Hahnemann employed Dr. Jahr in about 1834 to complete the second edition of the Chronic Diseases, and also to lay the foundations of a Repertory and encyclopaedia of symptoms. Jahr was a medical student, who had finished his medical course, but had not appeared in the final examination. Hahnemann was a hard-task master and whenever he entrusted any work to his pupils, he demanded an exactitude and sincerity, which could be found only in a person who was devoted to science.

Hahnemann, soon, began to complain of Jahr's hastiness and in exactitude. He had set high hopes on him and expected to finish a standard Homoeopathic lexicon. Jahr did not publish his first Repertory until 1835. It was in German in two volumes, containing 1052 and 1254 pages, followed by a third Repertory on the glands, bones, mucous membranes, ducts and skin diseases in 200 pages. This was, indeed, quite a voluminous work of Jahr. Earlier, Jahr under Hahnemann's guidance, had put symptoms from 'Chronic Diseases' in different sections alphabetically. Actually, he cut out a particular symptom from 'Chronic Diseases' and pasted it under the appropriate head alphabetically. These manuscripts are housed in the Hahnemann library in the Robert Bosch Hospital. Hahnemann also developed the Repertory idea still further but his later Repertories remained and are still in manuscript form.

One of the earliest Repertories was by Hartlaub published in 1828 in Leipzig.

In 1830, Weber compiled in German, a Repertory consisting of 536 pages 'SYSTEMATISCHE DARSTELLUNG der ANTIPSORISCHE ARZNEIMITTAL' with a Repertory of deteriorations and ameliorations in health, ranging from top to toe of the subject and ending up with sleep, and the mental symptoms. The later years saw different Repertories compiled by different authors, as outlined below.

1832 - Boenninghausen's **Repertory of the Anti-psorics** with a preface by Hahnemann

1833 - Glazor : First Alphabetical **Pocket Repertory** Leipzig - with 165 pages

1833 - Weber-Peschier : **Repertory of Purely pathogenctic effects** -prefaced by Hahnemann - 376 pages

1835 - **Jahr's Repertory** as assigned to him by Hahnemann consisted of three volumes containing 1052 pages in the first, 1254 pages in the second and 200 pages in the last volume

1835 - Boenninghausen : **Repertory of medicines which are not anti-psoric**

1836 - Boenninghausen : An attempt at showing **the relative kinship of Homoeopathic medicines (VERWANDSCHAFTEN REPERTORIUM)**

1837 - Ruoff : 236 pages. A Repertory published at Stuttgart

1838 - A Repertory published in English language in Allentown Academy by C. Hering

1840 - Ruoff : 254 pages. **A Repertory of Nosology** translated to German by Okie Humphry and published in English in America

1843 - Laffitte : One of the first Parisian Homoeopaths, who compiled- **A Homoeopathic Repertory of Symptomatology** - (first original repertory in French) Pages 975

1846 - Boenninghausen's famous **Therapeutic Pocket-Book.** Boenninghausen's Therapeutic Pocket Book was translated in English by Dr. Hempel and also by Dr. Okie. Later Dr. Allen published another edition with modification. The last and current edition was published by Dr. H.A.Roberts of Connecticut U.S.A. in 1935 and he edited it and made some modifications

1847 - Hempel's Boenninghausen - 500 pages

1847 - **Boenninghausen's Therapeutic Pocket Book** edited by Okie

1847 - **Jahr's Manual of Homoeopathic Materia Medica and Repertory** edited by P.F. Curie

1848 - Clofar Muller : 940 pages. **Systematic alphabetical Repertory**

1849 - Mure : 367 pages - Rio de Janeiro

1851 - Bryant : 352 pages. New York - an alphabetical Repertory- **A Pocket Manual of Repertory of Homoeopathic Medicine**

1853 - Possart : 700 pages. **A Repertory of characteristic Homoeopathic Remedies** published at Cothen

1853 - **Jahr's New Manual or Symptomen-Codex**- Vol.III (Repertory) translated and edited by Hempel and Quin

1853 - **Dysentery and its Repertory of Medicine** by Fred Humphreys

1854 - A Lippe - 144 pages. U.S.A. A Repertory of Comparative Materia Medica

1859 - **Cipher Repertory:** 600 pages - by English Homoeopaths Enlarged edition in 1878 containing 1030 pages by Drysdale, Atkins Dudgeon and Stokes

1859 - **Jahr's New Manual of the Homoeopathic Materia Medica with Possart's additions**- fifth edition revised and enlarged by the author and translated and edited by Hempel

About this time in England were known the following repertories:-

(a) Buck's **Regional Symptomatology and Clinical Dictionary**
(b) **Hempel's Repertory**
(c) **Repertory** by Curie
(d) **Hahnemann Society Repertory**, by Drysdale-Dudgeon

About this time the American Homoeopaths were also busy in making Repertories.

1873 - Berridge : **Repertory of the Eyes** published in England.
1874 - Granier of Nimes : **Homoeolexicon** in two volumes.
1876 - **Repertory of the New Remedies** by C.P.Hart published by Boericke and Tafel. Based on Hale's special symptomatology and therapeutics.
1879 - C. Lippe published his famous **Repertory of the More Characteristic symptoms of the Materia Medica** - Pages 322. (Indian Edition has 438 pages.)
1880 - T.F. Allen's **Symptom Register**
1880 - **Repertory to the Modalities** by Samuel Worcester M.D.
1881 - Hering's **Analytical Repertory** (Symptoms of Mind)
1883 - **Repertory of Intermittent fever** by William A. Allen
1884 - 1st Edition - **Cough and Expectoration** by Lee and Clark
1894 - 2nd Edition - **Cough and Expectoration** by Lee and Clark
1885 - **Alphabetical Repertory** by Father Muller (First repertory published in India)
1888 - **Pathogenetic and Clinical Repertory of the Symptoms of Head** by Neidhard
1890 - Gentry : **The Repertory of Concordances** in six volumes - 5500 pages

1890 - **Classified Index of the Materia Medica for Urogenital and Venereal Diseases** by Carleton M.D. and Coles M.D.

1896 - Knerr's **Repertory to the Hering's Guiding Symptoms**

1897 - Kent : **Repertory of the Homoeopathic Materia Medica** - First edition - 1349 pages

1900 - Boger - English translation of **Boenninghausen's Repertory of Anti psoric remedies**

1905 - **Boger's Boenninghausen's Characteristics and Repertory**

1908 - **Clinic Repertory** by P.W.Shedd M.D.

1920 - Repertory Section of **Bell's Diarrhoea**

1931 - **Synoptic Key of the Homoeopathic Materia Medic** by C.M. Boger

1935-1937-

Second and enlarged Edition of the **Characteristics and Repertory** by C.M. Boger -published by Roy & Co. **Times of Remedies and Moon Phases** - Published by Salzer & Co.,Calcutta

Recently a few repertories have been published with Kent's Repertory as the base.

1929 - N.M.Chaudhary's **Materia Medica and Repertory**
Piere's **Materia Medica and Repertory**

1963 - **Pathak's Repertory**

1963 - **Repertory of the New Remedies** by Stephens

1987 - **Synthetic Repertory** edited by H.Barthel in 3 volumes. It covers (1) Mental symptoms (2) Generalities (3) Sleep, Dreams and Sexuality

1990 - **Kent's General Repertory** by Kunzli

1993 - **Synthesis Repertorium Homeopathicm Syntheticum** by Dr. Frederik Schroyens

- **Clinical Repertories of New Homoeopathic Remedies'** by Dr. O.A. Julian
- **Index of Aggravations and Ameliorations** by Neatby and Stonham

Apart from the above Repertories, there were a host of regional and clinical Repertories, published in America and elsewhere, which have been listed later on.

The Main Currents

Right from the beginning, there were two schools of thoughts regarding the making of Repertories. There were two distinct movements, as we will see later, representing possibly two different temperamental reactions; two different currents uniting later on, to culminate in the best of all. Apart from these major movements, there were some repertorians, who laid more emphasis on the making of clinical Repertories than on the indexing of pure symptomatology.

Boenninghausen's Earliest Repertory

It seems, that about 1830 or so, Hahnemann was feeling acutely the need of a guiding index or repertory, but was undecided as to the nature or form of the index. That is why, we see him asking different disciples to prepare a suitable Repertory. Ruckert, Gros, Jahr and Boenninghausen were the four men, who set about helping in this project about the same period. While Hahnemann was fumbling with the development of a suitable form of index or repertory, Boenninghausen's keen intellect was already busy at finding a suitable repertorial index for guidance in his own practice. Hahnemann was quick to recognise his genius. He has been described as his ablest and most faithful disciple. Being disappointed in Jahr, Hahnemann gave him every assistance and encouragement. Like Hahnemann Boenninghausen was also thorough in his work and whatever he undertook, he did that with the exactitude of a true scientist.

Boenninghausen was one of the few remarkable men, without whom, the science of Homoeopathy might have been deprived of a vital link. He was 45 when he started his education in Homoeopathy. He was desperately ill in 1828. At that time, he did not know a word about Homoeopathy. About a year or two later, we find him hard at work with provings, writing and curing patients.

As early as 1830, he had already prepared an index or a Repertory for his own use. This hand-written guide was appreciated by others very much and he was constantly asked to get it printed.

In 1832, he prepared the first Repertory, which was the progenitor of the later Repertories. It was called the 'Repertory of the Anti-psoric remedies' and was prefaced by Hahnemann. The first edition was sold out in six months. The second edition appeared in 1833. In the introduction to the book, he said that his object was 'completeness, brevity and ease in consultation'. There was alphabetical order and systematical arrangement. Besides the extremely logical arrangement, the most useful innovation introduced by him, was the gradation or valuation of drugs for a particular symptom. Upto this day, we follow more or less Boenninghausen's standard of evaluation of drugs. Jahr, in his preface to the 4th edition of his Repertory in 1851, gave Boenninghausen the credit for the system of evaluating remedies, which he had begun to use. The Repertory of the Anti-psoric remedies was translated by Boger in 1900. This Repertory was the precursor of the Boger's 'Boenninghausen's Characteristics and Repertory', the first edition of which appeared in 1905. Later on, with the help of his manuscript of proposed second edition, and assistance from the wife of late Dr. Boger, second and enlarged edition was published, posthumously, in 1937 in India by Roy and Company.

One is, however, amazed at the genius and hard work of Boenninghausen to have produced such a work within two years of his taking up Homoeopathy. Even Hahnemann had started using this book for reference instead of Jahr's compilation.

Plan of Boenninghausen's first Repertory:

It will not be out of place to mention something about the first Repertory of Boenninghausen, because it was appreciated and used by Hahnemann in his daily practice, and it also formed the basis of many future Repertories, like that of Jahr, Allentown's manual, Lippe's Repertory and even the Kent's Repertory. Boger, as we shall see later, adopted this pattern and brought about a synthesis of Boenninghausen's early Repertories and Therapeutic Pocket Book in his Boenninghausen's Characteristics and Repertory. Boenninghausen in his first Repertory gave locations in general to comparatively fewer parts of anatomy. In section on Head, Internal, he gave Forehead and Sinciput, Temples, Sides, Vertex and Occiput. The only other region where he gave such locations' was under Abdomen, where he gave 'Upper abdomen', 'Lower abdomen', 'Umbilical region', 'Sides of the abdomen', 'Entire abdomen', 'Hips and the loin region'. He had kept Hypochondria separately - 'L' meant Liver region or right hypochondrium and 'S' meant Spleen or left hypochondrium. 'B' meant both sides.

Nowhere else has he given any location. Other arrangement was the same, as has been given in the Boger's Boenninghausen. Modalities were appended at the end of various sensations in a particular region or area and there were no particularisation of modalities for different sensations mentioned against a particular region. 'Concomitants' or 'Accompaniments' were given together in a generalised manner like modalities at the end after modalities, i.e. after giving complaints in the particular region.

The most valuable part was the 'Generalities' given at the end of the book, followed by general modalities, 'Aggravation' and 'Amelioration'. In his Therapeutic Pocket Book, he changed 'Generalities' into 'Sensations'. Kent, much later, combined Boenninghausen's Generalities and Modalities into one chapter at the end of the book. I think that earlier arrangement of Boenninghausen was much better from the point of view of greater ease in locating a particular symptom.

Boenninghausen was not, however, satisfied with his own work, and he went on from one form to another, in an attempt to condense space and lessen the arduous task of finding the indicated remedy. In 1835, he published a 'Repertory of medicines which are not antipsoric'. The next year saw the birth of another great idea of Boenninghausen in the publication of an attempt at showing the relative kinship of homoeopathic medicines. This was later to form the 'concordance' or the 'relationship' of drugs of his pocket Book. Between 1835 to 1845, he was hard at work to improve upon his Repertory. During this period, be studied the construction of Repertories. He must have made lots of trials and errors, before he gave the profession what he thought was the best arrangement for compiling a Repertory.

It was, indeed, a revolutionary approach compared to the thinking of repertory-makers at that time or even later on. By that time, there were a number of other repertories also, but this work of Boenninghausen caught the imagination of the profession, and one really wonders at the extent of the influence it exerted over the entire homoeopathic profession for the next 50 years or so. At that time. there were Repertories by Jahr and a few others, but this held undivided sway so far as the Repertories are concerned and there is no denying the fact that because of this Repertory, these wonderful cures were made by most of the master-prescribers of that era. His 'Therapeutic Pocket Book' was the answer to his attempt to produce a concise comprehensive index. I cannot help quoting Boenninghausen's own words, which sum up his way of making a Repertory better than I can attempt to do. "The defects of the Repertories, hitherto published, lay chiefly, in my opinion, in their being limited to the material given in the Materia Medica Pura, joined to the carefully tested cases in practice, but these have never been combined, so as to furnish the means of judging the value of each symptom, of completing those which were incomplete and of filling the numerous vacancies constantly met with, by every practitioner. Fearing to divide symptoms more than has been done hitherto, it was my first intention to retain the form and arrangement of my original Repertory, which Hahnemann repeatedly assured me he preferred to all others, and to condense it into one volume, making it clearer in every part as well as more complete from analogy as well as from experience. But after finishing about half of the manuscript, I found that it had increased on my hands, beyond all expectation, to such an extent that at last I gave it up as I saw that similar object might be attained in a more simple and satisfactory manner, if by bringing out the peculiarities and characteristics of the remedies according to their various relations, I opened a way into the wide fields of combinations which hitherto had not been trodden".

On studying the development of Homoeopathic Repertory, I used towonder why Boenninghausen changed the name of his Repertory to 'Therapeutic Pocket Book'. Originally he called his book as 'Repertory of the Anti-psoric remedies'. There must be a reason, although the homoeopathic doctors of his time and later on have continued to refer to his book as Boenninghausen's Repertory. Boenninghausen had a very analytical and logical mind. He could see that in this present form of his book (The Therapeutic Pocket Book), it was no longer a Repertory in the accepted sense of the word. It was a revolutionary departure in creating an instrument, which could help the prescribers tremendously in their search for similimum. It could not have been a whim or a theoretical or idle philosophisation. It was constructed after lot of clinical experience and verifications. His stand was vindicated by numerous prescribers of great eminence, both in United States and other parts of the world. Of course, as we shall see later, it had its short-comings, and could not always give a complete solution to our problems of search for the similimum.

It may be mentioned here that Jahr's work also underwent a number of editions, as his fourth edition was published in 1851, where he had appreciated Boenninghausen's contribution, especially with regard to the evaluation of remedies in a particular rubric and Jahr had adopted this innovation in his work. But, by and large, it was Boenninghausen's Repertory which was in the libraries of all the Homoeopathic doctors of those times. Boenninghausen was contemporary of Carrol Dunham and Dr. Adolph Lippe and both of them had appreciated the work of Boenninghausen. Dr. Lippe mentioned his work to be particularly noticed for his accuracy. I think both senior Lippe and his son worked on a Repertory based on Boenninghausen's earlier Repertory in a completed form. Unfortunately, the influence of Boenninghausen's Repertory had started waning towards the close of the 19th century. The two greatest exponents of this Repertory, who made the work of Boenninghausen better known, were Dr. Boger and, later on, Dr. H.A. Roberts. Of course, Dr. Allen, earlier, had added to the Repertory and Dr.Roberts, later, had modified the rubrics to some minor extent.

The Doctrine of Analogy

The philosophy of Dr. Boenninghausen's construction of a Repertory depends also upon his doctrine of analogy. According to his approach, he says that one can create order out of chaos, by combining the scattered fragments of symptoms, by making use of analogy. That is, we can fix the locality of one paticular symptom, by noting locality in other symptoms. Simlarly, we can fix the character of sensations by fixing a locality in one part, taking the character of the sensation from the symptoms expressed by the patient in relation to the other parts, and similarly conditions of aggravation and amelioration from an affection of some other part, or perhaps, from consideration of all the parts affected. By a wider application of the principles of analogy, he gathered all the affected localities of the sensations, and all the conditions, each, in its proper place, and thus erect an edifice of totality, which ultimately reveals the remedy. It appears extremely logical and has stood the test of time. We are all familiar with this work of generalisation of Boenninghausen. If you knock away this pillar of analogy from any sound Repertory, it rests on most unsteady foundations. In Repertory-making, it is not merely indexing of symptoms. Then it would be presenting skeletons without the virile qualities. In the evolution of Repertories, the highest contribution was bound to lead to generalisations deduced from the study of provings and vast clinical confirmations. Of course, Boenninghausen carried the ideas of analogy to an extent, which was not accepted by many of his colleagues and followers. Boenninghausen said that analogy is extremely important in the selection of remedy, and that is why, when he noted a particular sensation in a part of the body, he supposed that this sensation could be related also to the other part, which neither the patient expressed, nor it has been brought out in the provings, but from the analogy itself, one could ascribe this sensation to be present in other part of the body also. That is, he generalised that particular sensation belonging to the patient or to the remedy.

Hahnemann had promulgated that drug selected should correspond as closely as possible, both in number and character, to that of the patient. Character is more important than mere numerical totality. The grounds of totality of symptoms is a safe rule but which is usually disregarded. The reasons are:

(a) Exigencies of business
(b) Difficulty, because of lack of complete development of essential symptoms
(c) Imperfection of our symptomology; provings are insufficient in number to develop a complete parallel to the case in hand; or provers have carelessly observed and imperfectly recorded their symptoms. Incomplete symptoms are rather the rule in our Materia Medica.

Boenninghausen had learnt that the symptoms which existed in an incomplete state in some part of a given case, could be reliably completed by analogy, by observing the conditions of other parts of the case. If, for instance, it was not possible to decide what aggravated or ameliorated a particular symptom of the case, a patient could readily express a condition of amelioration of some other symptom. It did not take long to discover, that conditions of aggravation or amelioration are not confined to this or that particular symptom. But they extend to almost all the symptoms. Boenninghausen's approach was that provings are not complete and can never be really complete.

Similarly, case histories as given by the patients, are also not complete. He says that to make these things comparatively more complete so as to make the best of what can be found out, he wanted to complete the case and hence the character of the remedies by analogy, as learnt from actual experience and practice. So, he completed the case or a symptom by analogy from other parts or a sensation of other parts or modalities of symptoms from other parts as mentioned by the patient. This one thing which Boenninghausen brought to the notice of the profession, as already known, is the basic 'elements of symptoms'. These elements of the symptoms must be completed, before we can have a real totality of the case. And these he did by his principle of analogy. We have seen many remedies, which have comparatively greater preference for left or right side of the body. So far, in the provings or in the clinical confirmations, there are many symptoms, which have not been mentioned or clinically confirmed, but knowing that the remedy has got a greater preference or a marked preference for one particular side, we have cured, in our practice, certain complaints or symptoms, which were markedly present on one side of the body, although these symptoms have never been noticed before by anybody else. For example, we have cured cases of warts present only on the left side of the body by Lachesis. According to the existing literature in the provings, authentic journals or the clinical confirmations, we have hardly come across this peculiar thing. So, this location has been generalised, because we found that this left-sidedness was a very strong characteristic of Lachesis, although in Hering's Guiding Symptoms, the author has given symptoms in his chapter on

Lachesis, symptoms which are present both on left and right sides of the body. Only thing is, that the symptoms on left side are only slightly larger in number than those on the right side of the body.

Similarly, Boenninghausen deduced that if coldness is confined to left side, then possibly, heat or sweat confined to left side of the body could also be deduced from this particular analogy, and thus made a sort of generalisation. The problem arises when there are contradictory modalities. A part of the patient is worse from cold and the other part/parts of the patient is/are worse from heat. But according to Boenninghausen, if we take the history carefully, and work out the case properly, these contradiction or apparently opposite symptoms will not interfere in the final results. The advantages, according to him were too great compared to certain anomalies which normally would not vitiate the results.

In Boenninghausen's repertory, 'Lach' was given the highest evaluation for the 'Side Left'. One does not have to go to the Materia Medica to see if a particular symptom occurred in the left-side. One can predict and can utilise this knowledge for prescribing the remedy. These generalisations based on analogy are accepted today like our morning tea, but it took a genius like Boenninghausen to have these things crystallized.

Concept of Concomitant Symptoms

Apart from the elements of location, sensation and modalities of symptoms as defined by Boenninghausen, his introduction of the fourth element of 'Concomitants' laid the strong foundations of his repertorial system. The accompanying symptoms or secondary symptoms which are usually ignored by us, are sometimes the most valuable because these do not seem to have any connection with the pathology and are typical of the individual's reactions.

These fulfill the requirement of Hahnemann as laid down in the Organon. They are of the same class as the rare, strange and peculiar symptoms. From his study and experience, however, it became clearer to Boenninghausen that some remedies, more than others, tended to have concomitant symptoms and these do not consist exclusively of peculiar symptoms. Most often, concomitants of the symptoms was related to the conditions of aggravations and amelioration. He, therefore, introduced under each section, the concomitant symptoms together and indicating, at the same time, the varying values of the remedies by different types.

The introduction of concomitant complaints under various rubrics was indeed a masterly piece of logical brevity and, yet, covering all that was desired. The symptoms that occurred together or in a definite association, were considered to be more valuable for prescribing and more characteristic of the individual. They are of the same class as the rare, strange and peculiar symptoms. The doctrine of concomitants, plus the idea that group is of more importance than the single symptoms, no matter how peculiar the symptom may be, led Boenninghausen to pay special attention to this aspect of his research. He, like Hahnemann, accepted fully that totality must govern, but found the number of such symptoms increasing so rapidly that he adduced certain generalisations based on analogy. From his study and experience, it became certain that some remedies, more than others incline to have concomitant symptoms and that these do not consist exclusively of peculiar symptoms. He wrote, "this discovery tested by long experience led me to place the "concomitant symptoms" together under each section in which I have again pointed out the varying values of remedies by means of different types".

Boenninghausen, while writing about the treatment of intermittent fevers, mentioned that it was indeed very difficult to treat such cases with Homoeopathy. But, if one understood the value of these concomitant symptoms and paid more attention to the symptoms of the patient during apyrexia than only to the symptoms of paroxysm, one could notice that these accessory, associated or concomitant or secondary symptoms during apyrexia become more important and lead to the correctly indicated remedy. These ought to be considered exclusively and sometimes even in contradiction to the symptoms of the paroxysm, until a drug shall have been discovered in the course of provings upon a healthy man, which shall correspond to both these orders of symptoms.

During our personal experiences in the treatment of malarial fevers in Bengal, I found very often that signs and symptoms during apyrexia were found to lead us to the indicated remedies. The symptoms during the paroxysms were, at times, not of much help in the selection of the similimum.

Boenninghausen, in his short span of life as a physician, discovered so many things, which we have confirmed time and again during the history of our profession in the treatment of chronic and other diseases. The concomitant symptom is to the totality what the condition of aggravation or amelioration is to the single symptom. This is the differentiating factor.

Concordances or Relationships of Remedies

Apart from the main Repertory that is the Therapeutic Pocket Book, Boenninghausen also wrote about the Relationship of remedies, also called as Concordances. This is indeed a novel and a very useful idea and gave a better understanding of the drug and points of contact with each other with regard to specific spheres, locations, modalities, tissues, etc., so that by the working out of these relationships, you could find out the remedy which is likely to follow another one after the former has done its job, though partially. This way, the remedy, which was to complement the action of the first remedy, could be found out by working out the relationship with regard to the case in hand and not on any rigid preconceived basis. This chapter on the relationship of remedies has not been made use of, by most of the physicians. This has been rather considered as a sort of mystery and the people have not given the attention which it really deserves. This part of his Pocket-Book has helped many in solving chronic cases and especially in their search for the second prescription.

This section of the book was envisaged as early as 1836 by Boenninghausen, but at that time he had not done it properly and as completely. In the Therapeutic Pocket Book, he tried to make it as complete and as correct as possible. Unfortunately, most of us have not understood properly or utilised this section for practical application.

Boenninghausen wrote in his preface that he hoped that no one would consider this section useless and superfluous. He wrote "For myself, who for the last fifteen years had made the Materia Medica pura my chief study as one of the most indispensable works of Homoeopathy, this concordance has been of extreme importance, not only for recognition of the genius of the remedy, but also for testing and making sure of its choice, and for judging of sequence of the various remedies, so as to determine the order of their successive exhibition, particularly in chronic diseases".

Complementary or Antidotal Relationship of Remedies

Students of Homoeopathic medicine must have seen that many authors of Materia Medica, from Hering onwards, have appended some sort of relationship of remedies at the end of the chapter on a particular drug, but it was Dr. C.V. Boenninghausen who was the first one to bring out our attention to these relationships(or concordances). He introduced the word 'relationship' in the circumstances, when a remedy possesses the property of extinguishing the symptoms produced by another remedy by the similarity of its own action to that of the other. Hence, there is some 'affinity' between these two remedies and it was denoted by him as the 'relationship'.

His innovative genius made it quite clear that, in this

relationship, there are two factors which are inherent here. First, that of antidotal action, in which case it is intended to weaken or neutralise the deleterious effects in sudden poisoning, etc.

In the case of its beneficial relationship, it seems also to be fairly similar to the symptom picture of the patient and the remedy earlier prescribed has already benefited the patient and has removed curatively a number of complaints but has not fully cured him and if the second or later remedy is given, it seems to complete the cure.

The very similarity of the symptom picture in both the remedies has the potentiality of antidotal action as well as that of 'affinity', because the second remedy has also certain other symptoms, which may not have been produced in the pathogenesis of the first remedy, and hence, it seems to work as a follow up remedy and complete the cure. It has been found in actual practice, that the second remedy acts far more curatively, if it has been preceded by the earlier prescribed medicine.

For example, it has been found and proved that Calc carb showed better curative efficiency if it is given after Sulphur; Nitric acid after Calc carb; Caust after Sepia; Lycopodium after Calc carb; Nitric acid after Kali carb; Sulphur after Ars and Merc; Sepia after Silicea, Nitric acid or Sulphur.

It is quite evident that these actions follow the fundamental principle of homoeopathic similia.

Boenninghausen has, however, warned that we should not follow rigidly that it is the only order in which remedies should be prescribed, that Calc should precede Lycopodium and not vice-versa. He quoted cases where Calc was given after Lycopodium and produced curative results. He insisted that we should be governed by the law of similarity. If a case shows symptoms of Lycopodium, we may prescribe it and later we may give Calc if corresponded to the remaining symptoms.

Boenninghausen claimed that he saw quite frequently the beneficial action of Calc after Lycopodium in certain cases, especially when the symptom-complex at the beginning was indicative of Lycopodium, and after it had exhausted its action, Calc corresponded to the remnant of the case, which, however, does not always happen.

Boenninghausen collected the principal spheres of action of the remedies and then according to the similarities of different remedies in these regions, placed them in different relevant sections of the particular remedy whose relationships have been detailed. This is the basis of his chapter on Relationship or Concordances of remedies, as given in the Therapeutic Pocket Book. The basic logic behind his advocacy of these relationships depend on the following facts-

1. The related remedies are mutual antidotes.
2. Experience shows that the related remedies act far more curatively, when administered after each other, than the unrelated medicine can do.
3. The so-called one-sided diseases present an excellent opportunity for the utilization of relationships of the remedies. But the advantage of accurate knowledge of the relationships of remedies is even greater in the chronic than in the one-sided diseases, which nearly always require for their cure, several remedies in succession.

   Boenninghausen said that be, very often, found it very advantageous in such chronic cases as were poor in symptoms, and, therefore, difficult to cure, to so arrange the order in which the remedies should follow each other in advance, and, of course, they must be related ones, if symptoms did not appear during the cure which rendered a change necessary. In doing this, one remedy should correspond to the principal complaint, another to the concomitant ones. "In my recent practice, as a general role, the result is more favourable and more rapid if related remedies are given in succession, than to repeat."

4. In certain cases, when the first chosen or indicated remedy was given, the symptoms increased, as in a severe aggravation without improvement following. In such cases, the remedy related most nearest to the prescribed remedy, gave wonderful results, as it not only gave quick relief of the aggravation, but also gave considerable improvement to the original morbid condition.

During these years of his researches, Boenninghausen had invited all his colleagues to communicate to him their experiences in this area of relationship of remedies.

Thus there are three applications or uses of this section on Concordances or Relationships of remedies.

(1) Grasp of the genius of the medicines.
(2) Greater certainty in selection.
(3) Sequence in second prescriptions.

In the Concordances, all the sections of the Therapeutic Pocket Book are represented and the harmonious relation of remedy to others is given under each section. He has added apart from these. Antidotal remedies as the last paragraph.

1. **Mind**
2 **Localities**
3. **Sensations**
4. **Glands**
5. **Bones**
6. **Skin**
7. **Sleep and Dreams**
8. **Blood, Circulation and Fever**
9. **Aggravations: Time and Circumstances**
10. **Other remedies**
11. **Antidotes**

In the first application or use, evidently, it is clear to understand the genius of the remedy, when we are able to compare it with other remedies in different areas of the application and also the degree of nearness or contact of these remedies in different spheres. This is indeed a comparative Materia Medica in a nutshell.

The second use of Concordance is also quite obvious, as it helps us in selection of remedy for the case more certainly, as we are able to compare the remedy in mind with contending remedies.

The third and the most important use is the sequence of remedies i.e. the remedy or remedies which could follow the remedy already prescribed and found either inadequate or had finished its usefulness. This application, according to Boenninghausen, is very important in chronic cases, but I feel this could be as useful in acute cases also. The next remedy or the second prescription is thus indicated with a certainty, which no other Repertory or Materia Medica could offer us.

The almost always satisfactory result obtained from using one of them in indicating the remedy to follow is due to the wonderfully accurate and comprehensive manner in which they are compiled and not to there being anything concealed or esoteric. One wonders at the remarkable genius of Boenninghausen and at the amount of work and study involved in the formulation of the Concordances. I wish there could be another follower of Boenninghausen, who could have extended this work.

Having selected the first medicine for a case with accuracy and worked out its action in various potencies, or if the symptoms change substantially, new ones developing, either case demanding a change of remedy - it is here the difficulty comes.

To meet these new and trying conditions, there are

instructions in the Organon and directions given by Hering with regard to the importance of the new symptoms that have appeared. Besides that, in Hering's Guiding Symptoms as well as in various Materia Medicas, a short list of remedies follow the main remedy as its complementary or remedies that usually follow.

All this is useful, but it is not as specific as are the concordances in this respect, and besides, it takes much less time to use the concordance. Unfortunately, so few of us utilise this area of our Repertories.

Let us, for example, examine relationship of Aconite and Belladonna. Both have many points of contact, but on studying Aconite's relationship and sequences relations to Belladonna, we find there are many areas where Belladonna could have followed, but on studying Belladonna's concordances, we find that relationships are less marked. In practice also we find that Belladonna may be the indicated remedy after Aconite but hardly vice-versa.

Similarly, we find that under Aconite, Sulphur seems better indicated as the chronic remedy, while Calc carb is better indicated as chronic of Belladonna.

Dr. Som Dev, under my advice, took the trouble of giving the summation of intensity of contact points in actual numbers and published the relationships of Boenninghausen with numerical summations.

The last paragraph in Concordances of each remedy has been designated as 'other remedies', which is rather misguiding. Actually, the remedies given here give in general, the quantum of contact points of these remedies with the remedy where concordances or relationships are given i.e. the remedy under study.

This paragraph is actually the resume of all the earlier

paragraphs of relationships of the remedy under study. This paragraph, therefore, is the most important and can be used alone in most of the cases.

How are the Concordances to be made use of in relation to the sequence of remedies ? This depends upon the case and no hard and fast rules can be given. These relationships may even be used without assistance from the first part of Therapeutic Pocket Book.

Here, we can give an interesting example of a case cited by Dr. H.A.Roberts regarding the use of this particular chapter on relationships and its adaptability.

"Here is a case that seemed to be a simple cold in a child of three years, and in the hands of a good Hahnemannian prescriber the condition apparently cleared under Belladonna; but Belladonna failed to hold, and the child was running a daily maximum temperature of 105 degree F. The glands of the throat were involved, sore and swollen. In the meantime, another physician had been on the case. It still seemed as if Belladonna might be indicated, yet there were a few symptoms that seemed to contraindicate it.

After the child was looked over carefully and no definite outstanding indications were secured, the case was analyzed by the chapter on Relationships, under the remedy Belladonna. Only the remedies ranking 3, 4 and 5 under the rubric Mind were taken (with the exception of Chamomilla, because of its peculiar adaptability to child life) and the other rubrics under Belladonna were checked against them. The workout is given here-

Belladonna

(**M**- Mind; **L**- Locations; **S**- Sensations; **G** - Glands; **B**-Bones; **S**- Skin; **S** & **D**- Sleep & Dreams; **B**, **C** & **V**- Blood, Circulation& Fever; **A**- Aggravations;**OR**- Other Relationships)

	M	**L**	**S**	**G**	**B**	**S**	**S&D**	**B,C&F**	**A**	**OR**	**Total**
Apis.........	4	5	4	.	.	4	1	2	3	5	8/28
Bapt...........	4	4	3	.	.	.	1	1	1	4	7/18
Bry............	3	4	4	4	.	3	2	4	5	4	9/33
Can-i..........	5	3	3	.	.	.	2	.	1	4	6/18
Cham.........	2	3	3	.	.	.	2	3	4	3	7/20
Lyc...........	4	4	4	5	3	4	2	.	3	4	9/33
Op.............	4	3	3	.	.	.	.	.	3	3	5/16
Puls............	3	5	5	4	4	5	5	5	5	5	10/46
Rhus..........	4	3	4	2	.	5	2	4	4	4	9/32
Sulph..........	3	5	5	4	2	4	4	4	4	4	10/39

Suppose, we had taken first the rubric 'Glands' and selected therefrom, those remedies related to Belladonna in glandular affections. We should have found (in the 4's and 5's) Arnica, Bryonia, Lycopodium, Mercurius, Phosphorous, Pulsatilla and Sulphur. Checking these through all ten rubrics, we should have found Arnica ruled out; Mercurius 9/37 and Phosphorous 10/34 would have been added to our group coming through in sufficient degree for consideration, but even with these additions, Pulsatilla holds the lead over all others.

A casual study of Pulsatilla verified this brief analysis, and the remedy was given. In three days, the temperature was normal, having fallen gradually in the interval, the glands were normal in size and sensations, and the child was rapidly gaining strength and his normal lively interest in the world."

Generally, a Concordance is to be used alone, taking as first rubric, the one which covers the part affected. In a mental case, however, 'Mind' is to be used first. If the part is elsewhere in the body, then the rubric 'localities' is to be taken first.

Although, Kent criticised Boenninghausen later, but he, earlier in his study of Homoeopathic medicine, had appreciated his work on Concordances. In his article 'How to study Materia Medica', he has explained in great detail, the value and the use of Boenninghausen's contribution towards 'Concordances of Remedies'. In Boenninghausen, we are able to ascertain the general outline of drugs, that had been given in the Materia Medica and the Repertory, and carefully compare all individual symptoms to see their similarity.

Kent's said "Why is it that Boenninghausen's book is out of print; simply because Hahnemann's method has not been taught. Nothing would please me more than to see the republication of his grand work. This book enables men to know how to study it to cure the sick."

Kent said that the greatest of all comparers of Materia Medica was Boenninghausen. The concordances are the most important part of his book.

The Rise and Fall of the Therapeutic Pocket Book

Boenninghausen structured the basis of his Therapeutic Pocket Book on the principle of Analogy. Its value or useful application lies when there is paucity of symptoms; where there is no presence of marked mental, rare or strange symptoms; where modalities predominate; where particulars and concomitants are marked; and where there are more of pathological or objective symptoms.

Although, the Therapeutic Pocket Book was a wonderful contribution from Beonninghausen, it had its weak points also. It has run through many editions and translations. Hempel, Okie, T.F. Allen, Boger, among others, have given their time to perfect this little great book. Allen added 229 remedies, but most of them lacked modalities and subjective symptoms in as much detail as the original remedies. He added many symptoms of the eyes and was the first one to think of adding 'Sides of

Body' to the Pocket Book. In 1935, Dr. Robert brought out a new edition with minor changes. Roberts has criticized some of the arrangements by Dr. Allen, especially with regard to Sides. Roberts was, I think, one of the last great exponents of Boenninghausen and after his death, unfortunately, the Therapeutic Pocket Book has fallen into disuse, because of lack of understanding of the deeper philosophy behind it, and partly, because it has not been made upto date. Lack of proper additions and revisions has made it limited in its usefulness. Hence, its sphere of usefulness is limited. A revision of such a work should not be neglected. Boenninghausen planned such a book after intensive observations and study because according to him:

1. Cases taken, may be incomplete.

2. Materia Medica and Provings are also not complete. Modalities and Locations may be incomplete. He found that he could complete some of these things by analogy, by observing conditions or modalities in other parts. Hence, his later generalisations. He constructed his book in such a way, that study of one part could complete the deficiency of the symptom in the other part. He did the splitting up or breaking up of the symptoms for the purpose of classification. Later, a case could be worked out by combining the parts of the divided symptoms. His was a work "much in little". He held that a symptom could be considered complete, if the elements of location, sensation, modalities and concomitants are present.

To the historian of Homoeopathy, it would be seen that Boenninghausen's work was most popular in American Homoeopathy. The British Homoeopaths, somehow or other, never took to this work enthusiastically excepting Dr. Berridge. If one is familiar with his famous work of Repertory of the Eyes, one can see Boenninghausen's marked influence on the arrangement and construction of this Repertory. It would be interesting, really, to study the rise and fall of this Repertory, and to find out the causes, which led to its downfall. It is imperative, therefore, to evaluate critically, the basic or intrinsic value of this work. Does it have any relevance to a modern Homoeopath, or is it to be relegated to the waste paper basket? There were criticisms of this work right from the inception, because there were certain doctors who did not see eye to eye with Boenninghausen in his approach to the indexing of symptoms. Like Hahnemann, Boenninghausen was also a great student of logic and whatever he did, he did it with logical precision. Personally, I feel that we should not lightly brush aside his work. Unfortunately, his work has suffered from lack of proper revision; lack of proper additions and scientific study and research. Dr. Roberts has beautifully mentioned in his introduction to the Therapeutic Pocket Book, that for a brief and comprehensive classification of Homoeopathic symptomology for therapeutic purposes, no plan has ever been devised superior or equal to that of Boenninghausen in his Therapeutic Pocket Book. The plan is fundamental and probably final, because it is found on the principle of logic and has been verified by experience of a century. To the critics of Beonninghausen, one can say, that this Repertory, because of its intrinsic vitality and basic usefulness, was able to serve the profession for such a large number of years. No other book or work of lesser value, could have withstood the onslaughts of time for such a long period. So, there must have been vitality in the conception of this work. Recently, Late Dr. Dhawle in India, who was one of the great students and teacher of Homoeopathic medicine and philosophy, laid great emphasis on the study and use of Boenninghausen's way of analysing our case records. The value of Boenninghausen's Repertory depends upon the existence or absence of the following type of symptoms-

1) Paucity of symptoms in general
2) Lack of reliable mental symptoms; also lack of strange, rare and peculiar symptoms
3) Presence of modalities
4) Presence of concomitants
5) Pathological generals

Criticism of Boenninghausen

According to Kent, the Therapeutic Pocket Book has the modalities of the parts and those of the patient all mixed together; so the book is unsatisfactory. He, like some of his predecessors, wanted the particulars and their modalities to be kept apart from the general symptoms of the patient.

Boenninghausen, on the other hand, laid greater emphasis on the elements of symptom, rather than on the symptoms themselves. He said that the Materia Medica ought to be studied in the way, that the prevailing modalities should be noted, and also prevailing sensations and localities. But he complains, as we all complain, that the symptoms are imperfectly recorded, and in many cases the provings are so insufficient in number, that our fragmentary knowledge must be supplemented by clinical observation, and asserts that many of the imperfectly recorded symptoms may be fitted out by clinical observations of the curative effects of the remedy. He, therefore, combines Therapeutics with the Materia Medica, in his Pocket Book. He, then, studies the patient from the three fold point of view, obtaining the chief modalities, sensations and locations, recombining them in a drug, which has the prominent feature of all the three essentials. Thus, for a tearing pain in the left hip, aggravated during rest, he would select Lycopodium not because Lycopodium has ever developed such a symptom in its provers, for it never has, but because, it ought to, and doubtless will, in some future prover, because, Lycopodium produces prominently 'tearing pains' in various parts of the body. It affects the left hip most prominently, and its general symptoms are mostly relieved by motion; therefore, he recombines these three essentials of Lycopodium and manufactures a new symptom for Lycopodium. As a matter of fact, Lycopodium did remove sciatica with these symptoms in a case of ours. Here is a clinical verification of Boenninghausean concept.

The Boenninghausen's Repertory has been a very useful

instrument in the hands of pre-Kentian generation of Homoeopaths, who swore by it. Even in recent times Dr. Gladwin, Harvey Farrington and Elizabeth Hubbard, though Kentians, have admitted that Boenninghausen's Repertory is still supreme in obscure cases; cases with paucity of symptoms, without many mental or rare, strange or peculiar symptoms; cases where modalities predominate and concomitants are marked, cases having pathological and objective symptoms. Dr. Gladwin, once said, "Let us be broad with our school, giving each student, what best suits his mind, leading him from his present state of knowledge to what he needs, by the method best suited to him".

Boenninghausen had a genius for looking for things, where others could see nothing. He was practically the first to make the first general Repertory; the first to give evaluation to the remedies in a particular rubric; the first to enunciate the principle of analogy; the first to see that certain drugs tended to have more and peculiar concomitants than others; the first to develop the concordances of remedies. He, at once, raised the repertory from a mere index or dictionary to the pedestal of a system. Like Hahnemann, he was ahead of his times.

Boenninghausen comes in handy, if there is paucity of noticeable or dependable mental symptoms and generalities, but instead, there are a number of modalities, and too many particulars and associated symptoms. It does not require any complicated evaluation of symptoms, as is required in the working with Kent's Repertory. But, its disadvantage is, that it is not properly updated, and certain leading or characteristic symptoms are not to be found. It has a very poor function as an index to the Materia Medica.

Each case requires a different approach regarding the selection of Repertorial methods to be used.

Jahr's Contribution to Homoeopathic Repertory

Although, Jahr had fallen from Hahnemann's grace, in the preparation of Homoeopathic Repertory, because of his lack of consistence in his work, and because of his superficiality, yet, as students of Homoeopathic Repertory, it is desirable to know about his contribution in this field, and give him credit due to him. He was one of the first few, who took up the tremendous task of preparing a Repertory, as I have already mentioned. It will not be out of place, therefore, to give a brief description about his Repertory. He had written three volumes on Homoeopathic Materia Medica and Repertory. We have, at our disposal, only the English translation edited by Dr. Charles J.Hempel. It was called Jahr's NEW Manual or Symptomen-codex and its third volume was the Repertory. It was published in U.S.A. in 1853, and was prefaced by Dr. C.Hering. It took four years for Hempel to translate and edit this work.

Apart from Hempel, Dr. F.K.G. Snelling and Dr. A.Gerald Hull also translated Jahr's works and Repertories.

In 1859, Charles J. Hempel translated Jahr's New Manual, which was modified with additions from Possart's translation and editing of the 4th edition of Jahr's New Manual. Hempel followed Possart, by producing the American edition in English in one volume, and combined the Repertory section to that of the Materia Medica, which had been modified by giving briefer account of the remedies. The Repertory section of the book differed from Jahr's earlier work on it, and seems more to be precursor of Kent's Repertory. It was considered as the fifth edition of Jahr's New Manual.

In 1907, Dr. Freder K.G. Snelling edited and enlarged Hull's translation of the 4th edition of Jahr's Symptomen Codex, and was published by Boericke and Tafel as Hull's Jahr. The Repertory part of this book was called 'Clinical Index'. Unfortunately, this clinical section was done rather poorly. Repertory attached to the 5th edition of Jahr's New Manual was much better and is worth talking about.

Jahr wrote his New Manual and Repertory as early as in 1834. His later editions became more voluminous, but his last and the fourth edition, written in 1851, was more concise, and was sort of new edition of his original concise manual. It will be interesting to record Jahr's views regarding Homoeopathic Repertory. He wrote that he had arranged Repertory as an independent work, not necessarily connected with the text of symptoms given in the Materia Medica section, because the students might like to use the Repertory, without caring about a mere synopsis of symptoms given in Materia Medica, and thus, able to survey at a glance, the principal remedies required in a given case. In former times, a Repertory was merely a mechanical, literal index of the text of a manual. To be useful, the text of the symptoms has to be arranged differently from that of the Repertory. The former is necessarily much more diffuse than the text of the Repertory, and on this account, has to be arranged as concisely as possible, to save space. It is different with the Repertory. Here, nothing can be left to the mere judgement of the inquirer; every little fact, in the Repertory, is of importance, and has to be clearly expressed, lest, from the necessarily disconnected state of the materials, a fact, a symptom should seem wanting. The text and the Repertory should not, therefore, flow from each other, but each should be derived from original sources, independently from each other. Repertory and the text complete each other, without being they not found in each other, but in the common source from which both are derived.

The Repertory does not have to be a mechanical index, it has to be a logical and scientific guide.

"In imitation of Boenninghausen, I have adopted in my Repertory from different kinds of print to correspond with the signs adopted in the Symptomen Codex; symptom printed in the common type (small pica) being the least in importance; the symptom in *italics* being a degree above the former; the symptoms printed in **small caps** being the next in importance and the symptoms in **Large Caps** being the principal remedies.

This classification is not based upon absolute necessary principles, but depends entirely upon the value which the individual author attaches to the symptom.

The selection of a remedy should never be made upon a single symptom but upon the totality of the symptom."

According to Jahr, numerical value of the totality cannot always be relied upon. Its value is rather suggestive. Here, Dr. Jahr rightly mentioned that evaluation given by different authors may be different. For example, evaluation of drugs, as given by Boenninghausen in similar rubrics, is different from what Kent has given later on. This problem of giving gradation or evaluation cannot be absolute, because a particular drug which enjoys only the lowest gradation, might after some experience, be upgraded to a higher gradation. Moreover, nobody earlier had given proper directions for giving gradations except later on when Dr. Hering laid down specific conditions for grading of remedies for a particular rubric.

Although, Jahr's work of Repertory making, was not very much appreciated by Hahnemann in his times, but on going through his work and the various translations made by Hempel or Hart, one comes to appreciate the work done by Jahr. He was a prolific writer and revised his work frequently and brought out four editions of his Manual and Repertory.

In the beginning, his Repertory consisted of recording and translating the symptom as they appeared in proving or clinical cures, i.e. without breaking them, but later, especially, he modified his approach in the fifth edition by Dr. Hempel. Not only he introduced the gradation of the remedies, but also introduced Boenninghausen's concept of generalisation of locations. For example, in the chapter XXII for affections of the urinary organs, bladder, kidneys etc. he has given 'Bladder, affections of'. Similarly, under chapter on affections of the Larynx and Trachea, he has given 'Bronchial affections in general'. In the chapter on 'Affections of the Back', he has given

'Lumbar region, affections of'. Similarly, he has given 'Nape of the neck'.

Thus, he was the precursor of Boger in presenting integration of Boenninghausen's concept with that of Kent.

Let us now look .at the structure of Jahr's earlier Repertory. As I have already mentioned that the 3rd volume of Jahr's Symptomen Codex or New Manual formed the Repertory. It was divided into 29 chapters as follows-

(1) Mind, Disposition, Sensorium. The symptoms are given in alphabetical order and eighty-two pages were devoted to this area. The symptoms were given in unbroken form with concomitants and were listed against a drug or two.
(2) Head
(3) Eye
(4) Ears
(5) Nose
(6) Face
(7) Lips
(8) Chin
(9) Jaws
(10) Teeth and gums
(11) Inner mouth, palate, tongue
(12) Throat, pharynx and oesophagus
(13) Gastric derangements, appetite, thirst etc.
(14) Stomach
(15) Abdomen
(16) Anus, perineum, rectum, stool
(17) Urinary organs
(18) Male organs of generation
(19) Female organs of generation
(20) Air passages
(21) Thorax(lungs, pleura, heart, muscles)
(22) Back and neck
(23) Upper Extremities, axillary glands, finger nails
(24) Lower extremities

(25) Sleep
(26) Fever
(27) Cutaneous symptoms
(28) General symptoms
(29) Characteristic symptoms of the remedies contained in the Repertory

Unfortunately, the last two chapters 28th and 29th on 'General symptoms' and 'Characteristic symptoms' were very short and sketchy. Only a few remedies were listed.

The characteristic symptoms in the last chapter contained rubrics containing certain modalities of pain and sides of the body affected by certain remedies.

Kent later combined these two chapters in one large chapter under Generalities, but did so in greater detail, and followed Boenninghausen in grouping remedies in different rubrics and did not give detailed unbroken symptoms for different remedies.

But, in the last edition, translated by Hempel as mentioned earlier, he changed the arrangement of chapters and broke up the symptoms and tabulated them, as Boenninghausen had, in his early Repertories.It was the beginning of 'modernisation of Repertories'. The arrangement of chapters was as follows-

(1) First chapter consisted of 'General affections and conditions' which corresponds with 'Generalities' of Kent or with 'Sensations and Modalities' of Therapeutic Pocket Book, but has also given generality of location. For example, under alphabetical arrangement, he has given 'Females, diseases of, 'Fontanels remaining open'.
(2) Chapter 'Cutaneous affections and other affections of external parts'
(3) Sleep and Dreams

(4) Fever and feverish conditions
(5) Mind and disposition
(6) Sensorium
(7) Headache and other internal affections of head
(8) Integument and external parts of the head
(9) Affections of eyes and the visual powers
(10) Affections of the ears and sense of hearing
(11) Affections of the nose and the sense of smell
(12) Affections of the face, lips, chin and jaws
(13) Affections of the teeth and gums
(14) Affections of inner mouth, palate and tongue, saliva
(15) Affections of throat etc.
(16) Appetite and taste; desires and aversions
(17) Derangement of digestive functions, complaints after eating
(18) Gastric ailments, eructations, hiccough, nausea, vomiting
(19) Affections of the stomach and pit of the stomach
(20) Affections of the hypochondria, including liver, spleen and diaphragm
(21) Pains and other ailments in the abdomen, inguinal region
(22) Affections of anus, alvine evacuations, and symptoms of rectum and perineum
(23) Affections of the urinary organs, bladder, kidneys etc.
(24) Affections of the male sexual organs
(25) Affections of the female sexual organs and of infants
(30) Catarrhal affections
(31) Affections of Larynx and Trachea
(32) Cough and accompanying ailments
(33) Disorders of the respiratory functions
(34) Affections of the chest including diseases of the heart and Mammae
(35) Affections of the back, axillae, neck, small of back, nape of neck, scapulae and os sacrum
(36) Affections of upper extremities
(37) Affections of the lower extremities

In this Repertory, Jahr followed, in the beginning, Hahnemann's way of designing the structure and arrangement of symptoms. Here, Jahr did not place all the remedies for a particular symptom or complaint, and did not **break the** symptoms, but kept them as they appeared in pathogenesis, complete with their particular modalities and concomitants.For example, under the first chapter containing MIND, DISPOSITION and SENSORIUM, the first symptom taken up by him is 'Absence of Mind'. Kent has a similar rubric listed by him as 'Absent-minded' under Chapter MIND. Jahr has listed 45 sentences or short paragraphs giving conditions of absent-mindedness. I am giving below a few examples to make my point clear.

1. Absence of mind- (8 remedies) Acon., Agn., Am-c., Cham., Lach., Lyc., Rhus-t.
2. Absence of thought- Am-c., Cic.
3. Absence of mind , irresolution- Alum.
8. Absence of mind, he does not recognise his friends- Cocc.
12. Unable to be attentive- Bor.
14. Absence of mind, in paroxysms, with stitches in the joints of the fingers, on return of consciousness- Mosch.
15. Absence of mind, with uneasiness in the head and pit of stomach- Mag-c.
17. The children are sitting in the corners of the room and give wrong answers- Bar-m.
18. Makes mistakes in writing- Nat-c.
26. He looks through the window for hours without seeming to be conscious of anything- Mez.
36. Frequent vanishing of thoughts- Ol-an.

Kent, however, later lumped almost all the remedies showing indications of absent-mindedness in a single paragraph(total of about 50 remedies with suitable evaluations). He has, however, given 8 small sub-rubrics, which indicate modification of the symptoms, according to Time or Circumstantial modalities. Kent had to make his selection for sub-rubrics.

Jahr's arrangement of symptoms makes it very difficult to do repertorial analysis, but once in a while, some of the symptoms mentioned cannot be found in Kent, as they were included in generalised rubrics. Jahr, for example, has given under 'Anger' the rubric 'Anger at everything with asthma'- Cham. This symptom has helped us in relieving acute asthmatic attacks, especially in children. Kent did not introduce it as a sub-rubric in the relevant main rubric of Anger.

Hempel, who translated Jahr's works, was one of those, who condemned Boenninghausen's approach to Repertory-making, and tried to keep the various symptoms of a drug from the Materia Medica unbroken while indexing them in the suitable areas of Repertory chapters. To make this point clear, I give the following examples-

Let us take up the mental symptom- 'Restlessness'. In Kent, as you know, there are a number of remedies kept in a group, of course, given with suitable gradations. Later on, Kent has given remedies for 'Restlessness', where definite modalities have been observed. In the Hempel's Repertory, however, there is no group as such given. He has given 34 symptoms, where restlessness has been observed. From No. 1 to 34, he has given the full, complete symptoms of the remedy, which may comprise of concomitants.

A description of patients' or provers' expression of restlessness and even modalities has been given. For example-

(1) "He does a variety of things with great haste, runs about in the house" - Acon.

(3) "Went from place to place"- Hyos, Lach, Stann.

(4) "Restlessness"- Petr.

(9) "Restlessness, has to rise, then to be down, cannot bear walking" - Merc.

(10) "Restlessness, going from place to place"- Merc

(19) "Violent agitation in bed"- Bell.

(30) "He cannot do anything fast enough and is not satisfied with his efforts"- Aur.

(34) "Restlessness, with desire to work, he undertakes a great many things as soon as he began it"- Verat.

This arrangement cannot be utilised for usual repertorisation of cases but we can, however, have a more graphic picture of restlessness in a particular remedy or a patient. We can refer to the book for confirmations as we refer to Materia Medica.

Dr. Gentry, in his Repertory, has given the remedies for Restlessness in a similar fashion but has given, more often, more than one single remedy, and has given under two separate heads 'Restless' and 'Restlessness'. Although, Gentry also, has tried to give a complete unbroken symptom along with concomitants and modalities, but is less descriptive than Hempel. Both of them, however, belonged to the school of repertorians who did not want to break symptoms beyond recognition.

Gentry's examples-

(1) "Great restlessness and impatience"- Dulc.

(2) "Insanity, with mental, physical restlessness"- Cimicifuga.

(3) "Hysterical restlessness and anxiety"- Asaf.

(4) "Anxious restlessness"- Canth, Sabad.

So, it is obvious that Repertories like this, can be useful if one has to confirm a particular remedy or remedies, which have been indicated by Kent's or other repertorial systems. This gives a sort of short-cut for references to Materia Medica.

Jahr divided his book into 29 chapters as already indicated, which was different from the common divisions used now-a-days.

This arrangement can be more useful and faster in

locating the symptoms than the current arrangements used by Kent and others.

In the 28th chapter, he has given 'General symptoms', which correspond to Kent's Generalities. In this chapter, Jahr called it also 'General Internal affections'. Following his approach of not breaking the symptoms, he has given the description of the symptoms as they appeared in the provings or in clinical confirmations.

I have given the contents of Jahr's Repertories, so that students of Homoeopathic Repertory may see, how different workers looked at the body's regional divisions for the purpose of indexing the symptoms, and how Kent arranged his regional divisions with sensations, and how much he owed to the earlier workers. The repertorian of the future may modify even Kent's arrangement, and may draw something from Jahr and others, so that we have no difficulty in locating the symptoms or indexing them. In Jahr's arrangement, General Affections and Conditions have the first place, and Mind and Disposition follow later. Actually, Mind and General Affections should be placed one after the other.

Allen's General Symptom Register of Homoeopathic Materia Medica

One of the earliest major works on Repertories after Boenninghausen's Therapeutic Pocket Book, was the Herculean work of Dr. T.F. Allen known as the 'A General Symptom Register of the Homoeopathic Materia Medica', which was, actually, an index to his famous 'Encyyclopaedia of Pure Materia Medica' and was published in July 1880. It contains references to about 825 remedies. This is an important source book, but cannot be used as a daily tool for repertorisation, as Boenninghausen's book or Kent's Repertory. There are two problems with it; one is that its structure, though unique, and in certain ways a Hahnemannian concept, does not lend itself for easy repertorial analysis; the second is that Allen stuck rigidly to what was obtained from reliable provings and toxicological symptoms, and ignored the symptoms, which were confirmed and verified a number of times in the clinical use of the remedies, with the result, that the rubrics for use are left with much fewer remedies, compared with Repertories like Kent or Boger's Boenninghausen. The arrangement of symptoms does not lend itself for easy access and repertorial analysis.

Allen has followed a unique idea of listing and indexing the symptoms in his 'Symptom Register'. He thought of 'location' or part affected as the guide or starting point for search for a symptom. In this concept, he followed Boenninghausen to some extent. He did not follow the general Anatomical division, as was customary at that time. He located the regions or organs on absolutely alphabetical order, so that the search for a particular symptom can be made easier. May be, some day, computer programmers may design a software on a modified version of this type of arrangement. Allen had hoped, that this method of indexing symptoms can be easily used for classifying and indexing of future provings, as this will enable the future worker to do the job with greater ease and in shortest time.

He has taken first the General (the whole of the area or organ) 'locations', followed by various sensations or pains in the alphabetical order from A to Z. In the sensations etc., he has given first, the 'unmodified' sensations, followed by 'modified' sensations.

Time modalities are listed first, followed by other modalities in alphabetical order. The latter is followed by 'Extensions', which is arranged again in alphabetical order, and not in anatomical order.

For example, let us take the general location of 'cheeks', which Allen has given separately from face. Here, he has given 'Aching'; 'Abscesses'; 'Anaesthesia'; 'Bagging', 'Bitings'; 'Blood surges' etc. till 'Sweat'. After that, he has followed with parts of cheek like-

'Back of cheek'.

'Towards chin' (Chin. towards)

'Near Ear' (Ear, near)

'Inside' (He has given a reference to see Mouth walls under separate Heading 'Mouth')

'Lower part' etc. till 'Upper Part', of cheeks.

Each part of cheek is followed by sensations etc. relevant to that portion of cheeks.

Unlike other authors of Repertory, he has not listed sides of cheeks separately, but has given the sides (right or left denoted by 'r' or l') against different remedies in brackets. i.e. remedies, affecting the right side of part, are indexed with (r) in bracket, and those, affecting left side of the part, are followed by (1) in bracket.

For example-

Cheeks, swollen- Acon (1); Am-m (r) Baryta carb (1); Coca (r)

It may be mentioned that some locational indications are not very clear to a reader. Regarding the arrangement of sensations and locations, 'Cheeks' is followed by 'Cheerfulness' as the next rubric, following his strictly alphabetical order. Now 'cheerfulness', ordinarily, we consider to be located under Mind, but Allen does not give separate section on Mind, but refers us to see 'thoughts' according to alphabetical placement. Under 'MIND' he has referred us to 'Thoughts'. 'Memory' is listed under M after 'Membranes'. So, one has to be familiar with the structuring of this Repertory, before one can utilise this book for remedy analysis or researches in Repertory.

Another important difference from other Repertories is that Allen has made a clear distinction between symptoms, which appear only at certain times or under certain circumstances, or conditions from those symptoms, which are aggravated at certain times or in certain conditions, but are present otherwise also. Kent and many others have not made this distinction regarding the symptoms; they are all aggravated or ameliorated even if these symptoms appear only at specified times or under specific conditions or circumstances.

He has given under ‘Regions’, the sensations in general, followed by time incidence and other circumstance, which mark the appearances of symptoms. This section under general unmodified sensations is marked by capital letter ‘C’ on the left hand side of the paragraph.

Later on, towards the close of this paragraph, he has indicated remedies, which have the aggravation (Agg.) ‘<‘ and amelioration (Amel.) ‘>’ at specified time, or under specified conditions. Allen, in the paragraph marked by the letter ‘C’ (Conditions), has three main sub-divisions.

(1) General conditions associated with occurrence of symptoms.

(a)Time (Hours of the day).
(b) Circumstances (Alphabetically)

(2) Conditions of Aggravation.

(a) Time
(b) Circumstances

(3) Conditions of Amelioration.

(a) Time
(b) Circumstances

According to him, Aggravation or Amelioration of symptoms is different from, only mere association of symptoms with particular time or circumstances.

The third section is made up of rubrics or symptoms, which are classified by him as 'peculiar sensations'. They are arranged after main section of 'unmodified sensation' (e.g. Pain in general), along with their specific conditions of incidence, as well as their specific aggravations and ameliorations. This section is marked by letter 'P', kept on the left hand side of this section.

For example under 'Back' he has given-

P	Back	Pain (ache)	As in cold stage of ague
	-	-	Across back
	-	-	Alternating with tightness of Chest
	-	-	Arresting breathing
	-	-	Like a blow on stooping, > pressing against something hard
	-	-	Extending downwards etc.
	-	-	Wandering.

In this section of Peculiarities, he has included the extensions also. Even here, he has tabulated the symptoms alphabetically. I may mention here that, possibly, due to printing error, the letter 'P' in capital is missing at various places in this particular section referred to above.

These peculiarities are rather uncommon, and he could not place them elsewhere. Another feature of these symptoms in this section is that he kept the symptom without breaking it. He has kept the conditions and modalities alphabetically, even while including them in this particular section.

For example:

P (Back) (ache) Like a blow on stooping; ameliorated by

pressing against something hard- Sep.

Here, 'stooping' is the specific associated condition (not agg.), but modality is also given along with 'amelioration' pressing against something hard. 'B' letter of 'blow' follows the 'a' or 'ar' of the word arresting. This arrangement can be understood clearly by referring the pages 137 and 138 of the 'Symptom-Register'.

Since Allen is sticking rigidly to alphabetical arrangement, we see that after the section on Back-Ache is over, he has taken up Back- 'Acne rosacea' followed by Back- 'Anxiety in'; 'Asleep as if'.

After finishing with the sensations and signs on back in general, the last sensation being 'weakness', he starts with sub-regions or areas alphabetically. Before starting the sub-divisions and their sensations etc., the sensation etc. of Back in General is treated completely.

Even in the sub-divisions of back, he follows the same arrangements. Peculiar symptoms, which also contain concomitants, always follow after the Aggravations and Ameliorations have been listed. This order is followed also, where the author has given available, details regarding a particular sensation. For example, under Pain in Back in general, we find bruised sensations, which is recorded again in the following order-

Remedies in general- Time and other conditions of occurrence of this type of pain, which is indexed by 'C' on the left. This is again followed by peculiar symptoms and concomitants, denoted by 'P' on the left.

P Bruised pain, as if congested, < pressure- Nux-v.
\- - as after great exertion- Ol-an.
\- - as after a fall, at 1.30 p.m.- Hur.
\- - extending to nape of neck, evening after lying

down- Nat-c.
- - extending to sacrum- Gin.
- - extending to sacrum and abdomen- Caust.
- - extending to small of back and thence abdomen- Caust
- - shoulders to loins, on waking- Ox-ac.
- - shifting from place to place- Dros.
- - in one spot- Sulph.

As already mentioned, his so called 'peculiarities' are always mentioned after modalities, and are indicated by capital letter 'P'. These are the symptoms, which do not fit into the other broad sensations, but are consisting of concomitant sensations in the part, extensions of sensation to different areas or parts. The following examples will make it clearer. Let us take up 'Back' in general and the sensation of 'Cold' (page 140). He has given a number of remedies, which have coldness or chilliness in the back in general without any specific modalities. This rubric is followed by its time and circumstances, its occurrence followed by specific modalities of Aggravation and Amelioration. This section is denoted by 'C' in the left hand margin of the book. This main rubric is followed by symptoms or rubrics. Then comes a number of symptoms, which, as I mentioned above, are considered by him as 'peculiar' and certain concomitants and unbroken symptoms related to 'cold' feeling in the back in general. On page 141 of the Symptom Register, we see the following symptoms, which are denoted by 'P'.

P Back Cold Across back, darting, at 10 a.m.-Ere.; after sleep- Crot-t.
- - As from cold air, down back-Coff-t.; spreading over whole body-Agar-m.
- - Alternates with heat-Atrop., Verat; in evening- Thuja.; with flushes of heat- China.; with heat of head- Asaf.;of face, in forenoon- Lact.
- - Extending to abdomen-Spig; into arms- Gin, Verat; etc.

- - External- Coc-c., 5.30 pm- Lyc.
- - Mingled with heat- Coff., Com.

till it ends with the last symptoms, characterised by letter 'W'

- - As from a wet cloth, in afternoon, > after lying- Castor.

Although, Allen has mentioned, in his introduction, that he indicated such groups of symptoms by the letter 'P' on the left hand margin, but in the above group he missed to have it printed. There are many other examples where this has been missed.

For example

Back - Above anus (page 148)
Back - Arteries (page 148)
Back - Near axilla (148)
Back - Opposite bowels
Back - Dorsal region (which is again followed by sensations etc.)

In the rubrics indexed by 'P', as already stated, he has given more characteristic or descriptive definition of the general pain or sensation as given by the provers. Here, he has given unbroken symptoms and concomitants, which are considered peculiar. For example, under 'P', after Burning Pain External in general (page 188), he has given-

'periodic in spots'- Lyc;
'as from a mustard, plaster'- Kali-carb;
'in spots'- Ambra;
'better scratching'- Anac;
'wandering'- Arnica.

The Symptom Register of Allen is a very useful index to his Encyclopaedia of Materia Medica Pura, and is a useful piece of literature. It must have involved great deal of time, concentration and devotion, but cannot be depended upon as a tool of Repertorisation. As mentioned, symptoms which have appeared in our Materia Medica by breech presentation i.e. symptoms which were clinically verified and confirmed, have not been included. Hering, and later Kent, paid lot of attention to the latter class of symptoms and included them in the Repertories, with the result that the prescribers discovered that they had a better and more useful compendium of data to select the remedy from.

Although, Allen had tried to arrange all the symptoms alphabetically, but in working out a case from it, is very difficult and cumbersome. There is no logical group arrangement of symptoms pertaining to an organ, area or mental sphere.

It has, however, usefulness sometimes in providing clues to peculiar symptoms, local or general, which are not found in Kent's Repertory. For example, pain 'Burning in streaks' is not listed in Kent's Repertory. But in Allen's Register, it is mentioned in 'Burning streaks'- Carl. Similarly, 'Burning, tingling'- Vacc.

Such examples can be multiplied quite easily. For a serious student of Homoeopathic medicine, especially in Repertory, such sources cannot be neglected.

We came across a patient, who complained of burning of the feet(whole feet) which was extending to legs above ankles. He feared that it may not extend upwards and even extend to his heart. His burning was better by bathing with cold water. He did not stick out feet from under covers as is seen in Sulphur etc.

In Kent's Repertory, there is the rubric 'Pain- burning, foot', but there is no rubric mentioning extension. In Allen's Register, however, we find on page 474 'Foot- Burning extending above ankles'- Arsenic.

Dr. Allen wanted to add a separate chapter on the

'Conditions' but he could not do it'. He had planned to write a book called 'Book of conditions'. That would have been a very useful addition to our literature on Repertories.

The question, that is often raised by the students, is how to use the book? Is it any good for Repertorisation of cases? What place does it have in the Homoeopathic literature?

As I have already stated, it cannot be used for routine Repertorisation. It has very limited remedies, and no effort has been made to update the remedies. It is primarily an index to the Encyclopedia, and that function it does most admirably. The other important use for Research scholars is to make a thorough study of the book, and possibly make additions to Kent's Repertory wherever justified; additions regarding remedies, and additions where unusual concomitant symptoms have been mentioned by Allen. This book has to be made a part of study for Post-graduate students.

'Repertory of Hering's Guiding Symptoms' by Knerr, a student of Hering, did a yeoman's service by preparing a monumental index or Repertory of Hering's book, something like Allen had done by writing Symptom-Register to his Encyclopaedia.

Repertory of the Hering's Guiding Symptoms

Knerr's Repertory

Another Repertory, which was basically supposed to be an index of 'Hering's Guiding Symptoms (like Allen's Symptom Register as the index to his Encyclopaedia), was prepared by Dr. Calvin B. Knerr. Both Allen and Hering were prodigious workers, but Allen left more of his original works written by himself, whereas Hering's legacy was completed by his students and family members. Even 'Guiding Symptoms' were not completed in his life time, and some of the later volumes were completed posthumously, from his hand written notes etc., but the style and data were copied according to his own planning and design.

Knerr, in his Repertory, has divided the book into chapters, according to Hering's plan of regions in his Guiding Symptoms.

The main chapters are 46, but he added the 47th chapter based on Hering's stages of life and constitution, which he had appended at the end of all remedies, after giving their pathogenesis, including clinical confirmations, under different headings. The last chapter, the 48th chapter, is on Drug Relationships. The chapters are as follows-

1) Mind and Disposition
2) Sensorium
3) Inner Head
4) Outer Head
5) Eyes
6 Ears
7) Nose
8) Upper face
9) Lower face
10) Teeth and Gums
11) Taste and Tongue
12) Inner mouth
13) Throat
14) Appetite, Thirst; Desires, Aversions.
15) Eating and drinking
16) Hiccough, Belching, Nausea and Vomiting
17) Scrobiculum and stomach
18) Hypochondria
19) Abdomen
20) Stool and Rectum
21) Urinary Organs
22) Male Sexual organs.
23) Female Sexual organs
24) Pregnancy; Parturition; Lactation

25) Voice and Larynx, Trachea and Bronchia.
26) Respiration
27) Cough and Expectoration
28) Inner chest and Lungs
29) Heart, Pulse and Circulation
30) Outer chest
31) Neck and Back
32) Upper Limbs
33) Lower Limbs
34) Limbs in General
35) Rest, Position, Motion
36) Nerves (which includes Activity (strength). Catalepsy, Chorea, Convulsions, Fainting, Faintness, Hysteria, Lassitude(Fatigue) Malaise, Nerves, Neuralgia, Paralysis, Restlessness, Starting, Trembling, Twitching, Weakness, but sensations are dealt with in chapter 43).
37) Sleep
38) Time (Afternoon, Evening, Forenoon. Morning, Night Before Midnight, After Midnight); arranged alphabetically
39) Temperature and Weather (Air, Cold, Dark, Light, Seasons, Temperature, Warmth, Water, Weather).
40) Fever (Chill, Chilliness, Fever, Heat, Sweat, Temperature)
41) Attacks, Periodicity
42) Locality and Direction. (Laterality)
43) Sensations in General
44) Tissues (Adipose, Bones, Cancer, Cartilages, Decomposition, Degeneration, Emaciation, Excretions, Fibrous, Fluids, Gangrene, Tumours, Ulcers.)
45) Touch, Passive Motion, Injuries.
46) Skin
47) Stages of life and constitution.
48) Drug - relationships of

The basic difference of this index or Repertory from that of 'Allen's Symptom Register', is that it contains symptoms and remedies which have had not only provings and toxicological pathogeneses, but had also clinical provings and confirmations. Apart from this, it had four gradations of the rubrics or symptoms marked by vertical lines I, II, **I II,** which were appended before the relevant symptoms. These correspond more or less with Boenninghausean concept of evaluation. According to Hering, **I** and **II,** two heavily marked signs, correspond to remedies verified or confirmed in clinical practice a number of time, apart from their pathogenesis in the records of provings or toxicological records; **II** marks the most frequently verified by cures. The lighter vertical lines are indicative of occasionally verified symptoms; the single light vertical sign is less occasionally verified than the lighter double line.

This is one of the main Repertories (apart from that of Hale, Jahr and Hempel), where the symptoms have been placed unbroken, as far as possible. Let us take the example of a mental symptom 'Forgetful'. He has listed first, all the remedies which have forgetfulness in general. This is followed by smaller rubrics, which have special association with a particular circumstance or condition, or are related to a specific time frame. All these things are given alphabetically. In the above reference, for example, the general rubric is followed by 'Forgetful, loses **appetite'** (melancholy): Anac. The word appetite is specially given in bolder type. The alphabet 'a' of appetite gives it the right of placement in the first place. The second, sub-rubric is associated with **'business'**. The letter '**a**' of business naturally follows after **'b'** of appetite. But under this sub-rubric, there are further extensions connected with forgetfulness in business, as then this type of forgetfulness is modified or associated with other conditions also (concomitants). For example, the rubrics appear as follows-

Forgetful, in **business:** Fl-ac.; crept into a corner and said he must sleep, could not sleep but still remains lying down, Jamb.; remembers all he had forgotten, during slumber, Selen.

Forgetful of **dates: I** con.; Fl-ac

Forgetful, of what she is going to **do** : in post-partum haemorrhage, **I** Cann-s., II Carb-ac; what he has just intended to do, **I** Card-m.; what she wants to do or has done, **I** Chel.; from one moment to next what she wishes to do, **I** Manc; what he has done a short time ago, **I** Calc-p.

Forgetful of everything except **dream**: (melancholy after mortification), **I** Ign.

Forgetful in **evening** : Fl-ac., **I** Form.

Forgetful, of almost **everything** : Fl-ac. and so on.

Let us now study this example given above.

First of all, all the indications are given in an alphabetical order. I have marked the main circumstantial association by **bolder types**. For example, after 'business', comes 'dates'; then 'do'; then 'dreams', followed by 'evening' and 'everything' and so on.

Even in these sub rubrics, further extensions or variations also follow this alphabetical arrangement. Let us examine the rubric 'forgetful of what she is going **to do'** : in post-partum haemorrhage, **I** Cann-s.; II Carb-ac.; what he has just intended to do. **I** Card-m.; from one moment to next what she wishes to do. **I** Manc.; what he has done a short time ago. I have double underlined the letter or alphabet of the special word which indicates the special circumstance.

Here, it will not be out of place to mention that he omitted putting thin vertical lines before the remedies, which have been less frequently verified. He has, however, used double vertical thin lines, single and double bold vertical lines, to indicate the value.

If one studies Kent's Repertory under forgetfulness, there are comparatively much less number of sub-rubrics. Some authors have even criticised that Kent particularised very heavily in the section on Extremities where it is least valuable. But in the section on Mind, he omitted giving greater details, and made more generalisations. In his first edition, he had kept more of particularised details in the section on Mind. May be, someday, we may have to add to Kent's chapter on Mentals from these sources.

Unfortunately, in the Knerr's Repertory, the arrangement, though made very systematic, and after lot of hard work, is not amenable to quick and useful repertorial analysis. This data, however,. could be entered in computer software and utilised when needed. There is plenty of material in the book for research workers, and some of the sub-rubrics, though particular, could prove of great value. Of course, this Repertory also requires lot of additions, since it is based only on the symptoms given in 'Hering's Guiding Symptoms'.

Another area where it could be utilised is to gather the cross-references, and utilise them when revising and improving Kent's Repertory. For example, let us study the rubric 'Aversion' in Kent (Mind) and compare it with 'Aversion' in Knerr's book (Mind) page 25.

'Aversion to everything'- (Kent) Alumn., am-m. etc. But in 'Aversion to all things' (Knerr)- Bov. (in urticaria), is not there in Kent's Repertory and Calc. is again modified by 'as soon as he sits idle'. The following are not there at all in Kent's Repertory. For example-

'Aversion to **amusement'**- Ign.

'Aversion to **domestic** duties'- Citrus.

'Aversion to her **children'**- Plat.

'Aversion in women to opposite **sex'**- Raph.

'Aversion to **women'**- Puls.

In this context of aversions, Knerr gives a cross reference to rubrics like 'Company'; 'Dissatisfied' and 'Hate'. In his rubric on 'Hate', he has given 'Hates women - Puls'. Apparently, 'aversion to women' may extend even to 'Hate', and he has, thus, given them at two different places.

Knerr, however, has, at times, done too much of hair-splitting also. For example, he has separated fear symptoms into three areas- (a) Apprehension (b) Anxiety (c) Fear, where as Kent has referred to see Anxiety, Fear etc. in respect of Apprehension, and I think, it is rightly so. It is very difficult to differentiate the different shades or meanings of very closely related rubrics. 'Apprehension' denotes a mixture of Anxiety and Fear put together. Even 'Anxiety ' has an element of Fear, and Fear certainly has a component of Anxiety. For classification and tabulations, we have to make certain compromises. This difficulty is more compounded, especially, when symptoms and expressions collected from provers, is likely to be not very accurate or expressive, and may be misjudged. This is why, while repertorising, we are advised to see also, closely related rubrics or Cross-References.

In Knerr's Repertory, there is a mental rubric 'Depressed' (dejected despondent) and another 'sad' (dejected, downcast, low spirited). But Kent in his Repertory, has combined these two into 'Sadness'. Knerr has given a very short rubric in 'Discouraged', but Kent has given a fairly large rubric in his book. These difference have come about, because each author interpreted these expressions slightly differently or laid different emphasis.

In the section on HYPOCHONDRIA, Knerr has taken Diaphragm, Hypochondria, Liver and Spleen, although Kent has taken them under Abdomen in general. Knerr has, however, taken up general sensations and other organs under Abdomen which follows in chapter on Hypochondria. For example, the items taken here are Colic, Flatulence, Inguinal region,

Intestines, Perineum, Pubis. This division was followed in strict adherence to 'Hering's Guiding Symptoms'. None of them included 'Gall-bladder' as a separate entity or locational organ, but took it only as a part of Liver. Hence, indirect mentions were made. For example, there is no direct reference anywhere as 'Inflammation Gall bladder'. Knerr has given under 'Liver, **gall ducts**: catarrh' and 'Liver, **gall -stones** (biliary calculi)'. Kent has given under pain 'Liver- colic, gall-stones.

Kent did not keep jaundice in relation to liver etc. but kept it under 'SKIN' . But I think Knerr did it correctly and kept it under 'Liver, **jaundice.'**

Like the instances cited, there are many such examples, where something useful could be included in the Kent's Repertory from this great work of Knerr. There are remedies here and there, which should have found place in Kent, although, Kent borrowed a very large part of his material in his Repertory from 'Herring's Guiding Symptoms'. As I have mentioned elsewhere, his degree of valuation of remedies has been based almost entirely on Hering's works.

I have taken up rubrics and various sections, as it is not possible to review the whole book by Knerr. But, it is worthwhile for research workers and post-graduate students, to go through this literature deeply, so that Kent's work could be presented in a more complete and integrated form. This brings to my mind Knerr's chapter on OUTER HEAD, which has been kept as a separate chapter from chapter on INNER HEAD. (Kent has included both 'inner head' and 'outer head' in the same section) Here, the rubrics about Hair are given in more detail, and more extensively than in Kent's Repertory, although, Kentian rubrics have naturally large number of remedies because of later additions. With the increased problem of hair loss today, we are being approached by patients in large numbers. We should pay more attention to remedies, which have a bearing on hair loss etc.

Knerr's contribution contains a mine of information, which must be utilised fully in our relevant books on Repertory-making.

The Concordance Repertory of the Characteristic Symptoms of the Materia Medica by William D.Gentry.

Dr. Gentry published this Repertory in 1890, and the second edition appeared two years later in 1892. It was published in six volumes. He arranged the chapters of the Concordance Repertory as follows-

I Mind and Disposition
Head and scalp
The Eyes
The Ears
The Nose and Nostril
The Face

II Mouth, Throat, Stomach, Hypochondria

III Abdomen, Anus, Rectum
Urine and Urinary organs
Male Sexual Organs

IV Uterus and Appendages
Menstruation and Discharges
Pregnancy and Parturition
Lactation and Mammary glands

V Voice, Larynx, Trachea
Chest, Lungs, Bronchia and Cough
Heart and Circulation
Chill and Fever
Skin, Sleep and Dreams

VI Neck and Back
Upper Extremities
Lower Extremities
Bones and Limbs in general
The Nerves
Generalities and Keynotes

It must have been popular at that time, as the second edition had to be brought out within such a short time. His objective, in bringing out this kind of book in six volumes, was to enable the physician to find any characteristic symptoms with comparative ease and certainty, since, it was becoming more difficult to locate desirable symptoms, in the maze of symptoms, in the expanding Materia Medicas. In the preface of the first edition, the author wrote that in his effort to locate the symptom 'Constant dull frontal headache, worse in the temples, with aching in the umbilicus' he spent days in his search in different Materia Medicas and Repertories. He thought of planning a Repertory on the pattern of Cruden's Concordance Bible. For the above symptom, it could be placed and found under the letter 'U', under Umbilicus.

He has not taken all the symptoms of the remedies in the book, and taken only the symptoms which are (a) more characteristic with concomitant elements of the symptoms; (b) only symptoms which have been verified clinically repeatedly. He has described in detail, how to search such symptoms in his Concordance Repertory.

This book helps in locating symptoms, which are usually not found in the General Repertories which are being used for Repertorial analysis, as in these Repertories, complex symptoms had to be broken, and parts to be placed at the different relevant areas. Kent could not place all the concomitants in his Repertory. This Repertory cannot lend itself for usual repertorisation of case histories, but could help us tremendously in location of a particular symptom with a concomitant, as such a symptom even if 'particular' or 'locational' becomes characteristic or desirable for the hunt for the similimum. Apart from this, the author has placed the symptoms and the relevant words, expressing and describing it as they were found in the various Materia Medicas.

For example, if we were to locate fear of an accident, we do not find it in the rubrics located under the general heading 'Fear' in the Repertory, but in this symptom, the general idea is the accident. Hence it has to be searched under Accident (of course under Mind). It is placed there as follows- 'Accident- Trembling, anguish and fear, as if some accident would happen'- Mag-c.

Here is another example of a symptom with a concomitant, as found in the Materia Medica, but cannot be placed as such in the Repertories used by us.

Under Mind and Disposition- he has given 'Accomplishes- Indecision, never accomplishes what has undertaken but remains standing in one place as if senseless or intoxicated'- Nux-m.

In another example, Gentry has given under 'Employment (Mind and Disposition)- Anxiety, allowing no rest at any employment, as if she had committed a crime'- Chel.

But, looking at other page under Anxiety, we find- 'Anxiety- as if had committed great crime'- Cocc. (Chel., Ferr., Ign., Verat., verat-v.).
The remedies in the bracket are connected with this main symptom, but have other marked concomitants. For example, under Anxiety again-
'Anxiety- as after committing an evil deed, worse after dinner and evening'- Verat.
'Anxiety- as after committing crime'- Ferr.

From these examples, one can see that the remedies mentioned in the bracket above, are also connected with the feeling of having committed a crime etc. but in different context and with different mental state and concomitants.

This book could be useful for hunting a peculiar or a complex symptom, which has eluded us in the general Repertories and needs to be taken into account for solving our problem.

THE CROSS CURRENTS

Opposition to the Boenninghausen's ideas was felt by many workers and physicians of note and experience in the profession, because they felt that Boenninghausen had carried the idea of analogy to an extent, unpalatable for many workers in this line. For the purpose of classification and abbreviation, he split the symptoms, with the result that as an index or a dictionary to the Materia Medica, it was most unsatisfactory. It may be noticed that Boenninghausen was very clear in his mind, when be published that work. Earlier, he had called his books as 'Repertory of Anti-psoric Remedies and Repertory of Remedies not Anti-psoric'. That is why, he possibly called it 'Pocket Therapeutic Book' and not a Repertory, as he had done earlier for his Repertory of the Anti-psoric drugs. It was complained that he broke his symptoms into parts in such a way, that on reconstruction, unwarranted combinations of a drug could emerge, which have no sanction from the Materia Medica or clinical experience.

This other school of thought was very much opposed to Boenninghausen, as it did not like the breaking up of the symptoms according to Boenninghausen's concept of distribution and generalisation. They held that symptoms should be kept, as were found in the provings, and the Repertory should not distort or dismember these symptoms. The extremists holding this view were Jahr, Hering, Hempel and Hart. Dr. Jahr, though subscribing to this view, conceded, however, that no Repetory, however complete, can satisfy all the exigencies of practice, and that in many cases, advantage can be taken of the cases of concrete combinations, which the Repertory indicates. On the contrary, it will be necessary to make more combinations, founded upon the general character of the medicament, or on the analogies given in another organ, than that in which the symptom was sought.

This group held the view that in view of the almost universal tendency to dismemberment of the essential element of the symptomatology, "we feel called upon to utter our protest against such an absurd, not to say suicidal, policy. To analyse and classify the accessory and concomitant symptoms, is no less useful than convenient, provided the several parts into which the text is divided, and the relations to each other, are always preserved, and kept in view, so that their recombinations may not give rise to an infinity of imaginary symptoms having no existence in the pathogenesis, not even in the possibilities of the medicament".

Hering also was positively against Boenninghausen's generalisations, and wanted to stick to the combinations and character of symptoms, as found, either in the provings, or in the clinical confirmations. Even in his 'Guiding Symptoms', he has stated the symptoms as such, without deducing any generalisations. The example of Repertories of this school of thought are, (1) Jahr's Repertory, the last edition of which appeared in 1851. Later, Hull and Hempel edited the works. (2) Symptom Register by Allen, which was a sort of index to Allen's Encyclopaedia. (3) Knerr's Repertory, which was the index to Bering's Guiding Symptoms. (4) Similarly, Repertory of the Cyclopaedia of Drug Pathogenesis, as the fifth volume as its index. (5) Gentry's Concordance Repertory.

Jahr has been condemned for indicating remedies for diagnostic names in his Repertory. He was a prolific writer, and though, he had fallen from the grace of Hahnemann, yet his work was translated and improved by men like Hempel and Hull. Jahr was the father of Clinical Repertories. Hempel, however, checked and modified it searchingly. He was, of all people, a stickler for exactitude, and did not change or break symptoms given in the provings. The exact words or terms, used by the provers, were kept as such. To men like him, Boenninghausen and his followers were heretics. He was most uncompromising in this respect Gentry also concurred with Hempel, and classified the symptoms, without breaking the associations of the symptoms or changing the expressions or words of the provers.

As I have already mentioned, for about 50 years, Boenninghansen's Repertory had a complete mastery of the realm in the field of Repertory. But, from 1880 onwards, a large number of clinical and other Repertories started appearing, and there was some sort of unrest in the minds of the people that everything was not all right, so far as Repertories were concerned.

During about 25 years or so, between 1880 to 1905, there were born quite a number of small Repertories, regional and clinical. This seemed to be an era of Regional Repertories. For general information, they are listed below, but it is not possible to go into detailed account of these Repertories

1. 1873 - Repertory of Eyes- by Berridge.
2. Desires and Aversion- by Guernsey.
3. 1879 - Illustrated Repertory (of Pain in chest, sides and back)- by Rolin R. Gregg
4. 1880 - Repertory of Modalities- by Worcester.
5. - Repertory' of Haemorrhoids- by Guernsey.
6 - Repertory of Respiratory Organs- by Lutze.
7 - Repertory of Fevers- by H.C. Allen
8 - Repertory of Foot Sweat- by O.M. Drake.
9. 1883 - Repertory of the Intermittent Fevers- by W. A. Allen
10. 1884 - Repertory of Cough and Expectoration- by Lee and Clark.
11. 1888 - Repertory of the Head- by Niedhard.
12. 1890 - Classified Index of Homoeopathic Materia Medica for Urogenital and Venereal diseases- by Carleton and Coles.
13. 1891 - Headache- Concise Repertory- by King
14. 1892 - Repertory of Digestive System- by Arkell McMichell

15. 1894 - Repertory of Sensation as if- by Holcomb.
16. 1894 - Repertory of Rheumatism- by Perkins.
17. - Repertory of Therapeutics of Respiratory System- by Van Denbug.
18 - Repertory of Rheumatism- by Pulford.
19 - Repertory of Eczema- by C. F. Mills Paugh.
20 - Repertory of Headaches- by Knerr.
21 - Repertory of the Appendicitis- by Yingling.
22 - Repertory of Headaches- by Neatby Stonham.
23 - Repertory of The Labour- by Yingling.
24. 1895 - Repertory of Spasms and Convulsions- by Holcomb.
25. 1896 - Repertory of the Tongue- by Douglass.
26 1896 - Repertory of Neuralgias- by Lutze.
27 1896 - Therapeutics of the Eye- by Charles C. Boyle.
28 1899 - Repertory of Urinary Organs and Prostate Gland- by A.R. Morgan.
29. 1900 - Repertory of the back- by Wilsey.
30. 1904 - A Clinical Repertory to the Dictionary of Materia Medica- by John Henry Clarke.
31. 1906 - Repertory of the Uterine Therapeutics- by Minton.
32. - Repertory by P.F. Curie.
33. - Repertory part of Rau's Special Pathology.
34. - Repertory by Boericke.
35. - Repertory by Dr. Sarkar.
36. - Repertory of Respiratory Diseases- by Nash.
37. - Repertory of Mastitis- by W. J. Guernsey.
38. - Repertory of Throat- by W.J. Guernsey.
39. 1908- Sheds Clinical Repertory.
40. 1920- Repertory of Diarrhoea- by Bell.
41. 1931- Boger's Repertory of Times of Remedies and Moon Phases.
42. 1937 - Repertory of 'Sensations as if'- by Dr. H.A.Roberts.
43. 1945 - Repertory of Rheumatic remedies- by Dr. H.A.Roberts.
44. - Ward's Dictionary of 'Sensations, as if.
45. - Repertory of the Digestive Symptom- by Michell.
46. - Repertory section of Homoeopathic Therapeutics of Uterine and Vaginal Discharges- by W.Eggert.

48. - Leucorrhoea and its concomitant symptoms- by A.M.Cushing.
49. - Repertory of the Warts in Skin Diseases- by Drake.
50. - Homoeopathic Therapeintics in Ophthalmology- by J.L.Moffat.
51. - Repertory of Convulsions- by Sanlee.

Emergence of a New School of Thought

This quarter of a century, however, was a period of new awakening, and seemed to bring about the end of conflict of two schools of thinking about Repertory-making. The emergence of so many clinical and regional Repertories meant that there was something lacking in our Repertory-making. This was the period preparatory to emergence of Kent's Repertory. While the battle of different concepts was raging slowly and gradually, a stage was being set for making another kind of Repertory. The work of the purists was too rigid and lacked the elasticity of Boenninghausen's Pocket Book, where as, the latter was found at times, to lead to ridiculous conclusions, or in their analysis only the most prominent polycrests came out, and some of the remedies, which were really effective or really indicated, did not appear in the analysis.

Another weakness, pointed out by some of the exponents of the other school of thought, was that Boenninghausen paid too little respect for the mental symptoms, where as Hahnemann had laid the greatest emphasis on mental symptoms. Of course, Boenninghausen was conscious of the value of mental symptoms, but, he had given his own reasons, for not giving in minute details, the particularisation of mental symptoms. He was of the opinion that in a daily practice, it is difficult to extract reliable mentals. Very often, the psychic state has to be ignored, as it is only a mask for the true mental symptoms, which are exhibited through somatic symptoms. There also, he had made broad generalisations. So, now the time had come that there should be a work on a Repertory, which should combine both the concepts, and produce something, which could be elastic, where not only one could use it as a symptom and analyse a case in our search for the indicated remedy on definite principles, but also to locate a drug by its own peculiar, rare and strange symptoms, because, at times, a remedy is traced through a very peculiar symptom, and other symptoms are found to confirm the choice. Hence, doctors like Lippe, Lee and finally Kent, prepared their Repertories.

On seeing these things in the right perspective, one finds that in the Repertory-making; a sort of evolution was taking place which was very necessary for the culmination ultimately into the work of Kent. Kent's work can be said to be a desirable extension of Boenninghausen, and should be considered as complementing it. He has absorbed almost all of Boenninghausen except generalisations on locations, generalisations on concomitants and modalities of particulars. He has particularized them as given in the provings and Materia Medica, as Boenninghausen has done in his earlier works, but all the same, Kent made fullest use of Boenninghausen's 'Sensations and General Modalities' by incorporating them totally in its 'Generalities'. Kent, however, put the modalities of particulars at the appropriate sections dealing with the particulars themselves. As already said, Kent's work grew out of Lippe, and later out of Lee, and the latter grew out of the Repertory to the Manual of the Allentown Academy. It must be mentioned that the Manual of Allentown Academy had grown out of Boenninghausen's- Repertory of the Anti-psorics. So, ultimately, we find that we are all connected with Boenninghausen in some way or the other, and rightly he should be called the father of the Homoeopathic Repertories.

Kent, while using Lippe's Contribution to Repertory, rationalised many headings of the rubrics given by Lippe, but did not change the remedies. He constantly made additions to them.

For example, Lippe has given-

' Solicitude about futurity' (P 19)
'Solicitude about health'.

But Kent has given-

'Anxiety about future' (P 7)
'Anxiety about health' (P 7)

Similarly, Lippe has given-

'Locality, errors of' (P 14), but Kent listed it in the 'Mistakes'.

Lippe mentioned about 'Dreaming while awake' (P 7) but in Kent's book we find it as 'Dream, as if in'.

There are some rubrics, which are not found in Kent's Repertory. For example-

1. Anxiety in pregnant women- Con.
2. Anxiety at the approach of others- Lyc.
3. Anxiety from medication- Acon., Ars., Calc., Camph.
4. Anxiety with pain in abdomen- Ars., Aur., Cham., Cupr-acet.
5. Anxiety with pain in the head- Acon., Alum., Bell., Bov., Calc., Carb-v., Caust., Graph., Laur., Mag-c., Phos., Puls., Ruta, Sulph.

Of course, Kent changed valuation of the remedies in particular rubrics, and also added remedies, and sometimes changed them. He must have had some definite reason for doing so. But, research workers have to go through the original records and provings to confirm these things. For example, let us take the rubric 'Agg. from bread'. Kent has given 31 remedies (see Generalities under Food). In the Jahr's manual, there are 22 remedies, and Baryta carb has the highest value, but Kent has given it the second grade. China again is given the highest grade, whereas, Kent has given the lowest. Cina is there in Jahr's book, but it is absent in Kent's Repertory.

Boenninghausen, in his Repertory of Anti-psoric remedies, has given only six remedies, and Merc has been given the highest grade, although Kent has given it the lowest.

In my copy of Kent's Repertory, the following additions have been made-

Cina (from Boger's additions to Kent)
Zinc-p.
Verat.

Kent's Repertory

Kent began where others had left. It appears from Kent's writings, that he was torn between keeping a certain order and factual arrangement of symptoms as they occurred, and the 'doctrine of analogy' inherited from Boenninghausen. He held that Repertory was only a compilation at best, and all reliable symptoms were the property of all Homoeopaths. He gathered together, all that was in the earlier Repertories, and then added his own notes. He verified the symptoms, as far as possible. Doctors Gladwin, Milthon, Powel, Mary Ives and Dr. Arthur Allen helped him. Dr. Gladwin said that close scrutiny shows that Kent has the form of Boenninghausen's earlier Repertories, carried to the logical end. Kent's first edition appeared about 1897. Kent was strained financially and physically in bringing out this work. Kent had interleaved his Lippe's Repertory, to which he had added his own notes. Lee, who had been preparing a Repertory out of the manuscript of the second edition of Lippe's Repertory, was in contact with Kent and followed his suggestions. Lee, practically, lost his eye-sight by working for ten years. He was able to publish only the rubrics of MIND and HEAD. Kent owes quite a bit to the labours of Dr. Lee, that tireless, but comparatively, unknown worker.

One is familiar with the Kent's idea of a complete

symptom and its evaluation and classification for the purpose of repertorial analysis. He made greater study of classification of mental symptoms compared to Boenninghausen. I think, the section on Mind in Kent's Repertory is one of the most valuable introduction by Kent. However, Kent's evaluation of symptoms was much more complicated, compared to Boenninghausen's consideration of the elements of the symptoms. Kent's approach to the solution of a particular case, and its analysis, for finding a remedy was, indeed, complicated, and he laid down a system of evaluation, which could be followed only by a deep and conscientious study. It takes time and considerable patience before one can use Kent's Repertory properly and intelligently.

Kent had structured his Repertory according to the following divisions, unlike Boenninghausen's arrangements.

Each symptom had to be arranged in the order as follows-

1. Location
2. Sensation in general, which is unmodified or having many modalities
3. Sides of the body or organs
4. Time modalities
5. Other modalities arranged alphabetically
6. Extension of the sensation etc. from the specified location and other areas, arranged alphabetically.

Kent's final arrangement of his Repertory was novel in the respect, that he collected all the particulars with the modalities separately in their respective sections, unlike the previous Repertories or his own original planning, where the modalities were kept separately, and all symptoms, local or general, affected by a particular modality, were kept under it alphabetically. For example, 'Eating ameliorates' would have listed under it, say, pain in eyes, headache, irritability, pain in limbs, sadness, vertigo, etc. Dr. Jahr and Dr. Hempel had arranged the Repertories like this. Another thing that Kent borrowed from Jahr, was the arrangement of symptoms having no modalities, that is, sensation in general, and those having one or more modalities. The former, however, were arranged from the top, followed by sensation etc., with modifications in their alphabetical order. For example, 'pain in upper limb' will have remedies which will produce-

(1) pain of undefined nature or kind;
(2) confined to the whole or a number of parts of the upper limbs, not the individual parts of it;
(3) do not have any characteristic modalities or have many modalities.

Underneath will come, the sub-rubrics, sides, time, containing the particular modalities in regard to time and circumstances and last, the extension to other parts. After that, we follow the different parts of the upper limbs with similar arrangement. Then follow a different kind of pain with similar arrangements. Remedies in the sub-rubrics with various modalities may not be found in the main rubric. Hence, Kent's Repertory has been hailed as the best and the most complete Repertory compiled so far.

The publication of Kent's Repertory has a very interesting history behind it. Dr. Boericke, of Boericke and Tafel, had refused to publish it, because, the outlay required was too much in its printing etc. The figure in printing alone at that time was 9000 dollars. Kent did not feel like throwing away so much of good money. It was estimated that not more than 300 people would want to buy it. The pre-publication circulation list brought about 200 subscribers at 30 dollars per copy. It was issued section by section. After the second section was issued, all but 90 refused to contribute further and wanted the subscription to be cancelled. Kent wrote:

"Well, things went on from bad to better, not to worse and the repertory was born with much suffering in eyes and heads and bodies of both myself and my wife."

In the year 1914, about 1600 copies were in use throughout the world. Today, its circulation is many times, as this book has been published in India by a number of publishers and has run into various reprints. Kent, in his great book, tried to make it useful in both the functions of a Repertory, that is, as the index, as well as a practical instrument for elimination of non-indicated remedies.

Criticism of Kent

Kent, in his anxiety to be faithful in recording the symptoms as they have appeared, has posed difficulties for the practical analysis of the cases. There are a few things, which rather annoy the students of this Repertory. Dr. Pulford, for example, complained " that in some parts, the rubrics are over-generalised, and in some parts there is over-particularisation. There is a dearth of concomitant symptoms. It is undesirable that the extremities, though unimportant from our philosophical point, should occupy the largest section of the book, and be particularised to nth degree, while mental symptoms are over-generalised and yet supposed to be the most important guiding symptoms, is a fact that this person cannot understand."

The chapter on Extremities, though largest, is the least useful. It has been painfully brought home to everybody who works on this Repertory. In the various rubrics about pains and sensation 'in general', especially in Sections on Particulars, Kent has given remedies 'in general' having no modalities (or multiple modalities?). Underneath in the sub-rubrics, however, he has given remedies having a particular modality or so both in time and circumstances. Drugs mentioned in the sub-rubrics, are often not found in the large or main rubrics. Kent, has, however, warned us not to ignore the larger rubrics, as the sub-rubrics may not give you enough to choose from.

It seems, that Kent did not realise the problems posed by this arrangement in the beginning, and while writing the preface of the first edition, he wrote in the third paragraph -

"As is well known to older practitioners, the method of working out a case from generals to particulars (general rubric to particular rubric) is the most satisfactory. If a case is worked out merely from particulars, it is more than probable that the remedy will not be seen, and frequent failure will be the result This is due to the fact that the particular directions in which the remedies in the general rubric tend, have not yet been observed. Thus, to depend upon a small group of remedies relating to some particular symptom, is to shut out other remedies, which may have that symptom, although not yet observed. By working in the other direction, however, i.e., from generals to particulars, the general rubric will include all the remedies that are related to the symptom, and if after having done this, the particulars are then gone into, and the remedy which runs through the general rubric is found to have the particular symptoms, this will aid in its choice as the one to be prescribed. Take, for example, the particular symptom, 'blueness of fingers during chill'. If this symptom alone were consulted in a special work, we would be limited to Nat-mur, Nux-v and Petr. But if the general rubric 'blueness of fingers', regardless of the name of the disease be consulted, it will be seen that twelve remedies are to be noted. Even this is a narrow way of looking at the symptom; to be certain of finding the remedy, we may have to consult the rubric 'blueness of the hands', giving about forty remedies, among which the one sought may be found, whereas, it was probably not included in the groups of twelve and three. One object, then, of this Repertory has been to assist in obtaining good general groups of remedies. When pathological names are used, only the leading remedies in the condition referred to will be found in the rubric".

The above goes counter to the actual working of cases, because of Kent following Jahr in keeping in the major rubrics of sensation in general only those remedies which are not modified by a particular modality. Remedies, which are modified by time or circumstances and given in the sub-rubrics, are may be missing in the main general rubric. Similar distribution of pains or sensations in general and modified sensations over the different parts of a limb, makes the task of the student difficult.

For example, in Kent page 1023(American Edition), under 'itching of palm' there are a number of remedies, but Anagallis is not included. In the sub-rubric 'Itching palm, rubbing ameliorates', Anagallis is in the highest grade. Anagallis will be missed unless the modality is specially noticed in the patient and brought to the notice of the physician.

In another example - 'Pain in the ear on swallowing' (Kent page 305), there are thirteen remedies of first and second grade, but in the rubric 'sticking pain in the ear, on swallowing' there are two remedies, which are absent under the main rubric. It is not always possible to elicit the exact type of pain, both in the provings and in the patients. The concomitant of 'pain in the ear, on swallowing' is more important than the nature of pain.

On page 1064 of Kent's Repertory, in the main rubric 'Sciatica', Plat. is not mentioned, but in 'Sciatica, beginning in the ankle'. Plat. is given, along with Ars. and Cimic.

I am reminded of a case of Mrs. P.S., aged 58 years, who was suffering from extensive osteo-arthritis, but, under treatment improving in other joints, except ankle joints; especially the left ankle joint. There was drawing pain, worse on letting the leg hang down; worse in the evening and night, but better by external warmth.

There was no swelling, no varices, but tingling of the affected area, worse on standing. There was limping gait.

The lady had undergone severe mental tension and mortification, as her husband had left her.

On consulting the Kent's Repertory, under 'Pain in ankle'; there were 80 remedies. It was only when looking up the Repertory, in the rubric 'Pain in ankle, evening', we found Plantago. But Plantago was not listed in the main general rubric of 'Pain in ankle'. This remedy, of course, did the trick and removed her pains. If we had followed Kent's earlier instructions, we would have missed the remedy. This is why, I have recommended that remedies in the smaller sub-rubrics should be included in the relevant main general rubric.

Because of this inherent contradiction in Kent's planning of his Repertory, and, therefore, difficulty in the use of Repertory by beginners, usefulness of this great work has been diminished to some extent. It was because of this weakness in his Repertory that Kent deleted the third paragraph, mentioned above, in the Preface to the first edition, from subsequent editions. It would have exposed the contradiction.

The following paragraphs, apart from what is given in the foregoing, give the anomalies or mistakes in Kent's Repertory.

Kent page 454, under Throat is given - 'Liquids taken are forced into nose'.

Also, on page 340 under Nose- 'Liquids come out through the nose on attempting to swallow'.

Although, the majority of the medicines is the same, there are a few, which are present in one, and not in the other. There is a difference in evaluation also. In the same context, on page 465, study the rubric 'Paralysis'; the remedies are not the same. Arum Tr., which enjoys the highest evaluation in both the above rubrics, is missing in the rubric of paralysis in all its headings.

Similarly, the rubric 'Throat, swallowing, impossible, paralysis, from' (page 469), and the rubric 'Throat, paralysis' etc. (page 465) are not the same. They ought to be co-related. Also on page 465, in the rubric, 'Post-diphtheritic paralysis' and in the Generalities under the same heading, 'Naja', though highest in the former, is not included at all in the latter. So, in the particularisation of rubrics like that, there is bound to be some mistake and confusion.

In the symptoms about Oesophagus also, there is some confusion.

There is quite a confusion in the rubrics 'lack of vital heat'; 'chilliness in general', and 'aggravation by cold in general'.

On page 1233, Kent has given the generalised modality i.e. the rubric 'Wetting feet agg.'. It could very well be included in the generalities, as the rubric in the extremities does not indicate if 'wetting the feet' aggravates complaints in general, or the complaints only of the feet etc.

Kent, though, rejects Boenninghausen's methods and his rubrics about location; yet, has given in his Repertory on page 553, 'Liver and region of' (Remedies affecting 'in general' liver and region thereof - without indicating any complaints or sensations).

In Kent page 1390, in Generalities, 'Paralysis one sided, apoplexy, after' is a poorly represented rubric. A drug like Opium is absent. On page 1176, 'Extremities, Paralysis, apoplexy, after', is more representative of the condition, and contains Opium in the bold type.

A symptom or a rubric like 'Walk, impulse to' or 'Walk, must' is not given under Mind in Kent.

There is a confusion about spellings of 'Cainca' and 'Cahinca'. In the books on Materia Medica and other Repertories, 'Cainca' is given, where as, Kent has written 'Cahinca' at most of the places, excepting one or two place, where 'Cainca' has been given.

Kent, who, although, talked so much of Generals had given bewildering details about particulars, especially, in the section on extremities. This is the largest section of the Repertory and possibly the least useful.

In spite of Kent's criticism of Boenninghausen, he retained verbatim, certain rubrics from Boenninghausen, which the latter had included in the modalities after generalisation. On page 1009, 'Extremities, Hang down, letting arms, amel.', Kent has not mentioned in particular, any special complaint, which is aggravated or ameliorated by these conditions.

There are a number of errors of misprints and missing remedies or even lines. Dr. P. Schmidt of Geneva, had in his possession, a copy of Kent's Repertory, which has been corrected and added to by Kent himself. On Kent's page 1374, under rubric 'Motion agg.', Sumb is written instead of Samb.

On page 335, the following drugs are missing under the rubric 'Epistaxis'. They are - Ferr-ars., Ferr-m., Ferr-p., Gamb., Gels.

On Page 348, in the rubric 'Nose, Picking nose', the following drugs are missing - Nit-ac., Petr., Phos., Sil.,Thuj.

There are numerous places, where the alphabetical arrangement of drugs in the rubrics, is not observed.

On page 1390, under the rubric 'Generalities, Paralysis, painless' Chlor. is printed instead of Chlol.

On page 730, under the rubric 'Female Genitalia, Metrorrhagia, gushing'. Coca, an important remedy, which has this symptom, is not given, while Croc. has been given. In the rubric of 'Metrorrhagia, fibroids, from', there is need for addition of remedies, which have, in clinical trials, proved very useful. This is imperative, because this is a fairly common condition found in any practice. I have found, at least, in half a dozen cases, Thalaspi B.Pastoris, Ficus religiosa saving my repertorisation, and the life of the patient, when other remedies did not hold.

On page 1410, under the rubric 'Generalities, Undressing, after, agg.', Rumex is not given at all.

On page 278, there is a rubric 'Vision, Exertion of vision agg.'. It is not clear, whether it relates to the variation of vision by 'Exertion of vision', or does it mean aggravation of other symptoms also, by exertion of vision. This is again adapted from Boenninghausen's Repertory.

Anagallis has copious watery or yellow discharge from nose and violent sneezing etc., yet, it is not listed under catarrh or coryza, but given under discharge, yellow and watery only.

In the section on Chest, Back, Extremities, Head etc., Kent has not differentiated between subjective coldness, chilliness and objective coldness of the parts.

In the Generalities of Kent's Repertory, under rubric on 'Sides', Kent has listed Ant-t. in the 'Side left' in the second grade, but in the Guiding Symptoms, from where he has usually taken these indications, there are more symptoms listed on the right side. This needs to be investigated.

In the Kent's Repertory, we may add Ant-t. to 'Generalities, vaccination, after'. (See Hering's Guiding Symptoms page 406).

Similarly, Kent, under 'Generalities, Sides', has listed Manganum in the second grade in the right side, and in lowest grade in the left side, whereas, in the Guiding Symptoms, there are more symptoms recorded on the left side than on the right side.

Again, under the rubric on sides of body, Kent has given

Zinc. in second grade in the right side, but has omitted it in the side left. In the Hering's Guiding Symptoms, there are definitely more symptoms on the left side and in the right also quite a number of symptoms. In the Boenninghausen also, Zinc. has been given to affect more on the left side.

Similarly, Kent has given no preference for any side for Med., but Hering has given definitely more symptoms appearing on the left side.

In Kent, Mancinella has got burning pains, but it also has internal burning pains according to Hering's Guiding Symptoms, which could be added in Kent.

Mur-ac. has internal heat with desire to uncover etc. but it has no mention of this symptom in Kent's Repertory. Similarly, it should be added also as a remedy for eczema, Eczema Solaris, as it has been given second grade in Hering's Guiding Symptoms. Kent missed listing it under eczema or adding a rubric like eruptions from exposure to sun.

Similarly, in Kent page no 1194- Stiffness knee - Aesc is not mentioned but in Hering's Guiding Symptoms it is marked on left side.

Thus, it can be seen that Kent's Repertory needs to be made more complete and updated.

From the above, it is quite clear that Kent was torn between keeping a certain order and factual arrangement of symptoms as they occurred, and the principle of analogy as inherited from Boenninghausen. In spite of its shortcomings, it is the greatest Repertory planned and the most popular. No repertory can be perfect, and it will continue to be so, as long as man continues to be imperfect. Till then, it is a blessing to have as many Repertories as possible.

Kent and Boenninghausen

If we follow Kent during his career, we find that in the beginning he was very much influenced and impressed by Boenninghausen's Repertory. He had acknowledged the profession's gratitude to Boenninghausen. He himself had been brought up in the tradition of Boenninghausen's Repertory. But, later on, either, because of his own experience, or because of his plan for making a new and better Repertory of his own, he became more and more prejudiced against Boenninghausen and actually started criticising him bitterly. He wrote rather strongly about the harm done by Boenninghausen. He said:

"Nothing has harmed our cause more than the books that generalise modalities, viz., by making a certain aggravation or amelioration fit all parts as well as the general body states. Cold air may aggravate the patient but ameliorate the headache. Stooping seldom aggravates the headache, backache, cough and vertigo in the same degree. Yet, Boenninghausen compels you to look in one glance for all of them, and mark with the same gradings. The patient is often better by motion, but his parts, if inflamed, are worse from motion." (Kent's Lesser Writings p. 475 -American Edition)

Although, he himself has mentioned in his LESSER WRITINGS that whenever you have written down the case history, the beginner should write down the full general rubrics for exercise at least, and then from the full general rubric, he should write down the sub-rubric with a modality. But, he admits that many of the most brilliant cures are made from the general rubric, when the special does not help. With experience and practice, one can include many more remedies in the special rubrics, from the list of general rubrics. The special aggravations are of great help, but such observations are often wanting, and the general rubric must be pressed into service. Here, he mentions also that we must work by analogy, and in this method, Boenninghausen's Pocket Repertory' is of the greatest service. This is again a tribute by Kent to Boenninghausen's genius.

As an example, he mentions that menstrual pains ameliorated by heat are peculiar to Ars. and Nux-v., and by moist heat to Nux-m. But, all the cases are not amenable to these two or three remedies alone. In many cases with this modality, other remedies also come in. But here, we must take recourse to the doctrine of analogy, and, therefore, form an anamnesis, and thus make use of the general rubric, taking all the remedies known to be generally ameliorated by heat and warmth applied.

Kent, later on, in his writings, has mentioned that Boenninghausen had worked out generals very well, but rather much of it was overdone, as he generalised many rubrics that were purely particulars, and the use of which as generals, is misleading and ends in failure. The success coming from Boenninghausen's Pocket Book, is due to the arrangement whereby generals can be quickly used to furnish modalities for individual symptoms whether general or particular. He has admitted that this feature is observed in his Repertory, as all know who use it. But here, he departed from Boenninghausen by saying that it is only the general that can be used this way. A general rubric made up on the promiscuous particulars, none of which are predicated out of patients, is a hit or a miss, when applied in general and usually a miss. Kent cited examples like aggravation from writing. Now, does it mean that headache from writing, or depression from writing, or pains in chest from writing, could be taken as any of these symptoms, which could be worse from writing?

Towards the close of Dr. Kent's professional life, he had departed from the concept of Boenninghausen. Actually, he was rather unfair to him in repudiating some of the things which had been advocated by Boenninghausen, and which were approved and appreciated by Hahnemann himself during his own time. But, according to Kent, Boenninghausen's concept about Repertory was a departure from Hahnemann's own teachings. Kent criticised the method of Boenninghausen's case taking and analysis. He felt that in this method it is a serious departure from Hahnemann's teachings, as it does not give us the picture of the patient. Hahnemann never recommended concomitants of the part affected. Concomitants cannot come into consideration except as in connection with an objective condition. Concomitants of the symptoms in a part cannot really lead us to the picture of the patient as a whole, as taught by Hahnemann in his Organon.

Kent in the later period of his life, was strongly of the opinion that stressing only the elements of the symptoms tends to destroy the Hahnemannian concept; it is not in line with Hahnemann's method. "You are led away from the characteristic picture of the patient; you ignore the scientific approach of working from centre to the periphery or circumference." Later on, Kent went as far as to say that he started out to follow the Boenninghausen's plan in the treatment of his patients, but "it did not cure the patients. You can give different remedies in succession without holding to any one and after years the patient is no better. They are not curing the patient." "In the Boenninghausen's method, there is no opportunity to distinguish between the patient and the particulars. This method has retarded the development of Homoeopathy. It has obscured Hahnemann's Homoeopathy, based on the idea of the patient first, and focusing observations on things strange, rare and peculiar. These do not relate to the particulars, that is, the part affected."

Influence of Boenninghausen on Kent's Repertory

With all the bitter criticism of Boenninghausen by Kent, it is of historical, as well as practical interest to find out how Kent's Repertory was influenced by Boenninghausen, and how departures from Boenninghausen improved or affected adversel your techniques of repertorial analysis.

Although, Kent asserted that Boenninghausen's concept and technique of repertorisation departed radically from. Hahnemann's teachings, it must not be forgotten that it was

Hahnemann who wrote a preface to Boenninghausen's Repertory of the Anti-Psorics in 1832, and recommended it to his friends and students. They were in constant communication with each other, and Boenninghausen must have found encouragement and inspiration from the master. Kent could, however, have argued that Boenninghausen published his Therapeutic Pocket book only in 1846, 3 years after Hahnemann's death, and in this book he had made serious departure from his earlier Repertories, the last of which (Repertory of the Medicines which are not Anti-Psoric), was published by him as early as in 1836. The Pocket Book appeared after a gap of ten years. Hahnemann, possibly, could not have made a proper assessment of what Boenninghausen was preparing during his life-time.

But, what ever be the merits or demerits, Boenninghausen's Repertory dominated the scene for fifty years.

To study critically, the influence of Boenninghausen on Kent's work, we have to refer to the first edition of Kent's Repertory, when Kent was still under his spell to a great extent. Since, this book is long lost to most of us, I would like to quote some portions from its Preface, as it is very valuable from the historian's point of view. He wrote:

> "This work is offered to the profession as a General Repertory of the Homoeopathic Materia Medica. It is not calculated to take the place of the repertories on special subjects, such as Boenninghausen's Therapeutic Pocket Book; Guernsey on Haemorrhoids; Allen' Intermittent fever etc. but rather a connecting link between these special works--".

In the Preface to both the first and the last Edition, he has written:

> "....to those who have used Boenninghausen's Therapeutic Book, the working out of cases from generals is a familiar method....".

It will be of interest to find out how Kent's mind worked

in the early years of his Repertory-making, because that will give us a correct impression about Boenninghausen's influence on his work at that stage. In the first edition, we find that Kent has given us a general rubric 'Aversion to coition' in the section on Mind, and has not made any difference with regard to sex. Here, he followed Boenninghausen, because in the latter's Repertory of Anti-psoric remedies, he had put it as 'a general rubric, both for males and females, under sexual impulse'. He did not, however, keep it under Mind. It is interesting to find that in the Therapeutic Pocket Book this rubric was omitted.

Another interesting development that we find in the evolution of Kent's Repertory is that in the section on Mind in the first edition, he has given more of particularisation and details of modalities than in the later editions. This has happened in numerous places. These things were generalised later. For example, under 'Irritability' we find 'cough, before; epilepsy before.' etc. which is not to be found in the subsequent editions.

Similarly, under 'Confusion of Mind', there are modalities like 'catarrh during'; 'coryza during'; 'sneezing ameliorates'. These sub-rubrics are missing. Actually, one of the complaints by subsequent students of Homoeopathy was that Kent should have given more of details and particularisation under Mind than given under the Chapter on Extremities.

Under the chapter on **Vertigo**, we find that in a sub-rubric, under 'Afternoon, Walking, while', aggravation at-

1 p.m.	Phel.
2 p.m.	Hura
3-6 p.m.	Sep.
4 p.m.	Alum.
5 p.m.	Dios., Ptel.
5-6 p.m.	Nat-m.

(Reference Kent's Repertory 1st Edition page 101)

These sub-rubrics have been omitted and all the remedies mentioned here are kept under 'afternoon' and also under 'walking'. So, it is obvious that Kent realised the value of generalisation and not to split hair in the process of tabulating symptoms as they seemed to appear. This was of, course, the Boenninghausen's approach.

The following rubrics in the first edition will enlighten us further about Boenninghausen's influence:

(1) Under Head: 'Coition, complaints of head, after'
(2) Under Eye: 'Infants, eye complaints'
(3) Under Eye-'Vision, weak, old people'
(4) Under Nose: 'Nose external'
(Remedies in general affecting various parts of nose)
'Nose Dorsum' in general
'Nose Bones'
'Nose Roof'
'Nose Septum'
'Nose Tip'
'Nose Wings'
(5) Under Mouth: 'Ailment of the Mouth'
(6) Under Genitalia, Male: 'Male Organs in general'
'Penis'
'Glans'
'Prepuce'
'Scrotum'
'Spermatic Cord'
'Testes'

Also under Genitalia, Female: 'Female Organs in general'

'External Female organs'
'Ovaries'
'Ovaries Right'
'Ovaries Left'
'Uterus'
'Vagina'

The above rubrics are typically Boenninghausen's locations in general. Boenninghausen had given the modalities of aggravation and amelioration at full moon, new moon, in detail. Kent had, in his first edition, kept rubrics like

Cough aggravated
at full moon- Kali-n., Sabad.
at new moon- Sabad., Sil.

But, in subsequent editions, these rubrics were removed.

Under the chapter on Generalities, Kent gave some of the rubrics which were typically Boenninghausean:

'Adhesion of inner parts, sensation, of'
'Blondes'
'Brunettes'
'Children, especially'
'Dryness of Internal parts'
'Dryness, sensation of'
'Lying-in woman'
'Moon, new, aggravates'
'Moon, full, aggravates'
'Nasal, catarrh, suppression of'
'Stiffness and rigidity'
'Shortened muscles and tendons'
'Turning around aggravates'
'Turning over in bed, aggravates'
'Whiteness of parts, usually red'
'Women, for'
'Yawing aggravates'

Almost all these rubrics were taken from Boenninghausen's Pocket Book and were generalisations of particular symptoms, which were, later on, so vehemently criticised by Kent.

These rubrics were omitted in the later editions, although, some of the rubrics in these editions still bear the impression of Boenninghausen's concept, which were retained, and, as a matter of fact, form a very important part of it.

The most important are the sensations and modalities

of the Pocket Book, which have been taken practically in toto and combined together in one section under 'Generalities'. This is where Boenninghausen's principle of Analogy is accepted. 'Desires and Aversions'; 'Discharges' etc. have been built upon this Repertory, as well as additions from other sources.

Kent has not referred anywhere to the earlier forms of Repertory evolved by Boenninghausen which were in many ways closer to Kent's way of thinking.

The following rubrics are found in Kent's Repertory in all the editions, which are out of tune with his approach:

'Liver and region of' and
'Spleen, complaints of' in Chapter on Abdomen
'Menopause' in Chapter on Genitalia, female.
'Drawing up limbs aggravates'
'Drawing up limbs ameliorates'
'Hang down, letting limbs, aggravates'
'Hang down, letting limbs, ameliorates'
'Hang down, letting arms, ameliorates' in Chapter on Extremities

Kent's Repertory today, in spite of its shortcomings, is the greatest Repertory planned and the most popular. It is said to be the most complete Repertory and is the back-bone of the Homoeopathic literature. But no Repertory is complete. There is always scope for not only making as many Repertories as possible, but also to make the existing Repertories as complete and as perfect as possible. It is very unfortunate that the task of revisions and additions has been neglected. It is possible that some day some of research workers will make a better and more complete Repertory. Dr. Boger had tried to synthesize the approaches of Boenninghausen and Kent, in his BOENNINGHAUSEN'S CHARACTERISTICS AND REPERTORY in 1905 and later in 1935-37. Unfortunately, this task has not been properly done. We need a Repertory, which contains not only a complete and comprehensive index of symptoms of Materia Medica, but also an efficient and easily workable system for selecting the similimum. May be, Boger's approach if translated into action, might solve our problems.

Boger's contribution to Repertory

Boger was a keen student of Boenninghausen. He had an uncanny sense of selecting the right rubrics for repertorisation. He would conjure up solutions of repertorial problems in a remarkably short time and in his novel way. His contributions have not been fully appreciated. He published his Boenninghausen's characteristics and Repertory in 1905. This was built up on the basic structure of Boenninghausen's earlier Repertories, especially the Repertory of Anti-psoric remedies, which Boger had translated in English in 1900. The Repertory was still not complete and Boger continued to work on it, till he was snatched away from his earthly existence in 1935. The posthumous edition, under the guidance of Mrs. Boger, has been published by Roy & Sons of Bombay, India. Unfortunately, there have been many omissions and errors of evaluation and of missing remedies. The printing is also poor. In his first edition in 1905 by B&T, printing and arrangement is better, and could be made the basis for further additions or changes for its new editions. I wish that Boger had been alive to finalise completely this book. He has brought about synthesis between two opposite view-points more effectively from the point of view of practical repertorisation. But I am afraid, in the present condition, it cannot replace fully the Kent.

Boger, in his Repertory, gave certain generalisations, which are very important from point of view of Repertorial analysis. For example, in Kent's Repertory, under the rubric Irritability, menses, before' we find that only the following remedies are given- Berb., calc., caust., cham., kali-c., kreos., lyc., mag-m., nat-m., nux-v. and sep. Although, in actual practice, we come across this symptom in a fairly large number of patients, and remedies not mentioned in the above list, have been found to be curative and relieving this symptom.

Again in Kent's, the rubric 'Weeping, menses, before'

has the following remedies - cact., con., lyc., phos., puls., sep., zinc.

But, in Boger's Boenninghausen, all the mental symptoms, which are aggravated or appear before the menses, have been lumped together in one rubric under the section 'MIND-Genitalia, female, aggravation (Concomitants) before the menses'. Thus, there is less chance of missing remedies here, as according to Boenninghausean concept, it is the mind in general affected before menses. Here, we have remedies which have greater evidence of emotional and mental disturbances before the menses. Of course, there is also the General rubric of **'aggravation in general before menses'** which could be utilised for all general symptoms aggravated before menses, which has the following drugs-

Alum., **Am-c**., am-m., *asar.,* **Bar-c**., bell., bor., **Bov**., bro., *bry.,* CALC., canth., carb-an., **Carb-v**., caul., *caust.,* cham., chin., cina., COCL., coff., **Colo**., **Con**., croc., CUP., *dig., dul.,ferr., graph,* hep., *hyos.,* ign., *iod.,* ip., *kali-c.,* kali-n., **Kreos**., LACH., LYC., mag-c., mag-m., *mang.,* **Merc**., mez., mos., mur-ac., nat-c., **Nat-m**., **Nit-ac**., *nux-m.,* nux-v., petr., **Phos**., **Ph-ac**., **Plat**., psor., PULS., rhus-t., ruta, sabad., sars., *sep., sil., spig.,* spong., **Stann**., SULPH., sul-ac., valer., VERAT., *zinc.*

Also 'mentals' in particular before menses, Kent has Cact. listed under 'Weeping, menses, before', but it is not mentioned by Boger under the general rubric, although, under 'Heart' complaints before menses, he has mentioned it in a high degree, and under mentals he has included it, though in a lowest grade.

It will not be out of place to narrate a story about the repertorial analysis of a case to be worked out simultaneously by Dr. Boger and Dr. Gladwin. Dr. J.M. Green told this story in a meeting.

"The patient, a woman in the early fifties, much wrinkled and worn out by hard life of worry and work, sallow or pasty, lay in bed, tossing about somewhat from a headache, which fretted her to pieces.

Fever high, 102 to 103 F. Pulse high and weak. Chill every time she moved under the bed clothes. Sleep in short naps and a little better on each waking.

Headache worse in occiput; very severe. Worse any motion, noise, light; accompanied by nausea and vomiting of mucous. Aching all over body. Aching eyes. Photophobia. Cough loose, frequent; very painful head. No stool for three days and no desire. Urine very scanty, only 1/2 pint in 26 hours; dark in colour.

Dr. Boger picked out in his mind a remedy which had some of these symptoms prominently but which he did not regard as the similimum. My recollection is that he chose 'Bell.'. He looked up this remedy in Boenninghausen's Pocket Book which was all I had of Boenninghausen out at my house.

He turned to the caption 'other remedies' under Bell. and studied the list, thinking out those most nearly like the patient. Then he called for the Materia Medica, and I produced the Guiding Symptoms. He looked up one remedy after another, putting this one down saying "I do not like that" and taking up another.

After consulting three or perhaps four this way, he came to Nux-v. and soon said: "There is your remedy, right there".

Dr. Gladwin looked at the list of symptoms and chose a few for repertory working. The symptoms chosen by her were:

> after sleep
Chill on motion
Pain back, better lying on it
Headache < motion
Headache < light
Headache < noise

Urine scanty
Photophobia

She analysed the case on Kent's Repertory, using Repertory sheets, and came to three remedies- Phos., Chin. and Nux-v. After consulting the Materia Medica, she also chose Nux-v.

Dr. Boger's way presupposes a fine knowledge of Materia Medica. Dr. Gladwin's could be used better by novices".

Some of the best prescribers in the history of Homoeopathy have recommended familiarity and even deeper study of as many different Repertories as possible, if we have to analyse our cases properly.

Philosophy and construction of each Repertory is different, and very often, clinical cases present symptoms-complex which are more suitable for analysis on one particular Repertory. Even good prescribers have tended to work on different lines, some on Boenninghausen and some on Kent, according to their temperamental inclinations. Dr.Erastus E. Case, one of the greatest prescribers of all times, chose Boenninghausen for his chronic hard cases and used Kent for his daily acute and simple chronic cases. To shorten his work, he used Boenninghausen's slips, a sort of card repertory. Of course, the beginners must be given an over-all picture of our Repertories, defining as best as possible, the scope, usefulness, and limitations of each, but asking them to work on Kent to begin with. May be, some of the learners are better suited for working on Boenninghausen and could be guided accordingly. In the beginning of my studies of Homoeopathic Medicine, I used to work with Boenninghausen and did a reasonably good job.

The research students of Homoeopathic Repertory are expected to go through various editions of the same Repertory carefully. There are, at time, anomalies to be found. For example, in Boenninghausen's earlier Repertory of Anti-psoric remedies, we find that 'Aggravation awaking on'-CON. Conium is in the highest grade, but later, in his Therapeutic Pocket Book, he has down-graded it, but Kent in his Repertory listed the same remedy in the second grade.

Maybe, we do not require the need of consulting a Repertory in a given case. May be, it is a case for prescribing only on the keynotes, whose 'routine' repertorisation may take you away from the indicated remedy. May be, your intuitive perception and clinical experience, with a diligent study of Materia Medica, directs you to the remedy. (Here the computer in your brain does the repertorisation).

In actual practice, there are usually two kinds of cases seen by all of us. In one type, remedies can be prescribed with great degree of certainty of success when prescribed on the symptoms that are known as 'characteristic and peculiar' (organon 153) or on keynotes which point to the pathogenesis of the remedy.

In other cases, there are no such symptoms standing out. That is where, this remedy has to be hunted out; where the totality can be worked out through the Repertories, and frequent references made to the Materia Medica. These are the cases where there are a large number of symptoms or complaints and it is not usually possible to discern or to have a clear cut indication of the curative remedy. There are a number of possibilities which seem to be competing for the place of honour (of the indicated remedy). That is where, Repertorial evaluations come to our aid, provided we refer to the Materia Medica for final judgement.

A word of caution will not be out of place for those who always start the study of Materia Medica from the different rubrics of the Repertory and neglect the systematic study of Materia Medica. Too great dependence on the Repertory leads one away from constant and systematic study of Materia Medica. This practice is prevalent in the west, where a practitioner of Homoeopathic Medicine starts with thumbing of the Repertory, immediately or starting with a case. A proper and constant study of Materia Medica can make a short cut for us in our search for the similimum. As mentioned already, Repertory is necessary only for those cases where the characteristic do not stand out boldly or where memory fails. That is why, in India, Homoeopathic prescribers are able to take care of a large number of patients in comparative shorter time. Ultimately, Repertory is a guide and one cannot get the correct results by prescribing only on the numerical totality from a Repertory. Repertory is the outcome of Materia Medica, and not vice-versa.

In such cases, where only Repertorial evaluation is used, one has to be cautious on prescribing the drugs with the highest numerical value, because some of the polycrests have much greater representations both in provings and Materia Medicas and hence in Repertories. So, only a few polycrests like Sulph, Calc, Bry, Sepia, Nux-v, Ars, Lyc appear most often in the lead, compared to Silicea or Staph etc. Many other remedies hardly appear in the analysis at all. In some of the computer softwares, they have made provision for the appearance of small remedies with special characteristics and strange and rare remedies.

This precaution is all the more necessary when one is working with Card-systems or with Computerised Repertories. Why some of the remedies appear so often on the top is, because they had more extensive provings and clinical records than others. Let us keep an open mind and bank on a remedy, which in essence resembles the picture of the patient, and which is confirmed by reference to the books on Materia Medica Of course, Repertory gives us a suggestive list and brings to our notice some remedy or remedies, which we would not have thought of. Later, in this study, we shall give a number of repertorised cases, where it was not .possible to be able to think of the likely similimum.

Problems in Repertorisation

Treatment or selection of the indicated remedy is always very difficult in cases where the disease is expressed by local symptoms. It is in these cases, that local topical applications are so often resorted to, which may later, result in a disaster for the patient in more vital areas of his economy.

Hahnemann, in paragraph 197 to 204 (Organon), talked of 'Driving off' and not 'Driving in', and condemned this treatment with topical application in no uncertain terms. This is especially so in skin lesions. Suppression at that time seems so much easier both for the patient and the physician.

These partial or one-sided cases, as called by Hahnemann, were dealt by him in quite an emphatic manner.

It is in such cases that a thorough search should be made for the patient's symptoms; his mental symptoms; search for any guidance for his past history or family history. Therefore, the need for proper case-taking is emphasised again and again, so that we could ferret out the individualising characteristics of the patient. The fewer the symptoms, more difficult the treatment. This is so in chronic diseases.

To the beginner, the changes and sufferings appearing on the external parts of the body are often attributed to the local causes only; the general system supposedly is not participating in the trouble.

The local symptoms to be treated locally, are only those which have been produced recently by injuries.

The beginners are warned about certain unwanted results when they start working with Kent's Repertory. They tend to take almost all the symptoms of the patient and work through the Repertory, and later, work out the totality of the values. These values will give only a few well-known polycrests, and mask the really indicated drugs. One has to take up only the characteristic, peculiar and well marked symptoms of the patient as a whole, and then work out the case, keeping in view, the Kent's general philosophy and background of construction of the Repertory. The student must study the examples of case-analysis from the experts in Repertorial work, where, they have worked out cases, using different methods or techniques of selecting and utilising the data for working with Kent's Repertory. Physicians with experience, have used, what is popularly known as an artistic way of selecting the rubrics, using some rubrics as eliminative rubrics, so as to make short cuts to the laborious method of repertorisation. The introduction of computers in the process of repertorisation has become a tremendous help, both for the experts, as well as the beginners in analysing the cases. In conclusion, however, it must be borne in mind that Homoeopathy is absolutely inconceivable without the most precise individualisation.

Clarke's Repertory

Dr. John Henry Clarke's contribution to Homoeopathic literature indeed, is very valuable, as the information that he has packed in his three volumes of Dictionary of Homoeopathic Materia Medica cannot be found anywhere else. In his later years, he decided to add the fourth volume to the Dictionary, which was supposed to be his Repertory to the symptoms of his dictionary. It seems that due to lack of time, he prepared only an outline called 'Clinical Repertory'. It is, therefore, not a Repertory of the symptoms of the various remedies given in his dictionary, although, he had planned to prepare a Repertory of that kind. His clinical Repertory has, of course, great usefulness in its limited sphere of application.

Clarke was of the opinion that some remedies have a remarkable likeness to a group of symptoms in particular sicknesses or pathological conditions. Some remedies seem to have a specific affinity for an organ or for the functioning of a particular organ. In such conditions, these remedies can be primarily thought of, provided they cover other essentials of the patient concerned. For example, Card-marianus has a very positive action on the left lobe of liver. In conditions where the left lobe is enlarged, and if the patient suffers from jaundice or some malignancy or hepatitis, Card-marianus could be very useful. Similarly, there are remedies which seem to have special affinity for polypoidal growths, whether in the nasal cavity, the aural cavity or in the cervix of the uterus. These remedies have to be thought of, when we have to deal with such pathological conditions. For example, remedies like Teucrium, Phos, Sang or Sang-nitricum are often indicated in such conditions. Various such examples could be cited. Clarke was able to set apart such indicated remedies in certain clinical or pathological conditions. In his introduction, he mentioned, however, that his nosological indications are merely suggestive.

Clarke divided his clinical Repertory into 5 or 6 Sections-

I. Clinical Repertory- Here, we would like to mention that Dr. Boericke was another author, who gave more of clinical or nosological rubrics in his Repertory to his Materia Medica. Both Clarke and Boericke, were really the first ones, who tried to bring out such Clinical Repertory.

Some of the remedies given by Dr. Clarke for clinical conditions in his Repertory, are not mentioned anywhere else. They have to be clinically confirmed. These clinical conditions, mentioned by him in the clinical Repertory, have been indicated also in his Dictionary, right in the beginning of description of the remedies. Few examples of his nosological rubrics are given below-

(1) For '**Adenoids**' 9 remedies are given-Agra., (Calc.), Calc-f., Lob-s., *Psor.,* Sang-n., Spig., Staph., *Sulph.*

(2) For '**Adhesions**' he has given Thiosin.

(3) For '**Affections of antrum of highmore**' he has given 3 remedies-
Com., Mag-c. and Merc-c.
Diseases of- Kali-s., *Phos.*
Inflammation of- *Chel.*
Pain in- Euph-a., Merc-b-i., Polygonum
Tumor of- Hecla

Most of the rubrics have been treated very poorly and the remedies given are too small in number.

For example, for the rubric 'Arteries, affections of', he has given only Calc-hp. For 'Atheroma of arteries', he has given Cact. For 'throbbing of arteries', he has given Fago. Very often, he has repeated same rubrics under different nomenclature. Under 'bearing down pains', he has mentioned only Caulo. Going through deeply, one could pick out some remedies which could be very useful in the clinical application, provided we are able to confirm their clinical application in actual practice.

II. The second chapter of his Repertory deals with 'causation'. The students of Repertory know very well that at times 'causation' becomes very important and rules out any other symptom for application of the remedy. This is a fairly useful chapter and could be utilised for addition to other works of standard Repertories.

III. The third chapter is devoted to 'Temperament; Dispositions, Constitutions and States'. Some of the remedies are so pronounced in their temperamental expressions and behaviour that they cannot be mistaken for any other remedy.

IV. The fourth chapter deals with 'Clinical Relationships'. There are given, relationships of remedies showing what remedies precede certain remedies and what follow up certain remedies. He has also given remedies which are complimentary or compatible and remedies which are incompatible. These relationships have been given in a tabular form and seems to have been influenced by Dr. Gibson.

V. The fifth chapter is devoted to 'Natural Relationships'. He has given different remedies, belonging to different kingdoms of nature, which have been arranged in their order of natural relationships. It has been found that clinical symptoms follow natural relationships in many ways. The list of natural sources of related remedies comprises of -

1) Metals or elements;
2) Vegetable kingdom;
3) Animal kingdom;

4) Sarcodes; and
5) Nosodes.

In cases of metals or elements, we should relate certain remedies, especially, the elements in the order of their atomic weights. Of course, in the case of vegetable kingdom, we already know how remedies in a particular vegetable classification are similar in certain areas of their clinical application.

In the animal kingdom, we know how certain serpent poisons have similar actions, in spite of their own distinctive individualities.

Similarly, in case of sarcodes and nosodes, we should think of certain relationships.

No other author has gone so deeply into such matters of remedy, origin and their relationships.

Card Repertories

It is interesting to note that it was fairly early in the hay-day of Homoeopathy that some doctors started thinking of using cards, punched or otherwise, for the purpose of elimination of remedies in the repertorial analysis. The need for such a thing was obvious, because the time taken in noting down rubrics, remedies and their elimination was so much that it discouraged the very efforts at it. Especially, working on Boenninghausen, it would require two to three hours. On the Kent's Repertory also, if we work on the standard method, it would require one and a half hours to two hours. In the 'short-cut' method, which may be a dangerous one, except in the hands of the most experienced, time can be shortened very much, but even here, with the right kind of cards, it could be faster and easier. Even working with printed Repertory sheets, time taken and strain on the eyes is considerable. Most of us just thumb through the pages of the Repertory superficially and make a glancing analysis. We miss certain possibilities. We tend also to look up merely the particulars, finding it apparently easy and obvious, as working with generals would consume more time.

The use of card indices within certain limits is very desirable if we have to do our work scientifically.

It is of historic interest to find out who was the first to think of this type of mechanical elimination in the Repertory work. The earliest Card Repertory is that of Dr. William Jefferson Guernsey, nephew of H.N. Guernsey. Dr. W.J. Guernsey had already made substantial contributions to the literature on Repertory. His monograph and repertory on Haemorrhoids was universally appreciated. He prepared, also, short Repertories on Urticaria, Throat and Diphtheria and on Mastitis. He prepared what was known as 'Guernsey's Boenninghausen slips'. They were long cards or slips 1 1/4 X 12 1/2 inches. There were 2500 such cards and on each was printed, in alphabetical order, the names of the remedies used in Boenninghausen's work. On the top was given the code number of the rubric. There was a separate index, where the coded rubrics were given. On each card, the remedies had number 1 to 4 printed against them, depending upon the degree of evaluation of that particular drug for that particular symptom following the Boenninghausen's Therapeutic Pocket Book. The rubrics were chosen from the index, and the indicated slips were taken out, and made to lie side by side, so that name of each remedy ran in a straight line from left to right On adding up the exponent of the several remedies, the one securing the highest number is the possible remedy for the case. It was as early as 1888 that he made these slips, but made them available to the profession in about 1892. Dr. Chapman called it the "Perfection of method for managing our Materia Medica".

Later, Dr. H.C. Allen improved these original slips by adding more remedies, and they were known as Allen's Boenninghausen slips. These cards were used by some of the best prescribers in America. Dr. Erastus E. Case, that wonderful prescriber, used the Kent for the daily acute and chronic work, but for the harder solutions he went to the Boenninghausen's slips.

The editor of Medical Advance (1909) wrote- "We have used Guernsey's work since 1886, a great time saver, most correct and ready reference. But only 126 remedies have been listed. No other new remedies added --" It was later Dr. H.A. Roberts of Connecticut, U.S.A., who added more remedies, and it is his edited version which has been utilised for programs of software for Computers.

Dr. Margaret Tyler made a punched Card Repertory in about 1912, but Dr. Kent, her teacher discouraged her on this venture. She used large cards and hand punched them. She later said, " I went so far as to devise a card-trick system, every card a symptom, and the drugs that produced that, punched out. I deafened myself punching one thousand cards. I have them still a great cabinet full." They were based on Kent's work, incomplete but very carefully done.

About that time (1913), Welch and Houston also put out a loose punched Card Repertory. It was based on Kent's generals and gave 134 symptoms.

Field's Cards

The most heroic effort was, however, made by Dr. Field in this line. In 1922, he brought forward a gigantic Card Repertory at a great expense. He was deterred by the immense cost, but realizing that between the great things that we cannot do and the small things that we will not do, the danger is that we will do nothing, he undertook and finished the work. He included Boger's numerous annotations and corrections and also that of Dr. Skinners. There were approximately 6800 cards, the actual number being a little above 5000. He included some rubrics from Repertories other than Kent also, but mostly it was from Kent. But unfortunately, in almost all the rubrics, only the first and second grade remedies were punched, with the result that any working of the cases with these cards has usually disappointed me. He was possibly the first to code the names of the remedies into numbers. The cards were thick and blocked the remedies easily; hence the indicated remedy was more likely to be blocked out. It is a pity that a work like that was not properly conceived, and hence, did not earn appreciation at the hands of the profession. The number of remedies was about 360 with a provision for about 40 more.

Dr. Gladwin favoured the converting of Kent's Generals into cards and the particulars to be worked from the book.

Dr. Pulford ventured to convert most of Kent into cards, but they never finished it. Dr. Boger brought out his famous Card Repertory in 1928, which was later published by Roy & Co. with a foreword from late Dr. L.D. Dhawle.

This Repertory, in its own limited sphere, is a marvel of brevity and generalisation.

Dr. W.W. Young, also spent a lot of labour on a Card Repertory, which was, however, never finalised. Dr. J.G. Weiss of Detroit, and later Dr. RH. Farley, published a spindle Repertory in 1950. A year or two later. Dr. Marcoz Jamenez brought out a Card Repertory containing about six hundred large-sized cards. Most of the major mental symptoms and generalities were included in it. He was the first to introduce the evaluation of drugs on the cards. Recently, indefatigable, late Dr. P. Sankaran brought out a Card Repertory similar to that of Dr. Boger, but with more remedies and a larger number of rubrics.

Requisites of a good Card Repertory

Unfortunately, most of the Card Repertories were either very much limited in their scope, or were ineffective, because of lack of proper construction.

Many of them are too small and give only a broad general selection limited to a few polycrests.

The most important, and really the only legitimate use of the Card Repertories, is its 'eliminative function'. But, this elimination can be dangerous if there is any mistake in the philosophy and the process of construction of the Repertory, even after a very thorough case-taking and expert evaluation. A Card Repertory should lead us to likely possibilities, without much pain and ruthless or senseless elimination. Recently, Dr. Piertkin of Robert Bosch Homoeopathic Hospital, Stutgart, made use of the computer for the analysis of cases. The data was punched on certain cards and the analysis worked out by the computer. The whole process according to him took 16 1/2 minutes. During one of the International Homoeopathic Congresses in London, in 1965, he gave an illuminating talk on this subject. But, the computer is beyond the reach of many of us, but the author has felt for a long time that a fairly good Card Repertory can be made, which can go a long way in helping us.

During the past 10 years, a number of attempts have been made for programming the Repertorial information in personal computers. Mostly, Kent's important rubrics have been utilised by most of the workers. One in Britain has incorporated the Boenninghausen's rubrics also. But, some have the impression that a proper Card Repertory gives us more elasticity and purely a numerical summation may not often give the right answer.

The results should be as close as possible to the factual texts on Repertory. The cards of the Repertory should be of standard texture and thinness, so that they should be able to go through standard machines.

They should be strong as well as thin enough, so that one or two blocking cards should not shut off the light completely, when the approved cards are held against light.

The punching should follow the usual standard methods, so that machines should be able to punch or sort them automatically.

The card system should be elastic, so that new rubrics could be introduced, or new remedies added to rubrics, if needed. The user of such cards should have available to him facilities, so that he can get new data transcribed on the cards or get new rubrics introduced. The card system should be made as comprehensive and elastic as possible, so that the maximum demands of the repertorial analysis can be met. That is, different approaches can be made from that same system without distortion of results. It should have a definite plan with proper philosophical background.

The ideal cards should contain a reasonably large number of remedies so that additional data on the lesser proved remedies can be punched later on. The rubrics should be so arranged that there should be least time taken in selecting the rubrics from the index. There should be adequate cross-references also.

The punching on the cards should be able to indicate the degree or evaluation of the drugs if desired in a particular rubric.

The Kishore Cards

In 1959, the author published the Kishore Cards with about 3500 cards. It was considered that they were still not adequate and did not fully meet the demands of the repertorisation, especially that of the Kentian method. In the second edition, published in 1967, the number of cards or rubrics has gone up to about 10,000, and about six hundred remedies have been processed on the cards. The third edition has appeared in 1986, with a number of additions in both rubrics and newer remedies.

Although the number of rubrics is fairly large, one is not hampered in the analysis. One does not have to make unwarranted generalisations or substitutions. It is rarely that one has to go to Kent, and that too, for very small rubrics for final elimination or confirmation.

It is versatile enough to enable one in making one's choice in either repertorial method, Boenninghausen or Kent. While working on Kent's method, we can apply it in various ways i.e. (a) Kent's artistic or 'short cut' method of choosing a small eliminative rubric (b) Kent's hard way of working on all the symptoms, generals and particulars and total evaluation (c) working from mentals to physical generals (d) working with physical generals (when mentals are not marked) and using more than one rubric as the eliminative complex.

It can be used equally well by the less advanced students of Homoeopathy, because one can find the rubrics very easily, and can work out the totality from simple basic principles. The remedies are not blocked out completely, as some light shows through even if a remedy does not appear in two rubrics or cards. That means that even an apparently less indicated remedy has a chance of being considered for final analysis, if the Materia Medica and the case in hand, give greater indication for that. Any Repertory, at its best, is only a pointer or a suggestive for a group of likely remedies and cannot take the place of the Materia Medica. It is not always the 'all-through' remedy which is the indicated one.

One of the greatest drawbacks of our Repertories is that they have become static. No revision or additions are undertaken by individuals or groups. Even Kent, in his introduction to his Repertory, exhorted his followers to keep up this work. But, this is a very delicate task and has to be done very carefully. The author has made numerous additions to Kent from authentic sources and these have been incorporated in the cards. For example, Boger's additions to Kent, Dr. James Stephensen's 'Hahnemannian Provings' and numerous other provings published in various journals have been utilised for this work. Whenever thought advisable or imperative, he has included in the Kentian rubrics, the isolated remedies of the sub-rubrics (with one modality), in the main rubrics. It is all the more necessary in a Card Repertory, otherwise, unwanted elimination will take place. Some of the Boenninghausen's rubrics, too, have been made up-to-date by including remedies which have been neglected previously. But, this is still a very much incomplete task and needs lot of work.

Apart from enlarging data on various remedies like Pyrog., Calc-f., Kali-m., Cench. etc., some of the new remedies which have been included are Cad-m., But-ac., Bar-s., Glyc., Ichth., Par., Rauw., and X-ray.

One can also combine rubrics and keep a new punched card for them for ready reference and quick elimination in daily work.

Such a collection of cards can stimulate us to do more of Repertory work, instead of always prescribing by so called intuition. The dangers of the routine rut are economy. By repertorisation, one often comes across remedies which would not come to one's mind otherwise. This, therefore, stimulates further study of the Materia Medica. Intelligent repertorisation always makes one a better student of Materia Medica and vice-versa. One could not cite a better example than those of Boenninghausen, Kent, M. Tyler, Boger and Erastus E. Case.

The Card Repertory, however, has no future as it has become obsolete because of excellent computer softwares now available both for IBM and Apple Macintosh computers.

Computer Softwares for Repertories

Recently, lot of efforts are being made for programming suitable software for Repertory of Kent, Boenninghausen, Boger's Boenninghausen, Synthetic Repertory etc. both in India and abroad. For I.B.M. computers, Radar is the most exhaustive software. In India, Tata consultancy prepared a software, which later has been modified by Dr. Jawahar Shah. Another software that is available is Polycrest. For Apple computers, the best is the Mac Repertory, which is much easier to work with.

Reference Works is the brainchild of Dr. David Warkentin of SanFrancisco, U.S.A. It has a combination of all the Materia Medicas, Repertories and many journals, at one source. It is a computer program that enables you to find a patient's symptoms anywhere they may be in the Materia Medicas and Repertories. Subsequently, Reference Works can analyze the results to find a similimum. For example, if you type a symptom and 'Search' by pressing a key, it will display within seconds a list of every reference to your symptom ever written!

Synthetic Repertory

Synthetic Repertory is one of the most important and exhaustive compilation on Homoeopathic Repertory. Updating of Homoeopathic Repertory is a never-ending business. Kent, the author of the most complete and reliable work on Homoeopathic Repertory, had already, by the end of his life in 1916, added to his published Repertory copiously, in his own handwriting, the newer symptoms, which had been confirmed in relation to the already listed remedies. These additions had remained unpublished for a long time. Apart from Kent's own efforts, there were still newer remedies proved and confirmed by young authors, which had not been incorporated so far. There were, however, some areas covered by older authors, which had been omitted by Kent, and they too had to be reviewed and incorporated, since clinical confirmations had sanctioned their value. Dr. Horst Barthel and Dr. Will Klunker prepared a Repertory covering only the Mental symptoms and General symptoms. In their Herculean efforts, they were helped by Dr. P.Schmidt of Geneva, who had in his possession, Kent's Repertory with additions made by Kent in his own handwriting.

In the area of Mental and General symptoms, this Repertory is the most comprehensive and complete and has been utilised by the authors of relevant computer softwares for Homoeopathic Repertory.

This Repertory has reference to 1573 remedies, compared to Kent's Repertory with reference to only 591 remedies.

Various rubrics concerning mental symptoms have been enlarged and this has proved of great value in working out the indicated remedy in a case. Grading of remedies was done according to assessment of the authors, depending upon clinical verifications and accumulated experiences of the authors.

It has been published in three volumes-

1) Mental symptoms
2) General symptoms with modification
3) Sleep, Dreams and Male and Female Sexual symptoms

Integrated Repertory

In the year 2000, I published a repertory of the Mind which was an integration of Kent as well as the Boenninghausen's concept. This repertory contained additions from Synthetic, C.B. Knerr, Julian, Boericke, Vithoulkas and Pathak's works in addition to my own confirmed clinical experiences.

We decided to put the sections of **Mind** and **Dreams** together in the first volume. The second volume will be on **Generalities** which has been arranged as follows:

* Sensations and Complaints in General.
* Aggravation in general.
* Amelioration in general

Sensations and Complaints in general has some rubrics usually given under other sections of the major repertories. eg. in view of the growing cases of cancer, I decided to keep all the related rubrics at one place so that it's more convenient for the user. So you will find Cancerous affections with all the local forms of this disease in one place. Same has been done with Tuberculosis and Jaundice. This is done because these ailments are in a way general in nature and cannot be localized.

These two sections are being published shortly and should be available this year. We have done extensive additons from all of the above repertories. Plus more additions have been done from

Lippe, Jahr., Worcester Repertory to Modalities, Drugs of Hindustaan by Ghose, some works of CCRH. Although Lippe and Jahr are the original source books, but while working we realized that many of the rubrics and remedies have been omitted in the major popular repertories. The whole of Boericke's Materia Medica was scanned for more additions to the Generalities chapter.

This repertory comes from a basic need of a Repertory in 'total'. Great planning and thought of our whole team has gone in this effort of making this huge task possible. On many occasions, we were disappointed not to find certain rubrics in the Generalities section though so many efforts have been done to make the work more complete. I give here a few examples and leave more details for the preface of the actual book soon to be published. eg. joint pains in general; diabetes; jaundice etc.

Conclusion

A symptom as an expression of sickness in the human beings is a complex entity (as complex and differentiated as the man himself), hence, with all our ingenuity in classification and evaluation, we are constantly reminded of our short-comings. One thing is certain that basic tenets of the symptom remain the same; the sensation, location, modality and concomitant differentiate a symptom; less of these elements, less of its value, and more of its common-ness. As the disease advances, these elements tend to disappear and gross pathology appears. The diagnostic and common symptoms shaded by the general modalities form the ground colour of the picture, from which its special features portraying the individuality emerge with more or less distinctness.

If the homoeopathic doctor succeeds in extracting from the whole symptom-picture, those outstanding characteristics, which refer to the patient's reaction as a whole, and not merely to the local pain or inflammation, he will soon recognise four or five determinative or determining symptoms, mental, general or modified particulars, according to the patient under study; which will lead him to the exact diagnosis of the remedy.

It may be emphasised here that while writing and working a case for repertorial analysis, one must carefully translate the patient's symptoms into the repertorial rubrics according to the Repertory one is using. A symptom from a patient's case has to be carefully understood and then interpreted with the reference to the rubrics in the Repertory in use.

Very often, one has to take a broader or a larger rubric in place of a smaller one, provided the related larger one includes the smaller one. For example, a patient is very fond of 'pickles'. In this case, it is desirable to have the rubric 'Desire for sour things' as the rubric 'Desire for pickles' is a very small one, and we may miss the indicated remedy.

The other alternative in such cases is to combine the two, in case there are many different remedies in the smaller rubrics. Sir John Weir and Dr. Taylor, who were great students of Dr. Kent, often combined rubrics, so that in the process of elimination of unwanted remedies, the indicated remedy is not eliminated. This danger is very great when we are using eliminative rubrics, and more, so when we use Card Repertories or computer software for repertorisation.

In my Kishore Cards Repertory, I had done this at many places. For example, we had combined the rubric 'Aggravation, thinking of complaints, from' and 'Amelioration, occupied, when'. Although, Ignatia is better from occupation, and has been listed only in that rubric. Yet, I have come across its aggravation from thinking of complaints in Boericke's Materia Medica and verified it in practice.

A Repertory cannot replace the Materia Medica, nor can it restrict it. It should, on the contrary, extend our horizons of the Materia Medica; it should make the dry bones of Materia Medica spring up into a living character. If a Repertory fails to do so, it has not fulfilled its function.

A Repertory may be well-planned and really grand, but what matters is, that it is not what the author offers but what the reader gets.

Chpeter Two

CASE-TAKING (PATIENT AND PHYSICIAN)

Any Repertory will be useless if the case is badly taken. The basis of any repertorial analysis is the thoroughness of the case-taking. The case-taking is an art. It is the real art of medicine, rest of which is science. The art comes first, before the science comes. This art can be learnt after a certain amount of practice only, but thoroughness, which is an integral part of it, can be practiced right from the beginning. Right from Hahnemann's time, the great teachers of Homoeopathy have had something to say about this art. The Master has given very definite instructions in the Practical part of Organon i.e. Section 83 onwards to 103rd section.

When a case is well taken, our work is practically done. The Master has made strict demands on the physician for the proper case-taking and they are as valid and necessary today, as they were in his own time. No body has improved on his ideas about it. If one is negligent in case-taking or has taken incorrect symptoms, repertorisation will give one the wrong answers. It will be like the birth of a monster instead of a normal body. There might be the head of the Gelsemium, eyes of Phosphorous, liver of Lycopodium and face of Carbo-veg. It will not make much sense; it will not be a recognisable picture of the person you have to identify.

It requires all the alertness, intelligence, ingenuity, care, and circumspection on the part of the physician. Rudolph Rale, writing in an editorial say, "There is no procedure in homoeopathic practice more important than a thorough knowledge of the right way to take a case. The ability to do this, insures against humiliating mistakes and failure, prevents misconceptions of the sphere of Homoeopathic therapeutics and paves the way to relief or cure where either is possible."

Diagnosis, prognosis and treatment all have to be dovetailed in the process of case-taking. They cannot be separated.

Hahnemann laid down the following three basic conditions-

Unprejudiced mind (freedom from bias).
Sound understanding.
Attention and fidelity in observation, recording and tracing the image of sickness.

These are dependent on each other and together form

Unprejudiced mind
(freedom from bias)

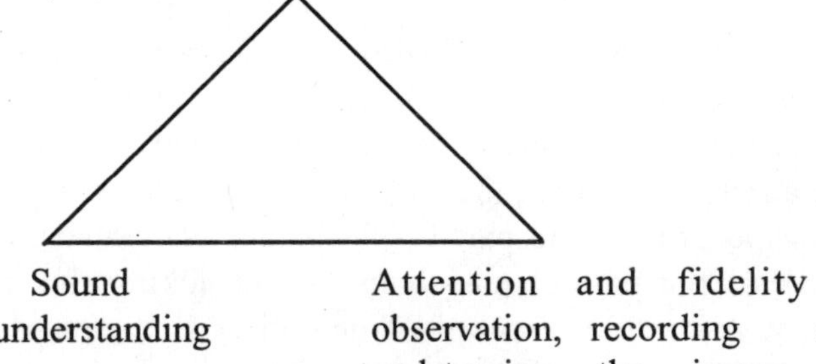

Sound understanding

Attention and fidelity in observation, recording and and tracing the image of sickness.

a Trinity which must be the basis of all case-records. Somebody remarked that good case taking is as rare as a chinaman with whiskers.

(A) Unprejudiced mind, i.e. there is absolute freedom from bias; there are no pre-conceived notions. It is very difficult for most of us to be completely objective and not to let preconceived notions or certain experiences influence our judgement. Very often, especially in the case of beginners or those who unfortunately lack the gift of balanced judgement, we see that they jump immediately to a particular diagnosis or a selection of a remedy. Not only that, but they continue to support their contention and not try to see other facets of the image of sickness or remedy.

The perceiving of the image of sickness and the corresponding drug requires, apart from basic knowledge, finer senses of perception and unbiased approach to a problem. Each case of sickness that is seen by us as Homoeopathicians, is a unique entity and should be explored as such.

(B) Sound understanding, i.e. the physician has the capacity for examining in every manner all and everything about the case. Senses are acute; thinking faultless. There is judicious approach and capacity for taking the best out of the patient This embodies also the capacity for laying down proper schematic arrangement etc. for recording.

(C) Attention and fidelity in observation, recording and tracing out the true image of the disease. Hence, there is no carelessness, no ignoring of even so called *insignificant or minute symptoms.* It requires complete alertness or aliveness and circumspection on the part of physician. Sometimes, a chance remark of the patient may help us in tracking the indicated remedy. A complete record of deviation from sound healthy state, felt by the patient, noticed by individuals around him and observed by the physician has to be recorded. It may be mentioned here that written records of the case histories are not only important from the stand-point of repertorial analysis for arriving at the similimum, but also for the follow up and prescription of the second remedy; for research and statistical analysis, for indexing and ultimately for additions to applied Materia Medica and Repertory.

Quite early in my practice I was asked to make a home visit and see a young girl suffering from a relapse of typhoid fever. In those days, Homoeopathy reigned supreme in the treatment of typhoid cases, as the modern medicine did not have antibiotics etc. for treating such cases. In this case, the patient had become afebrile after three weeks of fever, but she had a relapse after 4 or 5 days and the fever ranged between 104 degree F to 105 degree F, and the patient became drowsy.

On examining the patient and listening to the parents' account of her condition, I was rather no wiser as to the diagnosis of the remedy. I sat and observed her for half an hour and I found, however, that she laid with her face to the wall and did not turn and face my side. On inquiring, I was told if some stranger or visitor comes to see her, she turned her side to the wall as long as the visitor was there. Only on his or her departure, she turned back and talked to the family members.

She was given Sepia which aborted the fever in 24 hours and she recovered completely in a very short time. I had never heard or read about any case of typhoid treated by Sepia. But in Homoeopathic therapeutics, it is the patient which matters.

There is a difference in case-taking in both the schools of medicine. To the one, it suggests a name for its case; to the other, the points gathered are indices pointing to the curative agent. The one ceases its efforts the moment it has succeeded in justifying a name for the disease complex. It stops because it has no further use for the facts; with the few findings, it makes the diagnosis and outlines the treatment.

As opposed to it, the other school cannot stop inquiring further, till all the facts are brought out, because, if any part be omitted from the record (however trivial it may look), it may be that in the omission are the facts most important for the diagnosis of the remedy. This school considers the patient as a whole, the patient in general and see the patient in his totality and not in his parts; not the disease, not the pathology, not the diagnosis, but the patient, living, feeling and thinking

In other words, the aim of the orthodox school is to place the difficulties in a group class, classifying the symptoms under a 'group' head. With the homoeopathic school, the 'group' is never treated as a unit; the individual patient, into whatever diagnostic group he may fall, is treated as an individual unit. Hahnemann called it 'individualising examination' of each case of disease as it appears.

It may be emphasised that physical diagnosis is an integral part of our case-taking; it does not help us directly in the diagnosis of the remedy but indirectly it is of great use. 'It is not to the credit of a doctor to be intent only on his symptoms and prescription and to neglect the examination of, say, the rectum, where a patient comes complaining of piles and to leave it to the more conscientious practitioner to diagnose later an advanced carcinoma. The remedy-yes, but also the diagnosis.'

The diagnosis helps us in

(1) observing the course of disease and result of treatment (prognosis).
(2) preserving the reputation of the physician.
(3) in removing obstructions to cure.
(4) in choosing suitable potencies, as in advanced pathology or certain diseases of lungs, an unsuitable potency may start undesirable reactions.
(5) in finding out symptoms due to any mechanical causes or pressure symptoms due to tumours, growths or stones. Such symptoms, even though appearing very peculiar, may not be important.
(6) for the necessity of ignoring or discounting signs and symptoms which have origin in the gross pathological changes and cannot be diagnostic of the indicated remedy.

There are many conditions and symptoms which are due to mechanical causes beyond the scope of Homoeopathic remedy; for example, a large stone in bladder, impacted fibroid in pelvis or severely displaced inter-vertebral disc causing persistent nerve pain are all mechanical in nature and require mechanical means and the homoeopathic remedy may play only a secondary part.

The 'science' part of case-taking, is the institution of some standard procedure of Interrogation, Recording and Physical examination. A standardized case record has to be evolved. There may be individual variations but on the whole the best prescribers seem to follow practically a similar outline of case-taking. The most vital part is, of course, Interrogation. Individual departures from one's standard procedure may be dictated by individual patients and their special needs. Every case taken in the same stereo-typed or routine way may make us very prone to seeing great similarity in the past few cases that we saw and try to prescribe the same remedy.

The case-taking may be summarized into 'To listen, to write, to question and to coordinate'. Listening is quite an art. It should be an interested listening, because the patient is usually very sensitive to the physician's attitude; he knows immediately if the physician is attentive or is mentally somewhere else. While listening to the patient, one observes very carefully and assess the patient during the same process. A loquacious or a hysterical patient will be self-evident during the recital of his or her symptoms. One makes suitable notations for emphasising certain symptoms for evaluation and further analysis. After having listened to the patient and recorded the whole story as given by the patient, plus one's own observation, we come to the important task of interrogation. The patients often spin out long yarns but the physician brings them back to the subject proper by a judicious remark. The Interrogation comes only after the patient has told his or her story. 'It requires the wisdom of a savant, the knowledge of a sage, the acumen of the successful lawyer, tact of the trained diplomatist, the logic of the philosopher; the trained knowledge of the physician himself, last but not the least, rare insight into the human soul.'

The writing or recording part of case-taking is very essential and has been emphasised by Hahnemann. An omission of this aspect of case-taking is the greatest sin. Recording breeds confidence in the mind of the patient; it helps the physicians to preserve a cool and unprejudiced mind.

The clinical interview of the patient with the physician is quite an interesting study in itself. The late Dr. Dhawle once put it in a very interesting manner that it is the task of the physician to propose and set into operation the plan, but the patient disposes as per his disposition, abiding, abetting, distracting, countering, protesting. But the physician in his determination persists in finding the evidence despite the protestation of the patient and carries out the plan.

I remember the case of a very successful homoeopathic practitioner who was very popular, but in the later years, his practice started dwindling. The main reason that was found out was he started laying heavy bets on horse-racing. While taking a case, he seemed to be preoccupied and started asking same question twice or thrice.

While writing down the case history, the physician should write down the actual words of the patient and discourage the patient from using the so called medical terms.

While listening to patient during his or her narration, the physician continues to make his observations regarding mannerisms, the way the patient speaks or behaves, the way the patient enters the consultation room or the way the patient sits or fidgets. He makes notes of where the patient makes special emphasis in his or her narration. One can immediately perceive the tension, the anxieties, the fears or the depressions in a particular case, or one can note the arrogance or contemptuous attitude of the patient. Sometimes, the patient seems to have deep underlying fear or anxieties, but is not able to express except by laying undue emphasis on the physical symptoms. The physician is advised to have an attitude of watchful expectancy but apparently masterly inactivity. It may be mentioned here that observed symptoms are generally more reliable than those elicited by interrogation alone. Good prescribers feel that patients are potentially incapable of telling the truth regarding their innermost nature and personal character. A symptom which does not correspond with one's observation is of doubtful value for prescribing. Often, the way a patient responds to a question can be a guiding hint to the physician. An enthusiastic response with corresponding facial expression can be depended upon the reliability of the symptom.

For the physician who has his eyes open as well as his understanding, there are numerous mental symptoms that can be observed without saying a single word, as for example; timidity; loquacity; egotism; easily offended; embarrassed; exhilarated; easily startled; haughty; heedless; suspicious; laughing immoderately; even some memory troubles; quiet or hurrying disposition; sighing patients; restless; weeping when speaking about certain symptoms etc. During the interrogation, the physician must carefully watch the patient and observe the way he answers; the intonation of his voice, the play and expression of his physiognomy, especially, the mouth and eyes, must be carefully observed and grasped.

A good physician should be able, in the first consultation, to make his patient, laugh or cry, and in doing so, he is assured that the contact has been made, as he is able to put in vibrations in the living human being who was asking for help.

The following cases may illustrate our points. The cases were cited by Dr. E.F. Candegalue-

(1) BD, widower, 55 years old, has been suffering from headache for the last 22 years with complete failure of treatment. The attacks of headache are accompanied by nausea, vomiting and diarrhoea at the same time or alternating with them. Headache is localised in the forehead, bursting and ameliorated

by cold application. No apparent cause could be detected but on deep interrogation and discussion with the patient, the following points could be elicited.

1. Ailments from disappointed love.
2. Aversion to company.
3. Maliciousness
4. Pleasure in his own talking
5. Aggravation from consolation
6. Aggravation from warmth
7. Desire for sweets
8. Headache, forehead; bursting

The remedies that matched the case was Nat-mur. Two doses of Nat-mur 1M and then 10M, three months apart, cured the patient completely.

2) Mrs. D.F., 58 years old, complains from painful indigestion, acidity, sour belching, apthae in mouth, suffered from vertigo 4 years ago. She is exhausted, there is loss of weight, deep sadness, weeping, desires death and suicidal thoughts.

From the mental, general and the hereditary symptoms and the psycho-biographic history, the doctor culled out the following indications.

(i) Conscientious
(ii) Obstinate
(iii) Want of self confidence
(iv) Loathing of life
(v) Homesickness
(vi) Agg. from consolation
(vii) Agg. from heat and cold

Silica was discovered to bear the same tendency, and therefore, it could be the remedy that would bring about the true cure, 'modifying the minus-value that brought the patient and build so many pathological defenses.' One dose of Sil 200 set the order in the patient.

Let us mention another case from my own clinical diary, exemplifying the fact, as to how the germinating tendency unfolds itself with the passage of the time, while the remedy that can cure remains the same, or at most is complementary is called for.

(3) Mrs. N.G., 30 years old, has shooting pain in the right nates, with numbness of the part, extending in a sharp stitch, to anus on turning in bed. From the general symptoms and the psycho-biographic history of the patient, I selected the following symptoms as comprising the tendency of the psycho-biological make up of the patient.

1. Ailments from anger and vexation
2. Indignation
3. Sad tearful mood
4. Jealousy
5. Sexual desire insatiable, especially before menses
6. Menses copious
7. Leucorrhoea before menses

This tendency of the patient so strikingly corresponded to the innate tendency of the Calc-phos that a single dose wrought radical change. She got so much improved in a short time that she discontinued treatment. But, one day after a year or so, she again came into my office suffering with a gastric complaint. She had pain in stomach during and after eating. As is usual with me, cases of gastric disorders, I dismissed her with a few doses of 'placebo' and strict instruction as to change in diet. But on the 3rd day she came back, much depressed, to inform me that the pain had increased, and that she now felt pain not only in the stomach but the whole abdomen on the slightest attempt at eating. Now, there is one remedy in the whole Materia Medica which has the symptom well marked and that is Calc-phos. A single dose of Calc-phos 200 quelled all complaints before the next meal.

Modalities of symptoms are very important for the process of repertorisation. Often, time modalities are incorrectly perceived. Aggravation at night, actually, may have been something to do with sleep. One has, therefore, try to probe into other circumstantial activities etc.

The hysterical patients will give their narration differently. These observations perceived by the physician, have to be quietly recorded by him in the case-record sheet. Some of these things cannot be directly questioned. You can't ask a patient if he is very proud or over bearing. Some of this information which is perceived by the physician, will be very handy for interrogation later on. It not only brings the patient to be closer to the physician and have confidence in him, but also helps the physician in the discovery of signs and symptoms, which could be more reliable for our repertorial analysis.

During this narration by the patient, the physician makes a careful note of physical features of skin, eyes, etc. which could also be carefully noted down.

The art of clinical interrogation is the most important 'Art' part of our case-taking. No amount of rules or procedural outlines can teach it. It comes by constant practice and observation of sick humanity. In spite of this, there are certain basic observations about questioning a patient, which should be kept in mind in the interest of the patient.

In case-taking, the physician has to trace properly the evolution or development of the present complaints or symptoms. One never knows which link or chain of development may have played the decisive role and thus indicate the relevant part of history which may lead us to the curative remedy. This is most important, especially, in deep chronic diseases; diseases like cancer etc. One has to unfold the latent tendencies or genetical influences which have given rise to the present morbid picture. In other words, in Hahnemann's language, there must have been miasmatic rumblings in the past history and the evolution of the present pathalogy. The end-results of today do not give us any clue to the constitutional remedy.

A sign or symptom occurring in any person is not an isolated phenomenon; it may have multiple inter-relationships including causes, associated phenomenon, and effects. These may be often apparent or submerged, psychological components, sometimes of minor but often of major importance. The response of the patient to his disorder, his reactions to it and understanding of it, are essential and, often, deeply revealing parts of the history.

Therefore, the requirements on the part of the physician are-

a). Understanding, Sympathy
b). Intensely personal experience in medicine of the physician and his ability in sharing.
c). Embracing confidences and frustrations
d). Skill in eliciting bidden secrets in the history, using give and take method, especially, when one is engaged in coming to the most intimate problems.

It may be emphasised here, especially for the beginners, that it is not at all desirable for translating patients' conditions and symptoms into the medical terms of the present day, as it will make our task more difficult .Homoeopathy is all written in the simple language that accurately expresses what was actually felt by the provers. "This language is there for all times to come. Homoeopathy would have died out completely if these findings had been written down in the terminology of the science of Hahnemann's day. "This homeliness of expression causes wonderment in doctors accustomed to modem medical terms; but it is just this that has saved Homoeopathy."

Interrogation

Interrogation has to be a very tactful business. It will

be guided by the patients' story, and there cannot be any hard or fast rule, regarding the methods of interrogation, because every individual patient may require a special approach; for example, a secretive patient or a taciturn patient (introspection) will require entirely a different approach from that of a hysterical or a loquacious patient. Some patients will distort their symptoms and want us to see them as they would like to appear. But we want to see them as they are. The questions have to be at their level of intelligence or emotional maturity. Natural reserves of the patient must, however, be respected. Hence, questions about intimate and personal life have to wait till a suitable moment. Of course, every operator differs in the method of asking questions, but, there has to be a certain outline or a method to be followed by everybody.

There are three common mistakes made by us when we start the interrogation-

(a) frequent interruption of the patient,
(b) asking direct questions,
(c) making answers conform to some remedy in our mind

Therefore, the following directions should be kept in mind:

1. There should be no direct questions to which the answer may be 'Yes' or 'No'.
2. Avoid questioning in a manner when the patient is obliged to choose between two different alternatives. Leave the patient his own choice.
3. 'Torpedo' method of questioning is dangerous. Making answers conform to some remedy we have in mind, is a terrible error. A patient comes in, tells a few symptoms, and we immediately think of a remedy, and begin to ask questions, and see if we can get enough evidence to convict him of Pulsatilla or Sulphur, whatever it may be. It is surprising how well we can make the patient give us the symptoms we are looking

for, as well as, how little evidence it takes for some of us to make the conviction and give the remedy. Here, the mere writing of symptoms, helps us to keep cool and not to pass a hasty judgement.

4. The questions are worded and designed to unearth the therapeutic diagnosis and to elicit answers which correspond to the language of the Repertory and Materia Medica.
5. There should be some method in putting questions. One should not jump from one subject to another, without completing a particular symptom. The patient is likely to be confused.
6. Our questions should not make people more interested in Disease. There are people who are interested more in Disease than in Health.
7. In the clinical interview and when recording the notes on sensations or pains, we should try to elicit from the patient, as far as possible, the nature and description of the sensations. This has to be done very carefully without giving suggestions. Of course, one may have to keep in mind various kinds of pains etc. It is also imperative to note down the intensity of pains and sensations. The radiation and laterality of these pains and sensations should also be inquired into, as this information may give indication for certain drugs.

Since modalities are the natural modifiers of the sickness, they have to be obtained with accuracy and underlining those conditions or circumstances which affect the patient most forcefully. These modifying influences have to be investigated in all the areas of disturbed functions from head to toe.

One has also to find out the recurrence of these complaints, their periodicity. If so, why so? In the interrogation, one has always to keep in mind the words why, when, and how. While asking some of these questions, we should try also to get at anything strange, rare or peculiar, which some patients might have hesitated in talking about.

8. We should avoid making statements which could easily be adopted by the patient. Never ask "Do you like wet or dry or hot weather? What weather suits your pains in the joints?" Don't ask "Do you like cold drinks?" The patient will definitely say 'yes', and what he means is, that he likes cold drinks in hot weather. Actually, he takes hot tea also, and in winter he shuns cold drinks.

The most delicate moment in the clinical interrogation is, when you come to asking the mental symptoms. That is where the real acumen of the examiner comes into play. It has been suggested that all the experienced teachers never ask such intimate questions in the beginning of the Interrogation. They should be asked, either somewhere in the middle of the questionnaire or at the end. Dr. P. Schmidt was of the opinion that mentals should not be asked at that end because by that time, the patient is exhausted and is not able to give out his innermost feelings. Dr. Borland on the other hand, used to say, that the best time to ask such questions is when you are examining the patients physically; physical touch seems to bring the patient closer to the doctor mentally and emotionally.

One must try to elicit the mentals, especially his changed mentalities, due to sickness. If you open fire on these too soon, again he will probably take cover, and put up his defenses. First, the patient's confidence must be gained.

One thing is certain that mental symptoms should never be asked in the beginning; sometimes, it is worth-while waiting till the patient comes for the second interview.

While inquiring into chronic diseases, the ordinary occupation of the patient, his usual mode of living and diet, his domestic situation and so forth must be considered, to ascertain anything that may tend to produce or maintain disease, so that by their removal, recovery may be promoted. In such diseases, most minute details must be noted if a cure has to be established. Chronic patients are so used to their suffering that they pay little or no heed to the lesser accessory aymptoms, which are often of greater importance in determining the choice of the remedy. They can scarcely believe that these accessory symptoms, these greater or lesser deviations from health, can have any real connection with the principal disease.

Investigation of especially chronic diseases demands the greatest circumspection, tact, knowledge of human nature, caution in the conduct of inquiry and a vast degree of patience.

Our aim here is to indicate the value of case-taking in relation to the discovery of the Similimum, from the use of Repertories. From a properly taken case, we deduce also the diagnosis, hence prognosis and auxiliary measures like diet, general hygiene, nursing, environment, and obstacles to cure. To the orthodox physician, the diagnosis leads directly to treatment, but to the homoeopath, it is only a preliminary step. In the end, it must be emphasised that to the homoeopath nothing is so important and so difficult as the case-taking. *Almost all the mistakes in prescribing are mistakes made in case-taking.* While listening to the patient, we should be observant and ready to seize any opening that looks promising. Sometimes, the patient is able to give his case-history in very well-defined expressions, but, in most cases, the patients are rather vague in expressing their complaints, and are not able to define the nature of complaints they suffer from. In such cases, one has to give them certain suggestive hints, so that the patient can choose from the various expressions, the most suitable to his particular pain or complaint. But, impatience on the part of an examiner, may cause valuable information to be suppressed. We have to be tolerant towards the natural reserve which certain people show when details of their personal or family life are inquired. It is wise to ask firstly, questions which will cause no embarrassment; leaving questions of more delicate nature until patient's confidence has been won.

Patient and the Physician:

During case taking, when a patient presents himself

before the physician, we are primarily concerned with his disturbing signs and symptoms. But, we have to keep in mind all the time, the aim of studying his signs and symptoms. A sign or symptom occurring in any patient, is not an isolated phenomenon; it may have multiple inter-relationships including causes, associated phenomena, and effects. There may be inter-relationships, evidencing various types of disturbed physiology, but there is always a subjective psychological component; sometimes, may be, of minor importance, but often of major importance. The responses of the patient and his disorder, his reactions to it, and understanding of it are essential, and often, deeply revealing parts of the history.

Each illness has an emotional component. Sometimes, it is minor, sometimes amounting to emotional breakdown. The eventual health and well-being of the patient depend not only on his physical but also on his mental and emotional recovery. From the very beginning of patient-physician relationship, at the first interview, it is important to recognize that, no matter what the problem may be, every person has particular needs, according to his individual personality. The patient should, by the physician's approach, be given reason to know at once that doctor is interested in him as a person, as well as in his disease. The patient has the right to expect kindness and humane consideration as well as professional competence. The patient has to develop assurance and faith in the physician. As we are sizing up the patient, he is likewise making judgements about us.

The physician, as he starts to converse with his patient and elicits the story of his illness, becomes engaged in the most intensely personal experience in medicine. The narration of usual medical problems may yield, embarrassing confidences and more or less, pertinent information about past frustrations, present anxieties and hopes about the future. It must be kept in mind that we should not hurry the patient. Let the patient feel that the physician is having full attention and is not in a hurry to end the interview. Dr. Pierre Schmidt once said if you are able to make the patient weep or laugh during the first consultation, you have won him and he will stay with you as a very faithful patient.

As a beginner, the young physician tends to ignore such emotional and psychological manifestations or fails to understand the relevant value or relationship of the picture of the sickness.

In any case-taking, the mode of onset, history of development of symptoms or complaints, duration of symptoms and any special causation are very important. Of course, we must lay great importance on the symptoms, complaints which are most troublesome to the patient. We remember a case of acute pharyngitis, which looked like an Aesculus case and when given this medicine, throat became better but not quite all right. he had also intolerable cramps in the calf muscles. Cuprum-met has both the symptoms of throat and cramps of calf muscles and it put a very speedy end to both the complaints.

In daily clinical work, it has always seemed best, to first get a pretty full life history of the case in hand, then look over the objective appearance, and lastly, find out what the patient thinks and feels. These factors are then carefully built into a mental picture of what seems to be wrong. For sufficient reasons, all of its features can not usually be elicited at the first interview.

Hahnemann repeatedly pointed to the peculiar symptoms as being the real indicators for the curative remedy, and the successful prescriber is he, who can pick them out, and without losing touch with the essential diagnostic features, assign them to their proper place in the symptom picture. He links together and combines the essentials, with the singularities present in such a way, as to produce an harmonious whole. This is, perhaps, not easy to learn, but it can be done by avoiding a false start, but with persistence even to the point of seeming to be intuitional.

The number of such combinations is, of course,

unlimited, but we find that certain ones actually occur with relative frequency, giving rise to the idea of specifics, organ remedies, epidemic remedies, etc. all delightfully indefinite terms, full of danger and lacking in the accuracy which makes for correct and radically curative homoeopathic work.

In learning this art, it is needful to divest oneself of all speculative opinions as to the origin of such odd manifestations. These things belong to the obscurities of diagnosis, but this, however, does not mean that a diagnostic symptom can never be a major indicator, as witness the marked aggravation from motion, equally prominent in pleurisy and in the provings of Bryonia; or the 2 A.M. aggravation frequent both in duodenal ulcer and the effects of Kali-bi-chrom.

In case taking, all our effort should be to see, in what way we can discover the patient as he is, and not as he wishes us to see him. Dr. Gladwyn records, "Once, I visited one of the sensitive ones the other day. He described his dreadful headache, the terrible pain in the chest, which he thought could kill him every time he coughed or took a deep breath. But when I sat by him, the nurse accidentally struck him with a pin and he made just as much fuss over it as over his head and chest pains, leaving me in some doubt as to which was the most severe. Fortunately, for the patient, the remedies are also sensitive and are exaggerating also."

On the other hand, the good-natured happy-go-lucky ones do not take the trouble to notice their symptoms.

There are suspicious patients and patients with mistaken ideas about the meaning of symptoms. They will not acknowledge certain symptoms, fearing the physician will think ill of them. One can often obtain all necessary information about a denied leucorrhoea, after remarking that leucorrhoea is often the result of a cold. Similarly, false modesty will make a patient distort the truth by with-holding part of it.

One of my patients, a short time ago, told me such a good Pulsatilla story that I did not suspect that she was with-holding any truth of it. But as she was about to leave the office, she said, 'There is something else which I perhaps ought to tell you, though it is not very nice." Then she went on telling symptoms after symptoms, and when she finished, it was not Pulsatilla but Pulsatilla's sister Cyclamen.

Bashfulness is another stumbling block. You cannot do much with a bashful patient, until by acquaintance, you gain his confidence, and even then, you may never be able to get the whole truth. I remember a bashful boy of 14 years, who used to come to the clinic. With his mother's help, I managed to get enough symptoms to give him Nat-mur, but he would never tell he had trouble with nocturnal enuresis. Anyway, he had his mother's promise not to tell. One morning after receiving the remedy, he evoked surprise to find a dry bed. He accused his mother of having told the doctor. To reassure him, the mother came and asked how I had found it out. But the boy would never come for more medicine.

Patients with-hold symptoms simply because they forget to tell or because they think them value-less. They will say, "I forgot to tell you that the baby had a discharge from the ear." You may carefully take the things and among other things, ask, "What sickness the child had had" and the mother will enumerate them and assure you that 'that is all'. When you have had the baby under treatment for sometime, the mother will accidentally tell you that the baby has not been well since she was vaccinated. When asked why she did not tell that before, the reply was, "I did not think that had anything to do with it."

Then we have also the secretive patient. His sickness is the result of 'sin' and he wants us to cure the result without suspecting the cause. We have a patient here, who has been under our treatment for months. Each time he came to the clinic, he assured the physician incharge that there was nothing else about the case to tell. But finally, he became frightened and to one of the physicians, he confessed privately his sycotic history and symptoms, enough to cover seven pages of notes. He had so carefully hidden all his general symptoms that we did not suspect the nature of his trouble. It was an awful mistake.

Similarly, I remember a case of a man who had the symptom-picture of Rheumatoid arthritis with severe pain in the joints, and especially of knee joints and ankles. He was immobilised and confined to bed for years. He was admitted in the National Institute of Homoeopathy and he was given various medicines. Looking at the case, I suspected, he might have had some sycotic taint in the past .but he denied incessantly to all questions that our house surgeons put to him. But one day, during a fairly intimate conversation with him, I was able to find it out that he had contracted gonorrhoea 20 years ago and gradually his joints were affected. A dose of Medorrhinum 1M was given. Within 48 hours, he had disappeared from the ward. We learnt later on from the nursing staff, that he had gone home to attend some sort of important ceremony. Earlier, he was hardly able to walk at all.

In this context, we should remember that there are hysterical patients, who seem to have every kind of disease that they have heard of or seen. I remember one, whom I came in contact with, in the early part of my practice. Every time, a dose of sac-lac gave him immediate relief. The pretended hysterics are the patients to be avoided, if you can, not because they will deceive you, but because they will waste your time and disturb you. They will make up symptoms to fit the occasion.

Once, I had a female patient who one day became rigid and 'unconscious' while standing in the room in the presence of her daughter who had to support her for about 45 minutes right in the middle of the waiting room. The patient had taken such a position out of reach of everything, so that her daughter could not easily go for help. She bent her head back and elbows also with the result that the daughter failed to lay her on the floor lest she might be injured. The patient knew if her daughter managed to leave her even for a minute or two, she would bring boiling hot water to be applied to her feet or abdomen, which was often one thing that would stop the nonsense immediately.

Causation

One of the vital inquiries that has to be elicited during interrogation and examination, is the exciting cause or the circumstances leading to the origin of the main symptoms or sickness of the patient. Sometimes, 'causation' alone leads us to the anamnesis of the patient's remedy. Dr. Clarke in his Clinical Repertory, has devoted one whole chapter on causation. I remember the case of a young lady who had developed intractable eczema on the face and did not respond to the usual remedies. On deeper inquiry, it was discovered that she developed these eruptions after an attack of measles. Morbillinum 200 had to be given to set in motion the curative reaction. Many similar examples could be cited from our clinical case histories.

In the end, it may be emphasised that case-taking must be more than a list of the symptoms. The length is not enough. Indeed, it may confuse or tend to be a contradiction.

It is, therefore, obvious that the physician after writing down the case history, as presented by the patient, has observed things about the patient which he intentionally did not comment upon or inquire from the patient.

But now, at the end, the physician should note the behaviour of the patient during his visit; whether he was morose, hasty, quarrelsome, lachrymose, depressed or despairing, calm or slow in movements and in speech; whether he was drowsy or full of comprehension or he showed signs of fear and anxiety. He should also observe the condition of his eyes, skin etc., his posture of sitting, if he keeps his mouth open; how he sits and rises or walks. That is anything that the physician thinks is striking or abnormal and all these things should be put in writing at the end of interrogation.

Apart from obtaining the story from the patient, a physician must, if possible, try to interrogate relatives or persons, who are in contact with the patient. They may give information, which neither the patient nor physician's own observation at the interview could make available. Often, the persons tell us what the patient does not tell us or the patient does not realise it himself. For example, odors from the body, or odd little moods or the particular attitude and approach to events and things.

Physical examination

At the end of case-taking and interrogation, a physician has to undertake good physical examination. He has to know the physical disabilities, patho-anatomical results. With these findings and knowledge of medicine in general, one can differentiate between the rare, strange and peculiar symptoms and the symptoms which are diagnostic or which can be explained by physio-pathological findings or which can be called common symptoms.

For example, a patient suffering from painful ulcer on the foot feels better if he lets his leg hang down. This is something unusual, as we usually find that such patients with ulcers or inflamed varicosis are worse by letting the lower limbs hang down. They are better if the legs and feet are elevated.

Physical examination and diagnosis helps us in determining the prognosis. A patient complaining of bleeding from anus, may be taken as a case of bleeding piles, but after proper physical examination, it is discovered to be a case of malignancy of rectum.

All these findings condition our line of treatment, curative or palliative.

Diagnosis also helps us in research projects and makes our communication with other colleagues more meaningful.

It may be warned here that in an acute case, our approach in case taking is different. We should not confuse the acute symptoms with symptoms of the chronic ailment. Here, we have to confine ourselves to the symptoms which have been brought out by the acute illness. We should not spend unnecessary time on taking the case as outlined above, as that refers to chronic sickness. In acute conditions, we deal mostly with signs and symptoms of the acute conditions.

OUTLINE OF THE CASE-TAKING

One of the best outlines for case-taking is the one given by Late Dr. Elizabeth Hubbard Wright. The following outline is taken from her 'Brief Study Course', with some modifications.

I. The patient's story.

II. Locations and sensations, of each symptom with complete details after interrogation, especially with regard to the specific character of sensations, their location, laterality, extension and radiation.

III. Concomitants and alternations of these sensations.

IV. Modalities as applied to each of the above symptoms in the following order: Origin, beginning or causes of the sensations, their prodrome, onset, pace sequence and duration.

V. Modalities of Aggravation or Amelioration of the complaints and that of the patient as a whole.

   (a) Time (hour, day, night, before or after mid-night); periodicity; seasons; moon phases.

   (b) Temperature and weather: Chilly or warm blooded usually, chilly or warm blooded in present illness; wet, dry, cold, or hot weather; weather changes; storm or thunderstorm (before, during or after); hot sun, wind, fog, snow, open air, warm room, changes from one to other, stuffy or crowded places, drafts, warmth of bed, heat of stove, uncovering.

(c) Bathing (hot, cold or Sea), local applications (hot, cold, wet or dry).

(d) Rest or motion (slow or rapid, ascending or descending, turning in bed, exertion, walking, on first motion, after moving awhile, while moving, after moving), car and seasickness.

(e) Position: standing, sitting (knees crossed), rising from sitting, stooping; rising from stooping, lying; (on painful side, back, right or left side, abdomen, head high or low); rising from lying, leaning head backward, forward, sidewise, closing or opening eyes, any unusual position such as knee-chest.

(f) External stimuli: touch, hard or light pressure, rubbing, constriction (clothing etc.), jar, riding, stepping, light, noise, music, conversation, odours.

(g) Eating: in general (before, during, after, hot or cold food or drink), swallowing (solids, liquids, empty), acids, fat, salt, salty food, starches, sugar and sweet, green vegetables, milk, eggs, meat, fish, oysters, onions, beer, liquor, .wine, coffee, tea, tobacco, drugs etc.

(h) Thirst: quantity, frequency, hot, cool or iced, sours, bitters etc.

(i) Sleep: in general (before, during, on falling asleep, in first sleep, after, on waking)

(j) Menses (before, during, after or suppressed).

(k) Sweat: hot or cold, foot-sweat, partial or suppressed.

(1) Other discharges: bleeding, coryza, diarrhoea, vomitus, urine, emissions, leucorrhoea etc.; suppression of same.

(m) Coition, continence, masturbation etc.

(n) Emotions: anger, grief, mortification, fear, shock, consolation, apprehension of crowds, anticipation, suppression of same.

VI. Strange, rare and peculiar symptoms.

VII. The patient as a whole : Mental Generals (to be studied last for convenience), Physical Generals.

Physical Generals

(a) The constitutional type of the patient (endocrinologico-homoeopathic correspondences, lack or excess of vital heat, lack of reaction, sensitiveness etc.)

(b) Ailments from emotions (see also mental generals); suppressions (emotions; discharges such as menses, sweat, leucorrhoea, catarrh, diarrhoea; eruptions; diseases such as malaria, rheumatic fever, exanthema, syphilis, gohorrhoea etc.; of pathology such as haemorrhoids, fistulae, ulcers, tonsils, tumours, other surgical conditions etc.); from exposure to cold, wet, hot sun etc., from mechanical conditions such as overeating, injury etc.

(c) Menses- date of establishment, regularity (early or late), duration, colour, consistency, odour, amount, clots, membrane, pain (modalities of), concomitants, aggravation or amelioration before, during or after, both physically and mentally; menopause (symptoms of).

(d) Other discharges: cause, colour, consistency, odour, acrid or bland; symptoms from suppression of; symptoms alternating with; hot or cold, partial discharges as of sweat; laterality; better or worse from discharges (before, during or after).

(e) Aversions and cravings for certain articles of food; excessive intake of particular items of food or salt and spices.

(f) Sleep: better or worse from, position in, aggravation after, difficulty in getting to sleep, waking frequently or early, at what hour, somnambulism, talking in sleep, dreams (see Mentals), restless during.

(g) Restlessness, prostration, weakness, trembling, chill, fever etc.

(h) Aggravations and ameliorations applying to patient as a whole.

(i) Objective symptoms such as redness of orifices, superfluous hair, applying to patient as a whole.

(j) Pathology which applies to patient as a whole, such as tendency to tumours, wens, cysts, polyps, warts, moles; individual and family tendency to certain diseases or weakness of specific organs or tissues (also related to 'a' above and to physical examination); frequency of catching cold.

Mental Generals

In our efforts for obtaining the mental generals, we need to understand the Man behind the illness. Insomnia, restlessness, irritability etc. may point to some mental or emotional disturbances which is lying deep inside and that has to be brought to the surface as that 'causation' may unravel the indicated remedy. Tactful interrogation with establishment of rapport are required in abundance.

(a) Will: Loves, hates and emotions (suicidal, loathing of life: lasciviousness, revulsion to sex, sexual perversions; anxieties and fears; greed (in eating, and money); emotionality; smoking, drinking, drugs; homicidal tendencies, desire or aversion to company, family friends; jealousy, suspicion, obstinacy, contrariness, depression, loquacity, weeping, laughing, impatience, conscientiousness. Mental tensions due to anticipation or job situation; mental and emotional conflicts.

(b) Understanding: Delusions, delirium, hallucinations, mental confusion, loss of time sense.

(c) Intellect: Memory, concentration, mistakes in writing and speaking.

VIII. Quick review of condition of every system and organ, beginning with head and following the order of Kent's Repertory.

IX. Past history of patient.

X. Personal history; life situation.

XI. Family history.

XII. Physical examination and laboratory and other tests.

Here, diagnosis must be made, as far as possible, because it helps us later, in the assessment of the progress of the case; it instills confidence in the patient; it helps us later, in the use of right potencies; it may help us in removing the obo obstruction obstruction to the cure and also in giving some ideas of the prognosis. It will clarify the symptoms due to presence of mechanical obstructions like stone in bladder; fibroid impacted in uterus; large impacted stone in the pelvis of the kidney.

While writing the case-history and follow up of the case, it is convenient to write down symptoms and locations in one column where as the modalities are written down in the second column. Sometimes, the modalities are not given in the first meeting but the patient brings to our notice certain modifying circumstances in a subsequent meeting.

Chapter Three

EVALUATION OF SYMPTOMS

Symptoms and Their Grading

The Case-taking and Evaluation of symptoms are the two vital aspects of the same thing; they are interdependent and are-

Materia Medica
Case-taking & Evaluation
Repertory

entwined closely. Homoeopathic Case-taking has a very intimate relationship with Homoeopathic Materia Medica and Repertory. As indicated below, the trio of Materia Medica, Case-taking plus Evaluation and Repertory are the apices of an equilateral triangle. Sheetfuls of case-history may be useless, if we have missed the symptoms needed for making the correct prescription.

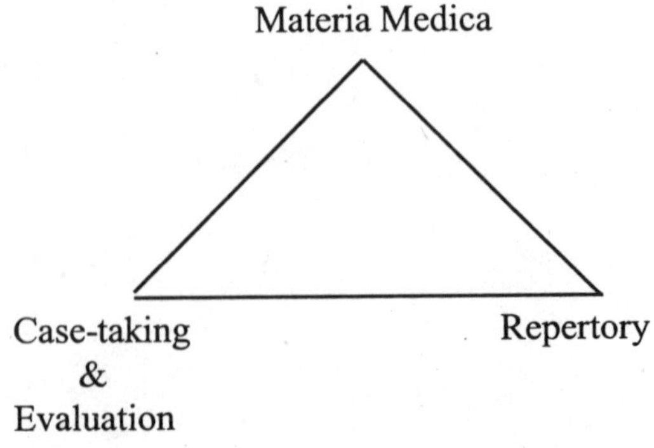

Without signs and symptoms, it is not possible to locate the curative remedy from our Materia Medica. The 'symptoms', therefore, are the most important data input for our achieving an objective. But the confusion arises, when we are faced with hordes of symptoms from our patient. Hahnemann, and later, Kent and others, tried to analyse this problem and gave fairly definite guidelines regarding the proper selection of symptoms, which only could be pointers for arriving at the indicated remedy.

Case Taking and Evaluation of Symptoms

Evaluation of symptoms requires maturity of mind, comprehensive knowledge of medicine including normal and abnormal structure, function and psychology, knowledge of Homoeopathic philosophy. Homoeopathic Repertories and the philosophical background of their structures. Without the previous knowledge of a sickness, as seen in majority of the cases suffering from it, one cannot differentiate the symptoms and signs which specifically belong to a particular individual suffering from that sickness, as compared to the 'herd' symptoms of that particular sickness. This is, of course, the first step. Later on, we have to see what are the signs and symptoms which belong to the patient as a whole, and those which belong to a part. Kent talked about 'Generals' as belonging to the patient as a whole, and 'particulars' or 'local' as belonging to particular part, organ or area of the body.

The earliest signs or evidence of sickness are usually subjective. There is, therefore, personal bias. Boger used to say that, "Individuality hides itself more and more as sickness advances and becomes more objective."

It is often seen that, earliest subjective symptoms are usually the mental symptoms and they are the most important for the detection of the remedy. As the sickness advances, there may be variations of these, and if the disease advances rapidly, the objective and local symptoms supervene; which take away the possibilities of the detection of the remedy. It is, therefore, not easy to see clear and definite image of the remedy, after the sickness has advanced to a great extent.

Hence, the 'quality' of symptoms is more important than the 'quantity' of symptoms, and the 'totality and intensity' of the 'quality' is what matters in the discovery of the similimum. Actually, case-taking is the first essential step towards differentiation of the individual case of sickness. The art of evaluation can be mastered only after years of study and practical application. Dr. Elizabeth Hubbard Wright, once said that she had been learning the art of evaluation of symptoms for the last forty years or so. I, too, even today, continue to learn and beginning to know more about the art of evaluation of symptoms after fifty years of practice of Homoeopathic medicine.

A student of Homoeopathic Repertory may, in the beginning, be confused by his inability to deal with large number of signs and symptoms collected by him in a single case and may spend lot of his time and energy and yet come to poor results. It is, therefore, very essential that he is given an understanding regarding the 'Grading of symptoms'. He has to know which symptoms are of vital importance and which may be completely ignored.

One of the most important task while applying the homoeopathic drug for curative purpose, is to understand and evaluate the different symptoms and signs as presented by the patient. Thus grading of symptoms not only economises our effort and time, but also saves us from failure and disappointments. The symptoms which have to be taken note of, or symptoms which can be used as eliminative ones, have to be marked out. To the beginner, it is very important to teach this valuation, as this is the very foundation for the process of repertorisation.

Disease is expressed in groups or combination of

symptoms out of thousands of symptoms, of both the phenomena of well-marked characteristics of certain diseases, as well as the individual's specific reactions to dynamics of disease. Of course, most of the symptom-groups are referable to particular diseases, organs and individuals, although, the former two remain constant But, at times, these exhibit very pronounced disease phases, thoroughly confusing the remedy diagnosis and leading to organopathic, pathological or diagnostic prescribing of a make-shift nature, ultimately, a most pernicious thing.

In the repertorial analysis, we are, however, concerned much more with the individualistic symptom groupings, for they generally show forth the real man, his moods, his ways and his particular reactions.

The final analysis of any case resolves itself into the assembling of the individualistic symptoms into one group and collecting the disease manifestations into another, then finding the remedy which runs through both, while placing the greater emphasis on the former. Therefore, the very large rubrics of our Repertories are likely to be more useful for occasional confirmatory reference than for the running down of the final remedy.

The place of *grading of remedies* in evaluation

As already indicated, the remedies were graded into five categories by Boenninghausen, and into three grades by Dr. Kent. For our Repertorial analysis, we sometime ignore the lower grade remedies in the larger rubrics by taking only the remedies of the upper two grades. The large rubrics usually indicate the commonalty of the symptoms, and hence, we can ignore the lower grade remedies. But, in the smaller rubrics of the related case, we take all the confirmed remedies, and then work out the similimum. This way, we can cut short the time taken for Repertorisation. Grading of remedies, thus, helps us in economising labor without compromising results. The intensity of symptoms should be matched with the higher graded remedies, which are usually indicated in Bold Capitals. Big types in the Repertory will never help you, unless symptoms are big type in the patient too. Grading of remedies in a rubric, indicates the intensity and frequency of the indication of the symptom for that particular remedy.

It may be noted that while using an eliminative or determinative symptom,(or combined eliminative symptoms) one caution is to be specially observed. A remedy or remedies, which are rare or unusual in the group, should be marked out separately for detailed study, as once in a while, such a remedy is the only one to unlock the case, but it may not appear in the usual analysis, where the extensively proved remedies may overshadow such a remedy.

While the grading or evaluation of symptoms largely depends upon their discovery and the extent of subsequent confirmation obtained for everyone of them, their sphere of action are also of vast importance, and may not be safely left out of the selection of the remedy. Of course, numerical summation may often mislead us from the choice of the right remedy. The relative standing of the individual symptoms always takes precedence.

In the abstract, the same symptom may have highest standing or importance in one case, but lowest in the next, all depending upon the general outline of the case, as delimited by the associated symptoms. Viewed from this standpoint, symptom-grading, as found in the Repertories, may be unsatisfactory, as well as of lesser importance, and yet, has great value. The relative value of a given symptom depends almost wholly upon its setting, therefore, changes from case to case; and is fully determined as to its repertorial standing by numerous clinical trials. If I apprehend the matter rightly, the original pathogenic symptom is really only a hint of what it may possibly develop in the future, as determined by successive testings.

As an example; 'Intolerance of clothes about the neck'

is found in the provings of quite a number of remedies, but it remained for Hering, to show that Lachesis decidedly outranks them all, and has only a few straggling followers. This is a particular which accentuates the value of Lachesis over Glonoine if the patient is intolerant of heat, but if sensitive to cold, Sepia takes the lead.

Experience leads to the conclusion, that the patient's actions, and of what he says of himself, are of the highest importance, and may not be lightly set aside. Just so, do drugs, in their general action, exhibit this or that predominant phase, and when one finds its counterpart in the other, the similimum has been discovered, provided the remedy contains the characteristics of the case in hand also. For example, we do not usually think of Phosphoric-acid for excitable, or Coffea for lethargic patients, unless the individualistic symptoms call for these remedies in the most positive way, an unlikely contingency. The quality of the general reaction greatly influence symptom values, be they pathogenic or clinical.

In a new proving, each prover reacts to only a part of the prospective picture and we properly sense the whole, only by seeing all the parts as a compound unit exactly as we see it in disease, the arrangement never being precisely the same, in either case.

Proper evaluation of signs and symptoms is required to reach the ultimate goal of finding the similimum, the remedy which will fit the patient in all his aspects of his ailments, and add accuracy and exactitude in our work. This process not only involves comparison of the symptoms produced by different remedies, to the symptoms of the patient, but also evaluation and comparison amongst the remedies, which have similar pathogenesis, and see which is the one which suits the patient the most.

Most of these processes naturally will be helped by Repertorisations, and later, by final study in the Materia Medica.

Very often, for this very achievement of the goal, we make use of key notes or therapeutic hints. They may, at best, be pointers in our search for the indicated remedy, but they cannot be depended upon. They might relieve some of the symptoms or palliate the condition, but they cannot be the proper similimum to the case. Therefore, one has to analyse the data and evaluate it properly, before we can really make the final prescription for the case.

The state of the patient's mind and temperament is often of most decisive importance in the homoeopathic selection of the remedy, since it is a distinct and peculiar symptom that should, least of all, escape the accurate observation of the physician.

Basic elements or traits of a symptom

1. Many workers have looked at symptoms from different angles and tried to use them in their own particular fashion. For the beginners, the various classifications and differentiations are rather bewildering. In spite of this, there are a few basic traits of a symptom, which are needed to make it complete. They were enunciated by Boenninghausen, and later propagated by Herring. Whatever be the type of symptoms, these features are needed to dress them up. The more complete these traits are, the more distinctive the symptoms become.

Elements of Symptoms-

SENSATIONS
in general
Complaints **objective** (pathological conditions i.e. pallor, cyanosis, anaemia, blackness, cracks, cracking of joints etc.)
&
subjective (includes also mental symptoms)

LOCATION (Includes also Laterality & Extensions) — **SIGNS & SYMPTOMS** — **CONCOMITANT** (Includes also the so called rare, strange & peculiar symptoms)

MODALITIES
(Includes also Causation; Effects of emotional upsets etc.)

LOCATION AND SENSATIONS :

The terms 'Sensations and Locations' are obvious. Location indicates the preferential sphere of action of a remedy on a particular part of the body.

(A) **Location**- The place of location in the evaluation of symptoms is, at times, very important and relevant for a case analysis. In the Boenninghausen's Repertorial approach, this is one of the vital elements of the symptoms and has to be utilised especially, in the cases where there are more of particulars and less of general symptoms or mental symptoms. Otherwise also, we have observed that certain remedies have a very specific affinity for a particular part of our anatomy. For example, Cardius-marianus affects very predominantly, the left lobe of the liver. Patients usually locate the pains or sufferings, and we have to see if that localisation helps us in the discovery of the indicated remedy. For example, if there is pain in the right upper chest, we can think strongly of Arsenic. The location of pain in the right middle chest will bring us to the remedies like Belladonna, Sanguinaria, Calc-carb etc. The pain in the left lower chest will indicate Myrtus, Pix-liquida, Theridion, Sulphur, Tub etc.

These pains and remedies are concerned more with lung troubles. But if such pains affect the external parts of the chest and not the lungs, then we think of Bryonia, Ranunculous-bulb, Arnica, Cimicifuga, Rhustox. The pains can be due to Pleuro-dynia, pleuritis, rheumatism of inter-costal muscles etc.

(B) **Sensation**- A patient will talk of pain, a kind of pain, or numbness or tingling, in relation to a particular part or whole body. The sensations of different kinds also are related in varying intensity to different remedies, and thus are an essential element of the data required for Repertorial analysis.

(C) **Modalities**- The Modalities are the conditions which modify a particular sensation or condition. Nausea may be relieved by eating; hence, 'eating' here is a modifying influence. The modalities make a symptom more distinctive and hence, essential for evaluation. All the conditions of Aggravation and Amelioration in relation to time, periodicity, circumstances, weather and temperature, position of rest or motion, pressure etc., are included in the modalities.

(D) **Concomitants**- The Concomitants are the accompanying symptoms which may seem to have no relation to the patient's main complaints, save that they appear at the same time; for example, a child with diarrhoea, who at the same time, has a nose bleed; and coldness with numbness of heels; or diarrhoea with overpowering sleepiness; involuntary urination while coughing etc.

There has been quite a controversy regarding concomitants or associated symptoms. Do these words mean the same thing ? In a broader context, it means only those symptoms which happen to accompany other main symptoms or complaints of patient. Boenninghausen's concept in utilising this class of symptoms was again wedded to this theory of generalisations and analogy and should be interpreted according to his philosophy and construction of his Repertory (Therapeutic Pocket Book). According to him, even aggravation or presence of certain complaints and symptoms, say, before menses, could be considered associated or concomitant symptoms, and are valuable for Repertorial analysis.

Boenninghausen kept a separate general rubric of concomitants wherever relevant; where the concomitant remedies were given in relation to particular locational symptoms or local functions, because he found that it was not possible to write individually all the concomitant symptoms in relation to that particular area. For example, a patient is having cough and while coughing he has got involuntary urination or vertigo or pain in the back. Now Bryonia and Causticum should be mentioned as one of the remedies in the group of concomitants under rubric of cough i.e. remedies associated with certain symptoms attendant on cough.

Let us study, for example, the concomitants or associated symptoms with cough. This is reflected in Boenninghausen or in Boger, after the main rubric 'cough'. In this rubric- troubles associated with cough- we find most important remedies which have largest and more characteristic symptoms of concomitants with cough are -

1) Bell.
2) Bry.
3) Caps.
4) Dros.
5) Ip.
6) Merc.

7) Nux-v.
8) Phos.
9) Puls.
10) Rhus-t.
11) Sep.
12) Spong.
13) Stann.

Let us take **Bryonia** for example. We find cough with gagging, with crawling and tickling in the pit of the stomach, vomiting of food while coughing, pain and bruised feeling in abdomen in hypochondriac region, bursting pain in the head, stitches in head, stitching pain in throat and chest, sides and epigastrium, sore pain in epigastrium, lachrymation, tooth pain, and cough with involuntary discharge of urine. You can see that it has got quite a number of symptoms which are associated with cough. Other cough remedies may not produce these associated symptoms. Therefore, Bryonia is considered to be one of the uppermost remedies which have concomitants to cough. Each prominent or important remedy has got its own peculiar association. That is where the differentiations exist.

Let us then take **Causticum**. In relation to this very rubric on concomitants, we find concomitants are less in number, less frequent, compared to those of Bryonia. This also has got involuntary urination when associated with cough. But elsewhere, we find intensity of concomitants is not as marked as in the case of Bryonia.

Let us get hold of another example. As a concomitant remedy with associated symptoms with cough. **Phosphorous** is again one of the most important remedies. Examples given below indicate its activity.

1) Cough with pain in head.
2) Cough causing soreness in the forepart of chest
3) Cough with tightness across chest.
4) Cough with trembling of the whole body.

5) Cough with stitching pain in epigastrium.
6) Cough with aphonia or hoarseness.
7) Cough with soreness and roughness in larynx.
8) Cough causing pain like smartness in throat.
9) Cough causing pain in root of tongue.
10) Cough causing constant pain in centre of lower chest, with sensation of weight there, and difficulty in taking a long and deep breath.
11) Cough with intolerable pain in larynx.
12) Cough with involuntary stool while coughing.
13) Cough with pain in sacrum as if broken.
14) Cough with pain in sacrum and trembling all over the body.
15) Cough with faintness.

Comparing with even Bryonia, we find it has larger number and more peculiar associated symptoms.

In contrast to these two remedies, if we take **Cantharis** for its value in the rubric on associated symptoms, it is the lowest.

For example
1) During cough, pain in abdomen.
2) During cough, erection.

Similarly, in the case of **Cannabis-sativa** there is only cough with blood spilling and stitches in right side.

Similarly, association of cough causing pain in inflamed knee joint, is a valuable concomitant and leads to remedies like Causticum, but cough causing pain in chest is more or less a common concomitant and does not lead to a specific remedy, but may only point to a large number of remedies.

Similarly, Boenninghausen has given a list of drugs as concomitants of mental symptoms. It might mean that the mental conditions are accompanied by other symptoms which apparently have no relationship with the main(mental symptoms). They are irrational intruders, and in this rubric they are more often found with drugs listed here.

Sometimes, these concomitants could be explained on the basis of pathology or physiology, but their importance increases only when they are removed far away from existing pathology or patho-physiology. In human beings, a disease appears in such different variations and combinations. We have to be ready to match these flexibilities or variations in the manifestation of the disease with similar capacity for flexibility and adaptation from amongst remedies.

Some of these so called concomitants or associated symptoms may not be valuable if they happen to be commonly associated with the main symptoms or complaint or are usually resultant of the same.

Such examples are numerous and only denote the diagnostic of disease and its pathology. For example, palpitation and vertigo with extreme pallor of face in a case of severe anaemia; or loss of appetite in the beginning of a case of acute viral hepatitis, are the associated symptoms of the main complaint or symptom like pain in abdomen and deep yellow urine. But consider the case of a lady who develops mastitis after childbirth, with fever, redness and swelling of breast and yet complains of no pain. This concomitant of painlessness of the usually painful condition of the inflamed breast, made us prescribe Stramonium, which brought about a very speedy recovery. Such associated or concomitants are of the utmost value. The concomitant of real value for remedy-diagnosis should have the following qualifications-

(1) It should not be indicative of any disease-diagnosis.
(2) It should be an unexpected stranger or intruder.
(3) We are not able to explain its existence.
(4) It should be a very uncommon and peculiar accompaniment of the main symptom.

Rarer and more bizarre the relationship of the attendant to the main symptom, the greater is its value for remedy diagnosis. If these are the unexpected intruders and their presence cannot be explained, then they are upgraded to Hahnemann's Rare, Strange and Peculiar symptoms.

It is the striking nature of the systemic effect that determines the value of a given symptom; a manifestation that is prone to occur without any obvious connection with the disease itself. In chronic cases, it is very apt to be a concomitant, while in acute ones, it often stands out like a freshly painted guide post. Such symptoms are utilised most profitably by using the Kentian method of Repertorisation.

Even in Kent's Repertory, many of interesting concomitants could not be entered, because of problems of space, and partly because many symptoms had to be broken for listing them in the Repertory. This process of division of the symptoms has cost us lot of valuable concomitants. Let us take the example of a patient who complained of pain in the arm, but with this pain, there was a sense of heaviness associated. There is no such rubric like 'Pain with heaviness in arm'. Cocculus-indicus has this symptom.

But we must, here, again emphasise that Boenninghausen had generalised all concomitant or associated symptoms, and the above mentioned qualification or distinction does not exist. According to his philosophy and structure of his Repertory, he emphasised that certain remedies have greater tendency for having associated symptoms in certain specified areas of function or location.

In a case of Rheumatoid arthritis, there were usual common symptoms of pain, swelling of the joints and stiffness worse in the morning on beginning to move, but another unexplained intruder was nausea which appeared whenever she had severe attack of these pains. The remedy which was curative in her case was Ipecac. We had hardly used this remedy earlier in arthritis of any kind. This strange combination of the associated symptom led us to the remedy.

Inflammation of tonsils just before menses, is again an example of strange association, and tonsillitis here is the valuable concomitant

One can cite innumerable examples of such concomitants, which have given us the clue to the right remedy. In actual practice, we have also come across peculiar concomitants for which no remedy has yet been known.

As a group, the concomitants contain many anomalous and peculiar symptoms. They are often so distinctive of a remedy, as to render the name of the disease, under which a peculiar symptom may occur, of little importance. Nevertheless, the modalities, mental concomitants and duration of an unusual symptom, govern its position. Where they go to make up a harmonious picture, it becomes a true characteristic; others only of negative value.

Sometimes the affected organ seems overwhelmed by the impact of disease, and the vital power can find expression through the concomitants only; there they become of supreme importance, as the almost sole guide for the selection of the remedy.

We often talk about the strange, rare and peculiar symptoms as a very important guide in the selection of the remedy, as even confirmed by Dr. Hahnemann, but actually, these rare and strange symptoms are indeed concomitants of the highest value. These are the symptoms which we are not in a position to explain on the pathology or in relation to the chief complaint of the patient, but they occur at the same time as the chief complaint.

A concomitant becomes all the more important if it is modified in the same way as the main symptom of the patient.

When a concomitant is a mental symptom in relation to usual complaint, i.e. the physical complaint of the patient, that also becomes very important. Of course, we cannot always explain the relationship of that mental symptom. For example, there was a patient who was normally very pleasant and calm, but during any fever with high temperature, he became very anxious and worried about the future and the other things. We could not explain this particular relationship, but then his anxiety during fever becomes a very important part of the symptom picture and is a great valuable concomitant.

Similarly, in a case of colitis, with mucus diarrhoea, a patient's transient feeling of anxiety and depression on waking in the mornings every day, becomes an important mental concomitant, and could lead us to the solution of the intractable colitis which is otherwise so difficult to cure. These mental attendants or associated symptoms become a very important guide to the indicated remedy. Dr. Roberts, in his Introduction to the Therapeutic Book, wrote that "the concomitant symptom is to the totality, what the condition of aggravation or amelioration is to the single symptom; it is the differentiating factor."

Both modalities and the concomitant symptoms are usually individual reactions of the patient and rarely diagnostic of disease.

For the working of the Boenninghausen's Repertory, the above classification is good enough to start the analysis.

Apart from Boenninghausen's classification of symptoms, we require more detailed distinctions when we have to work with Kentian mode of Repertorisation. Before we ear mark the relevant symptoms, we have to be very careful in assessing the symptoms given by the patient. Certain patients, especially ladies come again and again with a list of symptoms. They start with recitation of complaints which may be a recitation of the same or different symptoms each time. How do we evaluate them?

Is it loquacity?
Is it unsatisfied love?
Is it desire for sympathy?
Is it due to unhappy home?
Is it due to a domineering mother-in-law?

Symptoms and their evaluation

1. Uncommon and Common symptoms

Hahnemann tells us, "the symptoms which determine the choice of the remedy are mostly peculiar to that remedy, and of marked similitude to those of the disease".

In the section 153 of the Organon, Hahnemann has said, "In this search for a Homoeopathic specific remedy, that is to say in this comparison of the collective symptoms of the natural disease with the list of symptoms of known medicines, in order to find amongst these an artificial morbific agent, corresponding by similarity to the disease to be cured, the more striking, singular, uncommon and peculiar (characteristic) signs and symptoms of the case of the disease are chiefly and almost solely to be kept in view, for it is more these, that very similar ones in the list of symptoms of the selected medicines must correspond to; in order to constitute it the most suitable for effecting the cure."

In general, we may deduce that the symptomatic similarity has four Characteristics-

1. Striking i.e. surpassing; forcible; impressive, very noticeable; a prominent feature.
2. Singular i.e. out of the ordinary unusual; exceptional.
3. Uncommon i.e. not common, infrequent in such a case; not common to such a disease.
4. Peculiar i.e. belonging solely or especially to an individual; of private, personal or characteristic possession; not possessed in common but usually present

in the diseased condition; belonging to the patient as distinct from other patients with the same sickness; the individuality of the patient in the case.

From the above, it is quite clear that there are two groups of symptoms. Some belong to a particular individual and are not commonly found in others suffering from the same sickness. It is these symptoms which are important for the selection; others are practically useless. Hence, we call them 'uncommon' and 'common' symptoms. The common symptoms in a patient usually belong to the disease and common symptoms in a remedy are those which are found in the provings of many remedies.

The common symptoms help us the least in our selection of the drug, since they are the usual common part of disease or drugs. They will be present more or less in all patients of the same disease. The diagnostic symptoms or pathognomic symptoms are all common symptoms. They relate to the disease and its usual symptoms and not to the individual reactions of the patient.

Common symptoms are found in many patients, in many ailments and in many provings. For example, thirst in fever, pains in Influenza; flatulence, cough, inflammation, eruptions in eruptive fevers etc.

Sir Arthur Conan Doyle's character, Sherlock Holmes said that what is unusual or out of the ordinary, should always attract our attention. This applies to the hunt for the indicated remedy.

As a first preparation for dealing with diseases, the first essential is familiarity with their natural expression when their course has no interference. Each disease is characterised by special symptoms, by which it may be recognised, but in various human beings, these characteristics of the disease appear in a variety of forms. No individual is capable of exhibiting entirely all the symptoms of a disease; it is only a fragment of the whole; the full nature being portrayed by a large number. This individual fragment is yet, a sufficient part of the whole to present its nature. Many symptoms are so common to the disturbances of vital force that they are characteristic of nothing, e.g. Headache, skin eruptions, sweat, fever etc., but peculiar forms of the above complaints or modification of the same or peculiar grouping or combination of the same, makes them more out of the ordinary i.e. characteristic.

A symptom may seem to be infrequent, uncommon, definite and precise, but if it be a recognised symptom in a known disease, its value falls, so long as, at least, its intensity or order of its appearance is consonant with what we have known of the disease. The body has its normal orderliness, in disease as in health. The variability of such a symptom gives it a value, and its absence may be of peculiar importance. Likewise, a symptom - no matter what grade, when fully explained and accounted for, almost becomes useless.

Differences, not correspondences

Again, "Each medicine differs in its effect from all others." And here, remember that- <u>It is the difference and not the correspondences that concern us.</u> Hosts of symptoms may be common to a great number of drugs, and if you give equal prominence to these, you will find it impossible to make a selection. While, as regards indefinite symptoms, "Loss of appetite, loss of sleep, weakness etc., unless qualified, are useless in determining the remedy, because of being common to most drugs and almost every disease."

Characteristic features of a symptom

Hahnemann lays it down that, "In comparing the disease symptoms with lists of symptoms of proved drugs, the more prominent and peculiar (characteristic) features of the case are especially and almost exclusively to be taken. These should bear the closest similitude to the symptoms of the desired medicine, if that is to cure." Homoeopathy is absolutely inconceivable without the most precise individualisation.

In order to minimize labour, as well as to arrive at a more definite result, Kent has said- "When looking over a list of symptoms, first discover 3, 4, 5 or 6 or as many symptoms as exist that are strange, rare and peculiar: Strange, rare and peculiar must apply to the patient himself. When you have settled on 3 or 4 remedies that have these characteristic symptoms, then find which of them is most like the patient's symptoms, common and particular. Mentals are all important. The state of the patient's mind and temperament is often of the most decisive importance in the selection of the remedy.

When you have taken a case on paper, you will settle the symptoms that cannot be omitted in each individual. Get the strong, strange, peculiar symptoms, and then see to it that there are no generals in the case that oppose or contradict."

He further instances: "If you see the keynotes of Arsenicum, make sure that the patient is chilly, fearful, restless, weak, pale, must have the pictures on the wall straight, and Ars. will cure.

In order to get your key-symptoms easily, before starting work on a case, it is well to have a red pencil, and, again going through it, underline the 'strange, rare and peculiar' (i.e. the characteristic) symptoms of the case."

In the Kentian approach to the general evaluation of symptoms and working of the cases, one has to keep in mind both the scientific as well as the artistic analysis in case of repertorisation of symptoms.

As Homoeopathy includes both science and art, Repertory study must consist of science and art.

The scientific method is the mechanical method; taking all the symptoms and writing out all the associated remedies with gradings, making a summary with grades marked at the end.

There is an artistic method that omits the mechanical, and is better, but all are not prepared or competent to use it. The artistic method demands that judgement be passed on all the symptoms, after the case is most carefully taken. The symptoms must be judged as to their value as characteristics, in relation to the patient; they must be passed in review by the rational mind to determine those which are strange, rare, and peculiar.

In any case, one does not have to go through the elaborate process of repertorisation of fifteen rubrics or so, as in some of the cases, the cardinal or deciding symptoms of the case unlock this mystery of the indicated remedy. That is why, very careful case-taking and then proper evaluation of the symptoms and signs present is a must. It may seem paradoxical to advise the beginner that the proper case-taking and evaluation of the symptoms requires a fairly deep knowledge of Homoeopathic Repertory and, of course, the Homoeopathic Philosophy.

Symptoms most peculiar to the patient must be taken first, then those less and less peculiar, until the symptoms that are common and not peculiar are reached, in order from first to last

These must be valued in proportion, as they relate to the patient rather than to his parts, and used instead of ultimates and symptoms **pathognomic**.

The artistic prescriber sees much in the proving that cannot be retained in the Repertory, where anything must be sacrificed for the alphabetical system. The artistic prescriber must study Materia Medica long and earnestly, to enable him to fix in his mind 'sick images', which, when needed, will fit in the sick personalities of human beings. These are too numerous and too various to be named or classified. I have often known the intuitive prescriber to attempt to explain a so-called marvelous cure by saying: "I cannot quite say how I came to give that remedy but it resembled him."

We have heard this, and felt it, and seen it, but who can attempt to explain it? It is something that belongs not to the neophyte, but comes gradually to the experienced artistic prescriber. It is only the growth of art in the artistic mind; what is noticed in all artists. It belongs to all healing artists, but if carried too far, it becomes a fatal mistake, and must, therefore, be corrected by Repertory-work done in even the most mechanical manner.

The more each one restrains the tendency to carelessness in prescribing and in method, the wiser he becomes in artistic effects and Materia Medica work. The two features of prescribing must go hand in hand, and must be kept in a high degree of balance, otherwise, loose methods and habits will come upon any good worker.

Preference must be accorded to discharges from ulcers, from uterus during menstruation, from ears, and from other parts, as those are very closely related to the vital operation of the economy.

Next must be used the modalities of the parts affected, and frequently, these will be found to be the very opposite of the modalities of the patient himself. A patient who craves heat for himself, generally and for his body, may require cold to his head, to his stomach, or to the inflamed parts, hence, the same rubric will not fit him and his parts. Hence, to generalise by modalities of isolated particulars, leads to the incorrect remedy or confounds values placed upon certain remedies.

There are strange and rare symptoms even in parts of

the body, which the experienced physician learns are so guiding that they must be ranked in the higher and even in top class.

These include some keynotes which may safely guide to a remedy or to the shaping of results, provided that the mental and the physical generals do not stand contrary, as to their modalities, and therefore, oppose the keynote-symptoms.

Any remedy correctly worked out, when looked up in the Materia Medica, should be perceived to agree with, and to fit the patient; his symptoms; his parts; and his modalities. It is quite possible for a remedy not having the highest marking in the anamnesis, to be the most similar in image, as seen in the Materia Medica.

In the interrogation and evaluation of symptoms, domestic environment, personal life situations and the patient's individual reactions to such situation, are important and often indicate the individualising symptoms. Sometimes 'trivial things' or lesser symptoms' brought out in such interrogations or narrations by the patient are important from point of view of remedy-diagnosis.

One has to keep in mind that simple people express their complaints differently from the so called sophisticated patients. Hysterical patients will exaggerate or give free rein to their imaginations when narrating their story, some patients colour their symptoms; others misguide us because of exaggerated sense of modesty.

The Individualising Symptoms

An individualising symptom is one belonging to the patient rather than to the pathology involving a local part or the disease; the unmodified, unrestrained expression of the inner self of the patient; therefore, symptoms during unconsciousness are of great value, as in sleep; in delirium or when entirely alone, in infancy or early childhood when modesty, decorum, fashion or etiquette - all inhibitions have no restraining or perverting influence upon the patient's natural self. All such symptoms rank high. Earlier evidence of disease is to be largely subjective; it must necessarily have a decidedly personal bias, as already emphasised that Individuality hides itself more and more as the sickness advances and becomes more objective. The more firmly disease is established, the more objective are its manifestations; hence, ultimately there are grosser expressions of disease and that too in the 'parts' of the body.

General and Local Symptoms

Having defined the common and uncommon symptoms and their place in the remedy selection, we come to symptoms which are related to the patient as a whole, and those concerning only the parts of the body. The former symptoms are called 'Generals'.

General symptoms are those symptoms which are predicated of the patient, the symptoms which involve the patient as a whole or modify almost all parts of organism. Since the 'general' involves the whole organism, the particulars or local symptoms are, may be, only a part or aspect of the General symptoms. Actually, the general symptoms are often derived from the total sum of the particulars. The General will relate to the 'I' or 'Ego' of the patient. They indicate also things like sensitiveness to heat or cold, to storm, to rest or motion, to night or day or to time. They include general sensations or symptoms and modalities effecting the body as a whole. But 'General' symptoms in this context do not mean 'Common' symptoms; of course the 'General' symptoms can be common. For example, 'weakness during fever' is a general predicative of the whole patient, but it is so common and present in almost all the febrile states that it has no value for the prescriber. Unless we make these distinctions, we shall be lost in the maze of symptoms. Similar things are found in the provings also.

Against the symptoms of the patient as a whole, are

the symptoms which affect his parts only. They are called 'Particulars' by Kent. This is an unfortunate term as 'Particulars' may indicate something special. The local' symptom is a more appropriate term. Since 'Particular' is already in vogue, we shall continue to use this term.

It has been verified again and again that the 'Generals' are more important than 'Particulars' or Local; and uncommon Generals and uncommon Particulars are more important for selection than common Generals and Common Particulars.

Characteristic Particulars

Such unusual or characteristic particular or local symptoms acquire the status of Hahnemann's rare and strange symptoms when they are present in certain complaints but cannot be rationally explained. They may be present in only one or very few remedies. It may be a peculiar modality, or it is present as a concomitant, or it may be related to a particular causation. A clinician related a case that he had treated of a man aged 50 who had severe heart pain for more than three years and was unable to walk even a few yards and he had to sit down every few steps. He had been extensively treated. He was advised to take Cactus and Cratagus Q. But these medicines did not give him any relief. He found one unusual modality that his heart pain was relieved by the pressure of the hand. In the Kent's Repertory, only Nat-m. is given. This medicine was given in 1M potency, after which the patient reported great relief.

The particular or local symptoms become important when they cannot be explained, and may be an important pointer to the indicated remedy, provided the generals agree.

We do not usually find the prominent peculiar or uncommon in a particular. "Let us consider peritonitis; Arsenicum and Secale are seemingly indicated. How to distinguish? Both have violently distended abdomen, tympanitis, extreme sensitiveness to touch; motion or jar unbearable; the pains are likened to burning coals of fire; tongue dry with great thirst; vomiting of blood; running pulse. Both the medicines agree beautifully in their particulars, and hence, no distinction. On looking further, we find that the patient wants to be covered, kept warm even in the hottest of weather; wants warm drinks. These distinguish him from Secale who wants to be uncovered; wants cool open air and cold water to drink and is aggravated by heat and the warm room."

Here again, we may emphasise that the presence of a striking symptom unusual to the disease would constitute a peculiarity which relates to the patient - not to the disease.

Subjective and Objective symptoms

The subjective symptoms are known to the patient alone, of which the physician can take no cognizance, nor from any estimate, except as they are detailed to him by the patient as aberrations of mind and the sensual sensations; sense of pain, weight, lightness, fullness, emptiness etc.

The objective symptoms are those which are apparent to the clinician and of which the patient may or may not be conscious, such as appearance of tongue, eyes, skin, his gait and mannerisms, speech, proptosis, glandular enlargement, odour of the patient, warts etc. On the mental side, there are loquacity, diffidence, easy embarrassment, timidity, fearfulness, anxiety, tearfulness, suspiciousness, egotism, excitability, impatience, haughtiness, depression etc. Mind mirrors itself with great accuracy in the different modes and manners of physical expression. An intonation of voice may sometimes explain the source and meaning of a particular symptom; so intricate are the mental processes. The entrance of Platina patient always singles her out. The clinging affectionate Phos. child loves to sit in your lap the moment you call him; the Pulsatilla female bursts into tears the moment she starts her story of complaints. The fidgety hands of the Phosphorus patient and the fidgety feet of the Zincum patient are again objective pointers to the observing physician. Numerous examples could be cited where objective symptoms could be a most reliable help.

A patient may not be intelligent enough to express properly the innermost feelings; or a patient is a hysteric; too imaginative and exaggerates all his complaints. On the other hand, a patient may be so reticent as not to talk about his complaints.

But the objective symptoms, as observed by the physician and the attendants (though, often ranked as less valuable, especially, when expressed grossly in the tissues and parts), being exempt from self interpretation and allowing the largest scope for the acumen of the examiner, are withal the least deceptive. They should receive our first and best attention. They teach lessons not to be learnt elsewhere, and by their great utility have contributed much to the brilliant success of homoeopathy, particularly in the diseases of children.

The Place of Pathological symptoms

The pathological symptoms are those which pertain to the results of disease; end-products of disease. The objective symptoms of this class are usually not taken into Repertorial analysis because-

(1) they represent the ultimates of disease;
(2) they find expression in the local parts;
(3) they overwhelm the economy and refuse to let the organism give out finer symptoms for the selection of the remedy;
(4) they divert the attention of the examiner from more vital symptoms;
(5) few drugs have been pushed far enough in the proving to elicit such symptoms;
(6) we have as yet, no means of individualising these pathological changes in the living human beings.

There are, however, certain (objective) pathological changes which can be used for the purpose of selection. Dr. Boger stresses the value of pathological generals as opposed to the diagnostic pathology. He feels that these are the pathological conditions which become characteristic of the patient and affect him in many parts. For example, warts, naevi, keloids, polypi, fibroid tumours, corns etc., tend to show the constitutional tendency and are, therefore, valuable generals.

Dr. Stearns endorsed this view and was convinced that such objective symptoms are reliable as they cannot lie. He chose not more than five or six symptoms for analysis, of which one was a mental, one pathological, one objective and two physical generals. Boger laid more emphasis on general states and mental symptoms.

The place of Mental Symptoms

"The moral state and mental condition of the patient often determine the choice of the Homoeopathic remedy" (Organon). Mental symptoms, almost always, define a case absolutely when the doctor exercises the art and patience to extract them from a carefully taken case-history and to understand them.

Mental symptoms, though important when well marked, are at times difficult to understand or difficult to elicit from the patient. One has to refer to different Repertories often, and then interpret properly what the patient really means when he talks about his complaints. 'Fear of being alone', 'Fear of dark' and 'Fear of being alone at night' may have to be interpreted properly. In a young child or even in an adult, it may be really a fear of ghosts or robbers etc. and other relevant rubrics have to be taken into consideration. Similarly, the rubric 'Occupation ameliorates' may actually be 'thinking of complaints aggravate', and it may be desirable to combine these two when we resort to the process of elimination of not indicated remedies. To use a mental as an eliminative symptom, one has to be very careful and very definite about that particular mental symptom. Similarly, rubrics 'Fear of dark', 'Fear of darkness at night' may actually indicate 'Fear of ghosts'. We may have to combine all of them. One can see, how much careful and discerning we have to be, in assessing and evaluating the mentals.

Kent gave very definite guidelines regarding the mental symptoms. If the patient exhibits some noteworthy mental symptoms, they are to be taken in the following order-

First are those relating to the loves and hates, or desires and aversions. Next are those belonging to the rational mind, so-called intellectual mind. Thirdly, those belonging to the memory.

These, the mental symptoms, must first be worked out by the usual form, until the remedies best suited to his mental condition are determined, omitting all symptoms that relate to a pathological cause, and all that are common to disease and to people. When the sum of these has been settled, a group of five or ten remedies, or as many as appear, we are then prepared to compare them and the remedies found related to the remaining symptoms of the case.

Boenninghausen gave a very small place to mentals with a certain justification. He was of the opinion that in actual practice, it is difficult to extract reliable mentals. Very often, the psychic state has to be ignored, as it is only a mask for the true mental symptoms, which are exhibited only through the physical expressions. Boenninghausen did not under-rate the mentals but he felt that it was not practical politics. He, therefore, did not give the priority to the mentals which Kent later did. For Kent, it is the mental symptoms around which other symptoms revolve, because mentals express the inner-most of the man, and hence, the most characteristic of a sick individual. The mind is a subjective as well as an objective index which reveals the bias and rules the whole case.

Mental symptoms are truly 'generals' of the patient, but can be common as well as characteristic (uncommon). It is not always that mentals are given precedence because in certain mental diseases, the apparently characteristic mental symptoms are merely common symptoms of the disease. Here other physical generals are much more important The mental symptoms in the hysteric are not usually reliable.

Usually, earliest mental manifestations are decidedly the most important of all the symptoms. If we have the acumen to detect this very early, we will discover that the later mental phenomena are simply variations and that either will lead to the same remedy, which will, however, be found with increasing difficulty as the case progresses.

The mental symptoms pertaining to the will and emotions are more important than those concerning our intellect. Actually some physical generals may be more important from the point of view of remedy-selection than symptoms of intellect like forgetfulness, poor memory etc.

The Causations and 'its value'

Well marked causations, especially at the emotional level, may be considered equal in value to the mental symptoms. The Causation has a distinctive factor in the history of the patient and sometimes over-rules or dominates every other symptom. Sometimes, that may be our only thing to guide us and the remedy which is needed by the patient at that particular time. This is especially so when the patient says that he has never been well since a particular complaint or event like grief, fright, trauma or vaccination etc. Especially after an emotional trauma, grief, mental shock, disappointed love etc., we may have a train of symptoms both mental and physical which by themselves do not give any clue. These secondary symptoms lead us away from the remedy, as the patient emphasises only these symptoms. This is the psychosomatic expression. Similarly attacks of asthma ever since the acute infection of whooping cough, or chronic dyspepsia ever since excessive loss of blood, years ago, are striking examples. The 'causative' symptoms must be the pivotal symptoms. Similarly, a history of physical trauma may spark off a series of symptoms and here 'injury' becomes more important than the other symptoms. Very often, however, in our Repertorial analysis we tend to ignore its importance.

Any event or circumstance, which contribute to the onset of the present diseased condition, must be taken note of. Sometimes, the patient has forgotten or considers it to be of no importance. We have seen how Arnica unlocked the case, where there was an onset of disease since a physical trauma due to an accident. Boger mentioned that so much depended upon the knowledge of die causation of disease, that without it, the choice of the homoeopathic remedy cannot be made with safety.

A lady complained of severe pain in the sterno-cleidomastoid muscles of both sides; constant pain all the time, and had no sleep. She complained of fear of cancer and a host of other things. Any amount of repertorisation brought us to no results, until one day it was discovered that all the complaints dated from the mental shock that she received when her husband suddenly had to leave his house and property worth millions in Afghanistan and flee to India, and thus became virtually a pauper. The lady who was such a gay and carefree person, had now become abnormally sensitive, an extremely nervous person; always afraid of something.

We are reminded of another true story, when a prominent physician of the town complained that he had been having problem with his prostrate gland, as he had to go for urination very frequently, but passed very small quantities at a time. The frequent urge was very annoying. Detailed examinations had not revealed any cause or pathology. On deeper interrogation, it was discovered that this problem started six months ago, when he had gone out with friends on a hunting spree and travelled a great distance in the hot sun in search of his prey. He felt sudden urge for urination but was able to pass only a very small quantity of urine. He was suddenly alarmed and developed a fear that he had enlarged prostate gland.

On the basis of this discovery that the present train of symptoms were precipitated by the sudden fright, a dose of Aconite in high potency was administered. The results confirmed the Hahnemannian principle and he was free from this annoying complaint within a very short period.

Here is another case history, narrated by an experienced prescriber Dr. Ledermann, which testifies to the importance of causation in a case analysis.

'There is a case of a young boy, aged 12 years, who was brought to me. His visual acuity had diminished considerably during the preceding 4 years. The case was brought in September 1964. He stumbled on pavements, bumped himself on doors and had already several times been knocked down by cars. The child was passive, smiling vacantly all the time. He did not seem to understand what was said to him, and appeared to be very absent minded. The rough ophthalmologic examination showed bilateral concentric shrinking of the visual fields. In short, he behaved like a horse with closely applied blinkers.

The report of the ophthalmologist was that there was no functional sign of raised intra-cranial pressure. There was no headache or no vomiting. There was normal retinal arterial pressure and there is concentric narrowing of the visual fields on both sides. This could be accounted for by a deep lesion at the level of the optic chiasma.

This has been developing for over 4 years but without diminution of visual acuity; this does not suggest compression. During digital estimation of the visual fields, the child behaved as if he was blind which he is not. The picture is unlikely to be that of an authentic organic condition and one must suggest a neurotic complaint. Nevertheless to be on the safe side, an x-ray of the skull and sella-turcica was done and it was found to be negative. There was x-ray of the para-nasal sinuses which showed there was diminished translucency of the right maxillary sinus. Thus we have to deal with a non-organic case which had nevertheless a factor which could be objectively measured. That is, concentric narrowing of the visual fields in a simple young boy of 12 years.

On deeper interrogation of the parents, we came to know that this child came from Algeria, and his visual disturbances dated from the time when a bomb had exploded in the courtyard of his school. The family had noticed that there was something wrong about 20 days after the explosion, and his mother stated that after that, her son lost consciousness every time he heard an explosive sound.

Because of this traumatic experience, the boy, it seems, did not want to hear things, nor did he want to see things. He blocked his ears, blocked his eyes, to avoid the memory of this frightful experience. He seems to have turned his back on the external world and all its horrors. He used to be upset whenever he heard rifle shots close to his house where they were practicing shooting.

This was a case which required to be repertorised. The only remedies for the totality of the major symptoms in this case are complaints from fright and Aconite and Opium are the remedies which are most prominent for situations following frightful experiences. It may be mentioned here that Boenninghausen in his drug relationship has classified Opium as a remedy suitable for following Aconite. Although Aconite seems to be the first choice, as the remedy in this case. We considered the following symptoms, rubrics in Kent's Repertory which were:

1) complaints which follow a fright;
2) circumstances following wounds or psychic trauma;
3) absent-mindedness;
4) loss of vision.

Now the eliminating symptom 'complaints which follow a fright' have got 9 remedies in capitals, 8 in italics and 8 in small type- altogether 25 remedies.

Now the question is whether we give Aconite or Opium. You cannot give both remedies together. We have to see which one to select. He was given Aconite 30 ch. to be taken every eight hours for 24 hours, no other treatment for one month. At the end of 30 days, he was brought to the clinic and he was smiling and happy. There was, according to the Eye Surgeon, considerable improvement in the field of vision and his attitude of indifference and distraction had also gone."

I am reminded of a very interesting incident when I came across a middle aged and married patient who complained of very frequent night emissions, although he was having a normal sexual life. He had been treated for months by a very eminent teacher and colleague of mine, but without any result. On examining the patient, I found that he had excessive deposit of smegma and he did not clean it properly. On following my advice that he should clean it daily with soap and water, he found that he did not suffer any more from the night emissions and did not require any remedy.

In another interesting case, a gentleman complained of painful swelling of the left big toe, and told us that he was feeling miserable because he could not play golf. He was a very sensitive person and suffered very much from insomnia. His grandfather was one of the most prominent homoeopathic physician and was one of the pioneers of Homoeopathy in Calcutta. He presented a perfect picture of Coffea crudum and was prescribed a dose of Coffea 200 for his painful gouty swelling. He was able to play golf for about a fortnight but then appeared again with this complaint. I repeated the medicine in 1M potency, and he remained without trouble for about 15 days, but like a bad coin, he returned again with the same complaint.

This gentleman came from a place where people take lot of tea, but on further inquiry, he told us that he was taking 15 or more cups of coffee in a day. We asked him not to take coffee, and he was again given a dose of Coffea crudum. His complaint never surfaced again. Of course, it was a mistake on my part, not to have inquired in detail in the first interview, but the moral of the story is that such causation can lead us straightway to the indicated remedy. Coffea was actually producing a typical pathogenesis of its proving and he became a calmer person and had a more peaceful sleep.

The etiological factor, gross or subtle, may serve to differentiate one case from another, though they appear to be similar in other respects. A patient who develops a stroke after a long period of loss of sleep, may need a different remedy from another with the same condition but with history of suppressed anger. The pathology may be the same, diagnosis or nosological label may be the same, but the etiology(causation) may make all the difference to a homoeopathic drug diagnosis. Most fortunately, we have in our armamentarium, a variety of drugs, which cover a variety of such etiological factors.

Tubercular miasm in the family history, is one of the most frequent causative factor in the sufferings of some people. Such miasmatic background has to be kept in mind. One could cite numerous cases where 'causation' dominated in the selection of the remedy.

In the Kent's Repertory, we should really mark out the symptoms which follow certain suddenly depressed emotional or physical functions or symptoms.

In the Synthetic Repertory, the authors have given all these symptoms at one place under the heading 'AILMENTS from' in the chapter on Mind.

Now under the 'Mind', I am listing below important mental and emotional factors of causation, which have to be kept before us, whenever we see any relevant case.

1) ailments after **anger,** vexation;
2) ailments from **egotism;**
3) ailments after **embarrassment;**
4) ailments from **fright;**
5) ailments from **grief;**
6) ailments from **home-sickness;**
7) ailments following **indignation;**
8) ailments from excessive **joy;**
9) ailments from disappointment in **love;**
10) ailments from **mortification;**
11) ailments from **rudeness.**

Of course, in the generalities, you find- convulsions after anger; convulsion from fright; emaciation after grief; twitching after fright etc. Dr. Robert, once said, "let us now consider the external factors which suppress the normal function of the vital force and thus the normal functions of the body. Such conditions as fear, excessive joy, unsatisfied sexual desire, un-requited love, grief at loss of a dear one, social worries, frustrated ambition, excessive fatigue- all these factors have influenced vital energy and suppress its normal functioning and then a group of symptoms appear, which may vary very much in their manifestations, and which may result in a modification of the normal expression of vital force. We have even seen such cases in which pent-up emotions affecting not one individual but succeeding generations through the medium of the nursing mother.

We have found that psychological emotional stresses can bring down a patient's tolerance thresh-hold. They become more sensitive to allergic conditions than otherwise. Dr. Charcot noticed that whenever he went into a stable, when he was annoyed, he developed asthma. If he did so, in the normal state of mind, he did not have an attack.

So in these cases also, one has to find out the causative condition or factor, because by trying to repertorise the other symptoms, we may not get the right remedy. But when we are able to spot out the causation, a definite clear-cut one (causation), we have to tackle that aspect of it, and here in such cases both the remedy as well as counselling, or psycho-therapeutic aids will bring about relief and cure, as medicine alone may not do the trick.

There are many cases of dermatosis in which causative factors play more or less an important role. For example, urticaria, psoriasis, atopic dermatitis, nummular eczema, lichen planus, alopecia areata, a most commonly localised, generalised pruritus. The essential psycho factors in these patients seem to be emotional instability, stress, tension and anxiety and frustration. In these cases, these are the causative factors. But one has to understand and fish out these causative factors. Sometimes, of course, it is the other way round. A person who has dis-figuring lesion or lot of irritation, is subject to neurotic manifestations secondary to the eruptions. This is the other side of the picture."

Another case narrated by Ledermann, illustrates some of these points. Mrs. S., aged 42 years, attended the clinic in September 1965 and complained of desquamation of her feet. The minimal signs and symptoms made one wonder why she should attend the hospital with lesions which an average person would almost certainly disregard. On questioning, she admitted to being very worried about her husband who had a coronary thrombosis and now has severe attacks of angina. She had two sons, the eldest of whom was at university and she resented he fact that he frequently got into debt and expected help from them, although he knew his father was ill and they were worried about their financial state. Sometimes she brings along her younger son with some hypothetical feelings or scaling of feet. Repeated examination for fungus proved negative. She has been encouraged to talk about her problems. Remedies which were helpful to her, were Ignatia and Rhus-tox.

There are numerous examples of complaints dating from shell-shock or shock due to air-raids during the last war. All these have to be taken into consideration.

Under causation, we have to take note of aetiological factors also, like sudden exposure to cold dry winds, or getting chilled when overheated, or taking cold chilled drinks when overheated etc. Sometimes, these factors point to some definite remedy or remedies.

The Miasmatic background

Next to causation, we should consider the miasmatic background if it is definitely marked, as it is close to causation. In this connection. Tuberculosis or Tubercular miasm is very important, as this may overshadow other considerations, if its presence has been noted in the family history.

When the Common Symptoms change into Characteristics

A common general or a common local (particular) can change into a characteristic (uncommon) if:

(a) It combines with another symptom and forms a symptoms complex (concomitants of Boenninghausen).

(b) When it is modified by peculiar circumstances, for example. Eczema of 'Clematis' which is moist during the waxing moon but dries up during the waning moon. This raises the common eczema to the highest value.

(c) By the intensity of the symptom itself; for example, ordinarily 'burning' is a common symptom but if it is well-marked in the patient, its value is up-graded.

(d) Periodicity of a common symptom makes it a characteristic.

(e) Alternation of a common symptom with another symptom also raises the rank of the symptom.

(f) Absence or a lack of a common symptom which is usually expected in the circumstances, also makes it important and distinctive: for example 'thirstlessness in high fever'.

Positiveness and Intensity

Positive symptoms are more important than negative. What is present in the case matters. For example, a person loathing fats, may suggest Pulsatilla, but the fact that any patient who enjoys fat, does not rule out Pulsatilla from the consideration, should the rest of the symptoms, especially mentals, demand the remedy. Pulsatilla is usually thirstless in fever but it can still be indicated when there is thirst during heat if other symptoms call for it.

Positiveness of a symptom is indicated by the patient, by the 'spontaneity' in answering. As already mentioned, the intensity of the symptom upgrades it immediately. On interrogating, a hesitating or obliging expression on the face of the patient in relation to a symptom, takes away its value. On the other hand, if the reply is enthusiastic, it can be trusted, especially in desires and aversions. A patient may complain of dryness in the mouth; it is such a common symptom that we ignore it completely, but if this sense of dryness is very positive and constantly complained of, by the patient at every visit, it has to be taken note of, and it becomes an important particular; any modality might raise its value still further.

Hierarchy of symptoms

We are summarising below the grading of symptoms according to the value or importance for consideration for Repertorial analysis.

(1). Mental symptoms - provided they are definite and well-marked. Symptoms of emotion and will, loves and hates, aversions and cravings, indifference or abnormal affections, jealousy, suspicions, state of anxiety and mental restlessness, impatience, hurriedness in doing things, anxiety about health, future etc., irrational fears, fear of darkness, of being alone, of night etc., anxiety and fears may be followed by depressive thoughts or state, suicidal thoughts, loathing of life, weeping-abnormal or without any apparent cause, or while narrating symptoms. Depressive states may alternate with excitement. Mental and emotional excitement may follow or be incursor of somatic symptoms. It may be the result of interaction with people. Violent anger even with desire for hurting others physically. Impulse to kill others or break and destroy things.

Mental excitement may also be expressive in more pleasant way, like laughing inordinately without apparent cause. There may be abnormal loquacity. Another state of excitement may center in the sexual sphere, and the patient suffers from abnormal or perverse sexual thoughts or indulgence.

Mental irritability is a common but important mental symptom. Its importance is increased when it is modified by definite exciting or aggravating circumstances.

Symptoms of severe obsessive nature or conditions of other deeper psychosis are not as important with hierarchy of mental symptoms. Here, physical generals etc. may be more important.

The symptoms of intellect regarding memory, lack of concentration, forgetfulness are assigned, comparatively much lower positions in the mentals.

(2). Well-marked causation, especially at the emotional level- Causation may be considered equal in value to mental symptoms, by certain conditions, as has been explained already. Aetiological factors also may be considered here, for e.g. exposure to dry cold winds, getting wet, after being overheated.

Causation may originate due to physical factors, drugs, poisoning or chemicals; due to ingestion of the kind of food; mechanical cause and dynamic and psychological or emotional factors. It is, therefore, very important to have a clear idea about the onset of disease from homoeopathic point of view.

(3). Patient's reactions to physical and social surroundings- Next to the mentals and causations, we place in the hierarchy of symptoms, patients response or reaction to environmental conditions; seasons; to heat and cold; to wetness; to time, day and night; to smoke and dust; to change of position; to motion and rest. These are the physical generals which affect the patient as a whole. They have to be taken notice, if they are well-marked. These are also covered by modalities of the 'general' symptoms.

In the generalities, we consider thermal and meteorological conditions which affect the patients in their complaints in general; like wet weather; seashore; mountain air; thunderstorm; cloudy weather etc.; moon phases; metabolic conditions like eating; drinking; sweating; sleep and dreams; urination; stools; menses; environmental influences like exposure to air polluted by sulphur di-oxide Chronological and time factors and periodicity are also important for the selection purpose.

It may be mentioned here that chronology of symptoms helps us in separating the recent symptoms from the older or remote symptoms. Recent symptoms are of higher value and have to be taken first, because they are indicative of active disturbances in the body.

Remote symptoms are those which occurred in the past and only called to mind on careful inquiry. Sometimes they indicate a remedy which was possibly needed in the past, but may also cover the present picture of the patient, or it may be needed later on, when the dynamics of the movement of symptoms takes place after the current prescription.

Periodicity and recurrence of symptoms also indicate characteristics of certain remedies and may be that is happening because of some acute infection etc. which the patient suffered from, some time in the past.

Similarly, social and personal factors, like occupation, often affect the patient in certain specific ways. Of course, one has to consider the hunger and thirst, as well as sexual functions and discharges. Sometimes, odors of discharges makes the rubrics of greater importance.

Regarding pains, the intensity and character of pains, their mode of appearance and disappearance, their laterality and radiation and their modalities make them very desirable rubrics for analysis.

(4). Desires and Aversions- These reactions are followed in importance by 'Desires and Aversions'. Greater the craving for a particular item of food, the higher is the value of the symptom. Sometimes in actual practice, craving for extra salt helps us in limiting the remedies to a very small number, and may be that this rubric becomes the eliminative one. Cravings and aversions in the mental sphere are naturally much more important and should belong to Mentals in the hierarchy.

(5). Menstrual and other discharges- Later in value are symptoms connected with menstrual discharges in cases of females. The occurrence of some conditions or symptoms before, during or after menses are to be specially noted.

(6). Characteristic Particulars- Particulars and concomitants which are peculiar, unusual, unexpected or unexplainable.

(7). Local or particulars- which are strongly marked and have noticeable modalities.

(8). When common symptom changes into a characteristic one.

(9). Signs and symptoms markedly related to a particular organ or function.

(10). Miasmatic background in the family history especially to tubercular miasm. (See also causation)

(11). Pathological generals.

Varieties of names of different kinds of symptoms mentioned in our literature

In the Homoeopathic literature and especially when talking about symptoms, we come across various kinds of nomenclature of symptoms. There is a bewildering variety of about 50 kinds. I am quoting below, the various symptoms, but this list need not confuse us about the relevant symptoms which are required for working out the similimum, as we shall discuss only the symptoms which are commonly used for Repertorial analysis.

1. Objective
2. Subjective
3. Organic
4. Functional
5. Concomitants
6. Occasional
7. Characteristic
8. Uncommon; Bizarre, rare and strange
9. General
10. Common
11. Uncommon
12. Particular

13. Pathological
14. Mechanical
15. Reflex (e.g. wax in ears; spurs; errors in refraction)
16. Mental
17. Physical
18. Diagnostic
19. Determinative
20. Eliminative
21. Basic
22. Attending symptoms
23. Guiding symptoms
24. Positive symptoms
25. Negative symptoms
26. Keynote symptoms
27. Last appearing symptoms
28. Old symptoms
29. Suppressed symptoms
30. Metastatic symptoms
31. Alternating symptoms
32. Accessory symptoms and lesser accessory symptoms
33. Combination symptoms
34. Local symptoms
35. Pathogenic symptoms
36. Pathognomic symptoms
37. Direct symptoms (which bear a direct anatomical or mechanical relationship to some primary pathological or organic lesion)
38. Habit symptoms (Personal habits)
39. Ultimates
40. Pressure symptoms
41. Drug symptoms
42. Obstructive symptoms
43. Observed symptoms
44. Paradoxical symptoms
45. Changeable symptoms
46. Clinical symptoms
47. Generic or Common

48. Recurrent symptoms
49. Recrudescent symptoms
50. Reactive symptoms

Conclusion

A symptom as an expression of sickness in the human beings, is a complex entity (as complex and differentiated as the man himself), hence, with all our ingenuity in classification and evaluation, we are constantly reminded of our short-comings. One thing is certain, that basic traits of the symptom remain the same; the sensation, location, modality and concomitant differentiate a symptom; less of these elements, less of its value, and more of its common-ness. As the disease advances, these elements tend to disappear and gross pathology appears. The diagnostic and common symptoms, shaded by the general modalities, form the ground colour of the picture, from which its special features portraying the individuality emerge with more or less distinctness.

If the homoeopathic doctor succeeds in extracting from the whole symptom-picture, those outstanding characteristics which refer to the patient's reaction as a whole, and not merely to the local pain or inflammation, he will soon recognise four or five determinative or determining symptoms, mental, general or modified particulars, according to the patient under study; which will lead him to the exact diagnosis of the remedy.

We often talk of totality of symptoms as the basis of selection of symptoms. The students of Homoeopathy are reminded here again and again that numerical total of what the patient talks about or what the physician may interpret, is not the true totality. The 'gross' or so called total totality will often land us in trouble and indicate only remedies like Sulphur, Bryona, Bell etc. No Repertory or computer can help us in such a situation. It is only the totality of discriminating, individualising symptoms, which alone are the pathognomic of the sickness in a particular individual at that particular point of time.

Chapter Four

REPERTORIAL ANALYSIS WITH CASE-DEMONSTRATION

Boenninghausen's Method

Every case that needs to be repertorised has to be approached on its own individual merits. Some cases can be worked out beautifully on the Kent's Repertory only. These are the cases which present well-marked mental and general characteristics of the patient. Actually, particulars have a very poor standing, so far as working of the Kent's Repertory is concerned. But there are cases which lack the dependable mentals and characteristic generals. There may be a number of modalities, a large number of particulars and associated (concomitant) symptoms, where Boenninghausen's approach may prove very useful. It is, therefore, advisable to evaluate the case as a whole, to see which of the repertorial system is best suited to the case in hand.

Boenninghausen's Therapeutic Pocket Book is divided into seven parts which are as follows:-

1. **Mind and Intellect-** It is comparatively a very short section in the Repertory although, both Hahnemann and Kent, extolled heavily the mental symptoms. Boenninghausen, however, felt that these symptoms have to be very strongly marked in a patient and most of the times, such symptoms are very difficult to elicit. The patients that we see everyday in our clinics, do not bring out the mental symptoms. Such symptoms have to be observed and narrated by persons who have

observed the patient, but are not subjectively involved and they can give us also the mental reactions of the patient. Patient himself is not in a position to talk about it or he hides his innermost mental reactions and symptoms. That is why, Boenninghausen says quite early that instead of prescribing on so called mental symptoms, which may not be really reliable, it is best to couple it with the other elements of symptoms which can be definitely depended upon.

2. **Locations-** Parts of body and organs with their specific functions.

3. **Sensations and Complaints-** which include also the sub-sections on affections of (a) Glands, (b) Bones, (c) Skin. The sensations are not divided into sections but are given alphabetically.

4. **Sleep and Dreams**

5. **Fever**- which includes
   (a) Circulation of blood.
   (b) Cold stage.
   (c) Coldness.
   (d) Heat
   (e) Perspiration
   (f) Compound fever
   (g) Concomitant complaints.

6. **Alterations of state of health,** which includes-
   (a) Aggravation according to time.
   (b) Aggravation according to situation and circumstances.
   (c) Amelioration by position and circumstances.

7. **Relationship of Remedies.** This section requires detailed explanation.

This seventh section of the book on relationships or concordances of remedies was envisaged as early as 1836 by Boenninghausen. But at that time, he had not done it properly and as completely. In the Therapeutic Pocket Book, he tried to make it as complete and as correct as possible. Unfortunately, most of us have not understood properly or utilised this section for practical application.

Boenninghausen wrote in his preface that he hoped that no one would consider this section useless and superfluous. He wrote "For myself, who for the last fifteen years had made the Materia Medica Pura my chief study as one of the most indispensable books of Homoeopathy, this concordance has been of extreme importance, not only for recognition of the genius of the remedy, but also for testing and making sure of its choice, and for judging of sequence of the various remedies, so as to determine the order of their successive exhibition, particularly in chronic diseases".

Thus there are three applications or uses of this section on Concordances or Relationships of remedies.

(1) Grasp of the genius of the medicines.
(2) Greater certainty in selection.
(3) Sequence in second prescriptions.

In concordances, all the seven sections are represented and the harmonious relation of the remedy to others is given under each section. He has added apart from these, 'antidotal remedies the eighth section or paragraph of these concordances.

In its First application or use, it becomes clearer to understand the genius of the remedy, when we are able to compare it with other remedies in different areas of the application, and also the degree of nearness or contact of these remedies in different spheres. This is indeed a comparative Materia Medica in a nutshell.

The second use of concordance is also quite obvious as it helps us in selection of remedy for the case more certainly, as we are able to compare the remedy mentally with contending remedies.

The third and the most important use is the sequence of remedies i.e. the remedy or remedies which could follow the one already prescribed and found either inadequate or had finished its usefulness. This application according to Boenninghausen is very important in chronic cases, but I feel this could be as useful in acute cases also. The next remedy or the second prescription is thus indicated with a certainty which no other repertory or Materia Medica could offer us.

The almost always satisfactory result obtained from using one of them in indicating the remedy to follow is due to the wonderfully accurate and comprehensive manner in which they have been compiled, and not there being anything concealed or esoteric. One wonders at the remarkable genius of Boenninghausen and at the amount of work and study involved in the formulations of the concordances. I wish there could be another follower of Boenninghausen who could have extended this work.

Having selected the first medicine for a case with accuracy and worked out its action in various potencies, or if the symptoms change substantially, new ones developing, — either case demanding a change of remedy, — it is here the difficulty comes.

To meet these new and trying conditions, there are instructions in the Organon and directions given by Hering with regard to the importance of the new symptoms that have appeared. Besides that in Hering's Guiding symptoms as well as in various Materia Medicas, a short list of remedies follow the main remedy as its complementary or remedies that usually follow.

All this is useful, but it is not as specific as are the concordances in this respect, and besides, it takes much less time to use the concordance. Unfortunately, so few of us utilise this area of our Repertories.

Let us, for example, examine relationship of Aconite and Belladonna. Both have many points of contact, but on studying Aconite's relationship and sequences and its relations to Belladonna, we find there are many areas where Belladonna could have followed, but on studying Belladonna's concordances, we find that relationships are less marked. In practice also we find that Belladonna may be the indicated remedy after Aconite, but hardly vice-versa.

Similarly, we find that under Aconite, Sulphur seems better indicated as the chronic remedy, while Calc-carb is better indicated as chronic of Belladonna.

Dr. Som Dev, under my advice, took the trouble of giving the summation of intensity of contact points in actual numbers, and published the relationships of Boenninghausen with numerical summations.

The last paragraph in concordances of each remedy has been designated as 'other remedies', which is rather misguiding. Actually, the remedies given here, give in general the quantum of contact points of these remedies with the remedy, where concordances or relationships are given i.e. the remedy under study.

This paragraph is actually the resume of all the earlier paragraphs of relationships of the remedy under study. This paragraph, therefore, is the most important and can be used alone in most of the cases.

How are the concordances to be made use of, in relation to the sequence of remedies ? This depends upon the case, and no hard and fast rules can be given. These relationships may even be used without assistance for the first part of Therapeutic Pocket Book.

Generally, a concordance is to be used alone, taking as first rubric, the one which covers the part affected. In a mental case, however, 'Mind' is to be used first If the part is elsewhere in the body, then the rubric localities' is to be taken first. For detailed information and guidance on the use of this section of the Repertory, one is advised to study the introduction given by Dr. H.A.Roberts in his edition of Boenninghausen's Therapeutic Pocket Book. This will be of tremendous use to any body in his search for the second prescription.

Let us take an example or two. There was a case of sinusitis, which responded to Silicea, but was not completely cured. We looked up the relationship in the following sections, as they were the ones most relevant to the case.

1. Localities
2. Sensations
3. Modalities
4. Other remedies

We found that Calc was the remedy that was most prominent. Reference to Materia Medica seemed to confirm it. The case did respond to Calc which finished the cure.

Relationship of Silicea

Be=Bell, Ca=Calc, Cau=Caust, Co=Con, Gr=Graph, K-b=Kali-bi, K-c=Kali-c, Ly=Lyc, M=Merc, N-m=Nat-m, P=Puls. S=Sil

	Be	Ca	Cau	Co	Gr	K-b	K-c	Ly	M	N-m	P	S
Locations	4	5	4	4	4	5	4	5	4	4	5	5
Sensations	4	5	3	2	2	4	3	4	3	3	3	4
Modalities	3	4	3	4	2	3	4	4	-	3	3	4
Other remedies	4	5	3	3	2	4	3	5	4	3	4	5
	15	19	13	13	10	16	14	18	11	13	15	18
	4	4	4	4	4	4	4	4	4	4	4	4

Calc-carb has the highest evaluation in the relationship with Silicea in the areas selected. It was referred also to the Materia Medica which confirmed its indication for this case. The results of the prescription justified the selection.

There was another case cited by Dr. Turner. A case with mental symptoms of Hyos. responded to Hyos and which helped the case for sometime, but failed to improve the case further. The relationships (concordances) of Hyos were studied.

Pulsatilla was found to be highest in its relationship and was prescribed. It took hold at once and cured the case.

The section on 'other remedies' is often not properly understood, and hence, not utilised often enough. This gives the relationship of the remedy concerned to other remedies in general. Sometimes this section alone can lead us to the second prescription; especially, when other areas of relationships are not brought out or poorly present.

This chapter of Relationship can be utilised after a

remedy already selected has helped the case only partially or relieved most of the symptoms, but has not yet cured the case. The selection done earlier could have been on key-notes prescribing or based on analysis on any Repertory. The relationship is thus available to us, whenever there is a need for second prescription.

Before resorting to this chapter, one has to be sure of utilising the following options- (i) antidoting the remedy given earlier, if needed, (ii) repetition in different potency. The last option for second prescription is, of course. Concordances or Relationship.

It may be useful to mention that working with this chapter on relationships, one can utilise also, wherever feasible, the various rubrics which are given in the main part of the book and labeled under associated symptoms or concomitants. Some of the symptoms which are actually concomitants are given under the aggravations. For example, symptoms which appear or are aggravated before the menses or after the menses or during the menses, are really associated symptoms or concomitants, as they are not directly related to the rubrics of genitalia.

The following list will indicate the concomitants or associated symptoms given at different places in Boenninghausen's Repertory.

1). Mental - concomitants
2). Nose - Nasal discharges - concomitants
3). Stools - Complaints associated with -complaints before, during or after stools
4). Urine - Complaints before during and after urine
5). Menses - before, during or after
6). Leucorrhoea, associated symptoms
7). Respiration- Breathing and associated symptoms
8). Cough- concomitants and associated symptoms
9). Yawning- associated symptoms; aggravations

10). Sleep - complaints preventing sleep
11). Waking - concomitants
12). Sleepiness - concomitant complaints
(associated complaints with sleepiness, or caused by various things)
Sleep- concomitants (see also aggravation on waking)
Sleeplessness - concomitants causing
(symptoms causing sleeplessness in general)
13). Fever - cold stage - concomitants
14). Heat - concomitants
15). Perspiration - concomitants
16). Compound fever - concomitants before, during, after.

These rubrics of concomitants are useful conjuncts of concordances and can be utilised where applicable and where the latter does not help us completely. Of course, ultimately the Materia Medica is the final judge.

Many of us come across many chronic as well as complicated acute cases, where characteristics and keynotes are not available or obtainable in spite of our best efforts at examination and interrogation. At such times, the concomitants or the concordances are of great help to us.

Some of our best prescribers have utilised Boenninghausen's Therapeutic Pocket Book for repertorisation and achieved brilliant results. Boenninghausen has simplified the procedure and taken into account the symptom-totality as a whole; for him the four elements of a symptom are enough to proceed to the task of selection. For illustration, a few cases are worked out following this method. Since it takes lot more time in working out the case, even by using the Repertory sheets, most of the cases here are worked on 'Kishore Cards Repertory', as this Card analysis system has included all the Boenninghausen's rubrics. Now, such cases could also be worked out with suitable computer software.

After taking the history of the case, the elements of the

symptoms are separately marked. At times, the symptoms of the patient have to be translated into the language of the Repertory. The relevant cards are selected from the Index of the Rubrics given in the second part of this book. The cards representing the selected rubrics are arranged one above the other so that the corresponding holes synchronize. The opposed cards are held together against the light, so that one could see the holes which show the light all through. The code numbers are noted from the cards. We can also note the second group of remedies which are not all-through but are most trans-illuminant.

If need be, we can also note the remedy or remedies which are less trans-illuminant than the former ones, so that we do not take any risk of blocking out the likely remedy. This has to be done especially in cases where the number of rubrics is large. If we elect to use Boenninghausen, the number of rubrics is usually larger than when we use Kent, especially in the latter's short-cut or artistic method. A few cases worked on Kishore Cards (Boenninghausen's method) are given below. Since the cases were worked out at the time when proper computer software on Repertories were not available, I have recorded the analysis only on Kishore Cards in a number of cases.

Kishore Cards may not be available after sometime as the computers are likely to replace the punched card system. In our clinics, we still use the card system, although we have three kinds of software for Kent's and other Repertories. But at times, punched card system is advantageous. The following illustrations, worked out on the Kishore Cards system, just give an idea to the readers that Boenninghausen's and Boger's Boenninghausen still have an important place in the repertorisation and case analysis. These can be analysed on computerised Repertories and the results should be the same, although some of the rubrics have been updated in certain Repertories, as in the Kishore Cards, a number of additions had been made. Anyway, the following are examples of right selection of the rubrics and their analysis from the Repertorial data based on Boenninghausen in most of the cases.

N.B. The author has avoided giving his own cases(except one), so as to eliminate the personal bias as far as possible.

CASE I

Boenninghausen's Method

(Adapted from Dr. H.A. Robert's case in his introduction to Boenninghausen's Repertory)

Case history:

A young woman, 35 years of age, was brought in by her family physician who felt he needed help on the case. She was greatly depressed, cried a great deal, and felt so unlike her cheerful self that she "felt frightened at herself. She has a "mad desire to walk" although she is averse to any work, mental or physical. She "faces the day with dread"; feels as if alone in the world; music of which she has been very fond, is now extremely distasteful. She admits there is no reason why she should not be happy and content, since she has pulled through some hard times and now the road has been smoothed out. She has not slept for several days. Previously, she would awaken from sleep with a general quivering, especially in the pit of the stomach. She feels "weak in the knees" and has an "all-gone" sensation which is better after 4 P.M. She has developed an aversion to being with people, especially crowds.

There is a great deal of headache, dull pain that comes and goes across the forehead, in the morning: it becomes throbbing on stooping. There is a ringing in the left ear and sense of pressure in the ears as if they were stopped. Her tonsils are enlarged.

She is eating poorly and has recently lost 15 pounds.

She sweats all over. Her feet blister, and sweat. The nails are brittle.

Rubrics for Repertorial Analysis:		**Kishore Card No.**
1.	Aggravations, morning.	0051
2.	Aggravations, music.	0241
3.	Aggravations, stooping.	0298
4.	Ear, Noises, ringing.	1018
5.	Ear, stopped sensation.	1021
6.	Emaciation.	1024
7.	Emptiness, sensation of.	1028
8.	Eruptions, pemphigus (bullae or blisters).	1094
9.	Extremities, lower, foot.	1229
10.	Extremities, nails brittle, finger nails.	1286
11.	Head, internal, forehead.	1678
12.	Mind & intellect, sadness (mental depression).	2106
13.	Motion, desire for.	2200
14.	Pain, dull.	2447
15.	Pulsation, internally.	2531
16.	Sleeplessness.	2926
17.	Stomach, epigastrium.	2935
18.	Sweat, exertion, during slightest.	3033
19.	Sweat, single parts, on.	3044
20.	Throat, Internal, tonsils, enlargement.	3185
21.	Trembling, internally.	3197
22.	Weakness, nervous.	3478

Remedy Analysis

1st Grade (All through)

1.	164	-	Calc.	47/22
2.	543	-	Sep.	50/22

IInd Grade (Not 'all through' but most trans-illummant)

1.	393	-	Lyc.	45/21
2.	417	-	Merc.	46/21
3.	544	-	Sil.	44/21
4.	567	-	Sulph.	51/21

The Materia Medica confirmed the choice of Sepia which did help the patient satisfactorily.

Regarding the evaluation of the remedies or their grades for particular symptoms, they can be taken from the books, after selection has been reduced to 3 to 5 remedies.

It may be mentioned here that while using Kent's Repertory in a case like this with 22 rubrics, the results may be misleading. Then we have to take the task with a different approach.

To show the aberrations of Repertorial analysis if it is done on Kentian approach (withcertain adaptations of rubrics), let us see what the results are. This is done through Macintosh software on the computer.

See the next page for Mac Repertory graph.

Note- It may be mentioned that we adapted the rubrics on locations as 'Pain in general' on the particular part. Patient had dull headache, and we kept it as Pain dull in head in the place of General pain, dull.

I 8/1/97 Jugal Kishore, D

Analysis Options: Totality, All Remedies

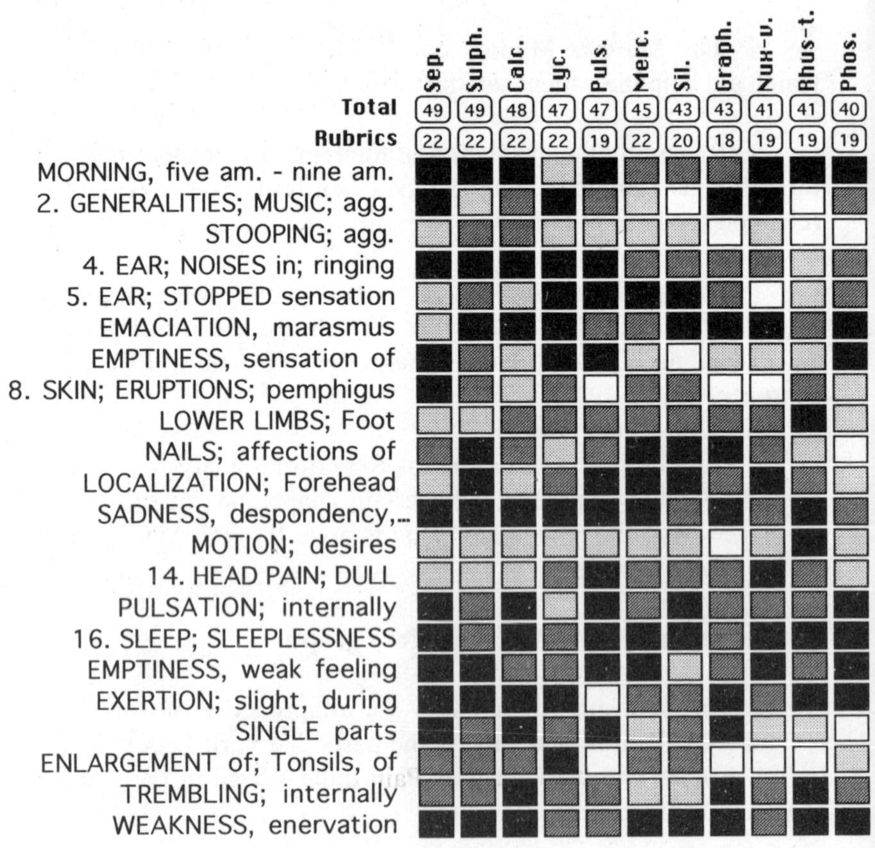
Sep.
Sulph.
Calc.
Lyc.
Puls.
Merc.
Sil.
Graph.
Nux-v.
Rhus-t.
Phos.
Total
49 49 48 47 47 45 43 43 41 41 40
Rubrics
22 22 22 22 19 22 20 18 19 19 19
MORNING, five am. - nine am.
2. GENERALITIES; MUSIC; agg.
STOOPING; agg.
4. EAR; NOISES in; ringing
5. EAR; STOPPED sensation
EMACIATION, marasmus
EMPTINESS, sensation of
8. SKIN; ERUPTIONS; pemphigus
LOWER LIMBS; Foot
NAILS; affections of
LOCALIZATION; Forehead
SADNESS, despondency,...
MOTION; desires
14. HEAD PAIN; DULL
PULSATION; internally
16. SLEEP; SLEEPLESSNESS
EMPTINESS, weak feeling
EXERTION; slight, during
SINGLE parts
ENLARGEMENT of; Tonsils, of
TREMBLING; internally
WEAKNESS, enervation

CASE II

Boenninghausen's Method
(Dr. H.A. Robert's Case)

Case History

A woman 65 years of age, complained of a pain which began as a soreness in the epigastrium and hypochondrium, increasing to a sore pain. The pain was > while sitting; > belching; < lying on the back; markedly < lying on right side; < on motion, especially on turning over in bed. There was a constant sensation of pulling in the right hypochondrium, < lying on the right side. The pain causes sweating. There is pain as of repeated blows in the region of the right scapula. The mouth is exceedingly dry. There is a great aversion to food or drink; and the odour of food or any other strong odours are very offensive and cause nausea. The patient vomits as soon as water becomes warm in the stomach; there is no thirst. Although there is much flatus, none passes. The urine has an offensive odour.

Rubrics for Repertorial Analysis:		**Kishore Card No**
Abdomen, Hypochondria, right	(Location)	0011
Aggravation, lying on back	(Modalities)	0217
Aggravation, lying on right side	(Modalities)	0222
Aggravation, motion of affected parts	(Modalities)	0234
Aggravation, odours, strong	(Modalities)	0246
Aggravation, turning over in bed	(Modalities)	0328
Amelioration, eructations	(Modalities)	0401
Amelioration, sitting while	(Modalities)	0440
Dryness of internal parts (usually moist)	(Sensation)	0960
Flatus incarcerated	(Concomitant)	1618
Mouth, Affections in general	(Location)	2205
Pain, sore internally	(Sensation)	2475
Pulling, sensation of	(Sensation)	2529
Stomach, epigastrium	(Location)	2935
Sweat, with associated symptoms	(Concomitant)	3075
Thirstlessness	(Sensation-concomitant)	3128
Urine. odour offensive	(Concomitant)	3368

Remedy Analysis:

Ist Grade

1.	456	Nux-v.
2.	484	Phos.
3.	506	Puls.
4.	567	Sulph.

IInd Grade

1.	058	Acon.
2.	156	Bry.
3.	191	Caust.
4.	354	Kali-c.
5.	442	Nat-c.

After referring to the Materia Medica, and finding that the patient vomited water when it became warm in stomach, Phos. IM was given. The patient became more comfortable and two days later, the white blood count had drooped to 11,200. The whole condition subsided within a few days.

See the next page for Mac Repertory graph.

CASE III

Boenninghausen's Method

(Adapted from the Homoeopathic Recorder 1928)

Case History

The patient, a woman in the early fifties, much wrinkled and worn by hard life of worry and work, sallow or pasty, lay in bed, tossing about somewhat from a headache which fretted her to pieces.

Fever high, 102° to 103°F. Pulse high and weak. Chill every time she moved, even under the bed clothes. Sleeps in short

I **8/1/97** **Jugal Kishore, Dr**

Analysis Options: Totality, All Remedies

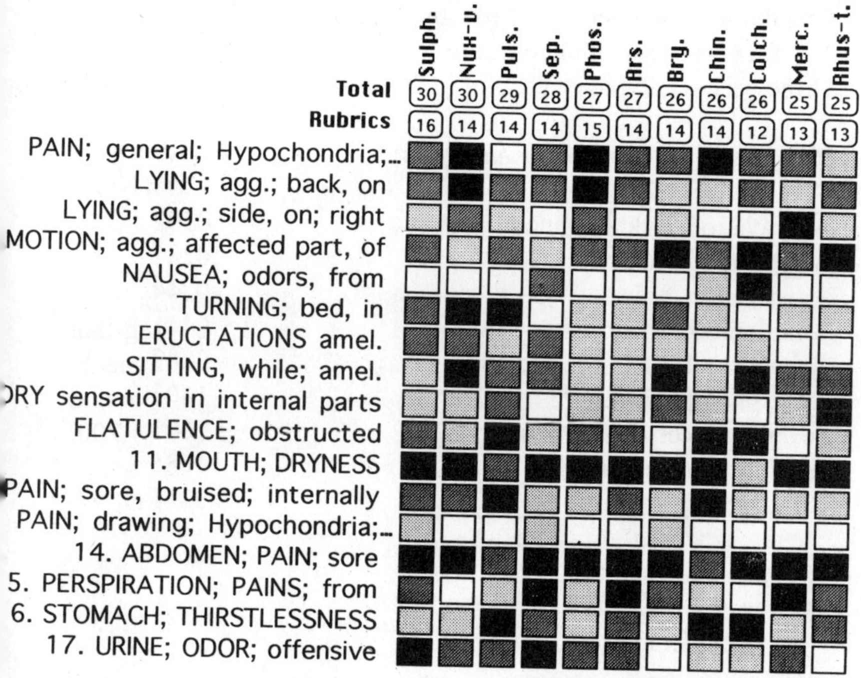

	Sulph.	Nux-v.	Puls.	Sep.	Phos.	Ars.	Bry.	Chin.	Colch.	Merc.	Rhus-t.
Total	30	30	29	28	27	27	26	26	26	25	25
Rubrics	16	14	14	14	15	14	14	14	12	13	13
PAIN; general; Hypochondria;...											
LYING; agg.; back, on											
LYING; agg.; side, on; right											
MOTION; agg.; affected part, of											
NAUSEA; odors, from											
TURNING; bed, in											
ERUCTATIONS amel.											
SITTING, while; amel.											
RY sensation in internal parts											
FLATULENCE; obstructed											
11. MOUTH; DRYNESS											
PAIN; sore, bruised; internally											
PAIN; drawing; Hypochondria;...											
14. ABDOMEN; PAIN; sore											
5. PERSPIRATION; PAINS; from											
6. STOMACH; THIRSTLESSNESS											
17. URINE; ODOR; offensive											

naps and a little better on each waking. Headache worse in occiput; very severe.
Worse any motion, noise, light
Accompanied by nausea and vomiting of mucous.
Aching all over body.
Aching eyes. Photophobia.
Cough loose, frequent; very painful to head.
No stool for 3 days and no desire for stools.
Urine very scanty, only 1/2 pint in 26 hrs; dark.

Rubrics for Repertorial Analysis:	**Kishore Card No.**
Aggravation, light in general	0202
Aggravation, motion	0231
Aggravation, noises	0244
Amelioration, sleep, after	0441
Cough, troubles associated with	0889
Eyes, photophobia	1403
Fever, uncovering, aversion to	1607
Head, internal, occiput	1685
Urine, scanty	3371

Remedy Analysis:

1st Grade

1.	058	Acon.	13/9
2.	164	Calc.	15/9
3.	235	Con.	17/9
4.	417	Merc.	19/9
5.	442	Nat-c.	11/9
6.	456	Nux-v.	25/9
7.	485	Ph-ac.	11/9
8.	507	Puls.	17/9

Nux vom 1 M set the curative cycle in motion.

See the next page for Mac Repertory graph.

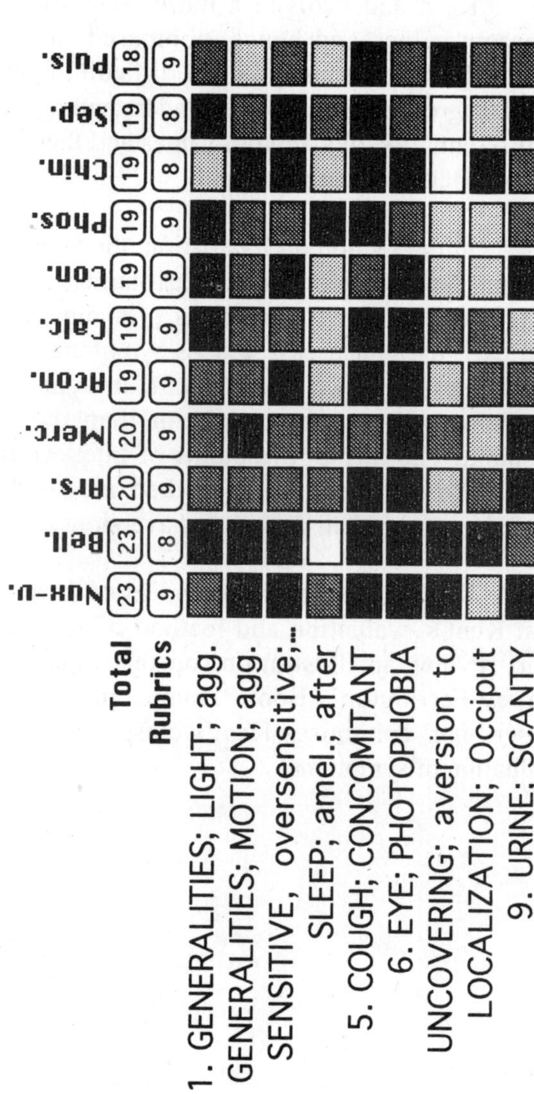
8/1/97
Jugal Kishore, Dr
Analysis Options: Totality, All Remedies
Nux-v. Bell. Ars. Merc. Acon. Calc. Con. Phos. Chin. Sep. Puls.
Total 23 23 20 20 19 19 19 19 19 19 18
Rubrics 9 8 9 9 9 9 9 9 8 8 9
1. GENERALITIES; LIGHT; agg.
2. GENERALITIES; MOTION; agg.
SENSITIVE, oversensitive;...
SLEEP; amel.; after
5. COUGH; CONCOMITANT
6. EYE; PHOTOPHOBIA
UNCOVERING; aversion to
LOCALIZATION; Occiput
9. URINE; SCANTY

KENT'S METHOD

Kent had evolved a more sophisticated hierarchy of symptom-values and hence, compared to Boenninghausen's method, his is more complex and difficult to grasp. It takes more time and greater application in understanding the various shades of differentiation of symptom-values and then to utilise the same for the repertorial analysis.

In the section on Evaluation, the value of different types of symptoms has already been explained. Kent, however, has laid rather rigidly the gradations of symptoms. As a matter of fact, each individual case and its symptoms require evaluations according to its own requirement. In some cases, a physical general may be more important than the so called mental symptom. The mental symptoms of intellect are comparatively useless compared to well marked modalities and physical generals or to marked desires and aversions.

It is expected that any student of Repertory is conversant with Kent's evaluation and method of Repertorisation. For a short review, an illustration (on the opposite page) from Dr. Harvey Farrington's Book 'Homoeopathy and Homoeopathic Prescribing' epitomises Kent's classification and hierarchy of evaluation of symptoms.

Kent's classification of symptoms may be illustrated by the following chart

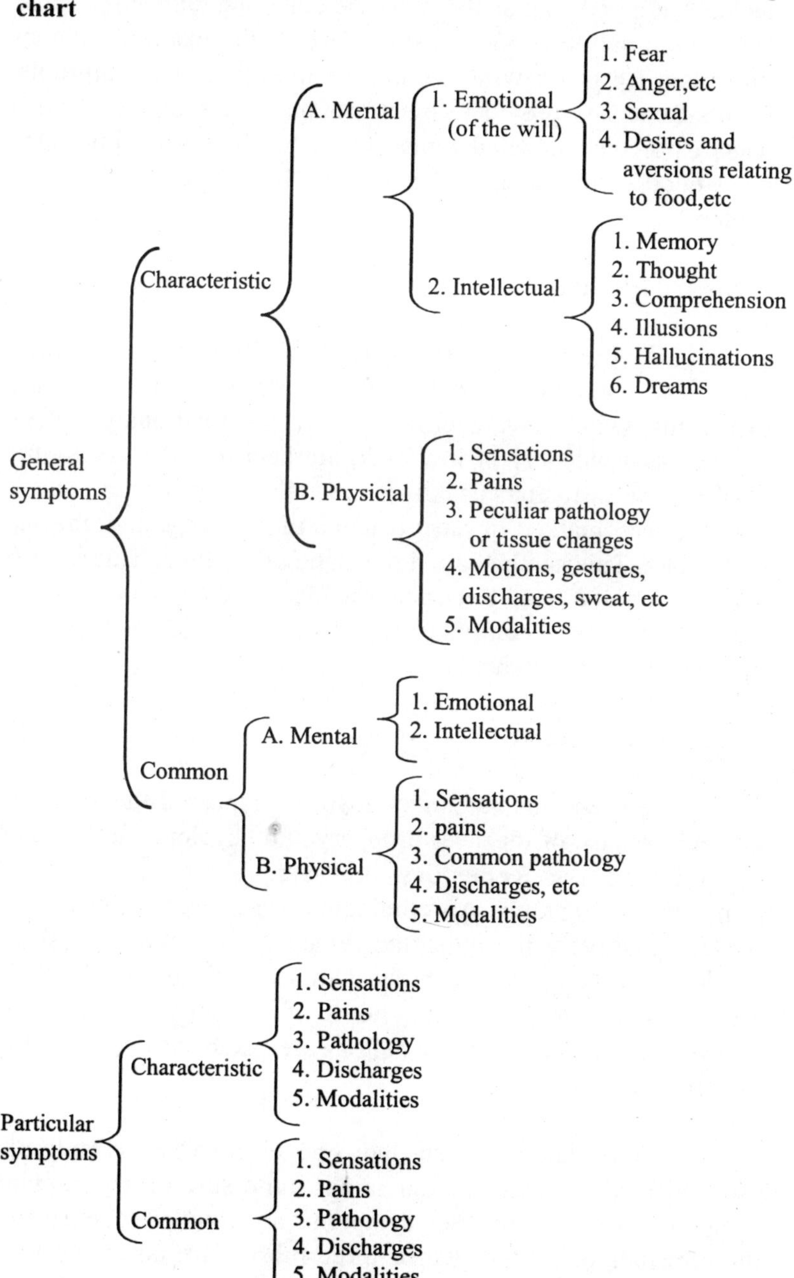

Kent's Repertory is a fine instrument in many ways and hence, the repertorial analysis can be done in a number of ways. Here, the analytical and artistic sense of the examiner comes into play. He has a wider scope for his repertorial solutions. Kent's Repertory provides sometimes peculiar symptoms which leads us to the indicated remedy in a much shorter time. One must necessarily refer to the Materia Medica to confirm the choice.

Standard Method

For the beginner, the best method is that of total numerical evaluation of the competing drugs, indicated in the symptoms, which have been chosen for the final analysis. The particulars, especially of low rank, are kept out of it. In Kent's analysis, the particulars usually are not taken into account, unless they are well marked or have become rare, strange and unusual particulars. This can be called the standard method. This is time consuming but a Card Repertory enables us to cut short the toil. Today, however, a computer can cut short the time further in the retrieving of evaluated data.

The Artistic Methods

Kent and his students, however, bypassed the standard method because of its sheer drudgery and developed a different approach to the Repertory-analysis. They made use of Eliminative symptoms. An eliminative symptom is expected to contain positively the indicated remedy. It is usually a short rubric and belongs to the highest ranks in Kent's evaluation. This symptom is the pivotal point of the case and only the remedies indicated in this symptom are taken into account for further elimination.

There can be more than one eliminative symptoms, especially when the examiner is not quite sure of a particular symptom. Here two or three symptoms are counted together i.e. the remedies of all the two or three rubrics are taken together for the further elimination. For example. Dr. Margaret Tyler, would combine 'fear of robbers' and 'fear of darkness' for the purpose of avoiding undesirable elimination. This method is also known as Kent's 'short cut' method.

Other Methods of Quick Elimination

If the mentals are well marked and there is a good sprinkling of physical generals also, it is better to start first with mentals, then physical generals and then particulars. The elimination can be done in this order. Of course, one can use here the totality of numerical values also.

When the mental symptoms are not as strongly marked, and in the opinion of the operator, the physical generals are more important or prominent, then it is safer to relegate the second position to the mentals, and take the important physical generals to the first position.

There is another method where the work of elimination is helped by using Dr. Gibson Miller's idea of differentiating the patients and the remedies into two main classes i.e. Hot and Cold. Dr. Tyler used this method of elimination but sometimes there cannot be such a rigid division and the likely remedy may be blocked out. I, personally, do not use this division for elimination.

There are cases where neither mental nor any other general symptoms are so well marked or distinctive. We have to use great caution in using such symptoms as eliminative symptoms, otherwise, we might never come to the correct drug.

The following case shows how a short but characteristic mental symptoms taken as the eliminative symptom gave the correct prescription.

CASE I

A case adapted from 'Post-graduate Course in Homoeopathy'.

A mentally deficient boy of 21, developed a new phase of very trying symptoms. He became very tidy, not only in regard to his own clothes, but he would go around the bed-rooms of the family, tidying up and putting things away in drawers (this was not at all appreciated). Also, from having been afraid to be alone, he developed a craze for walking, and would escape and go off at a great pace, so that his poor mother, who dreaded mischief or dangers for him, could not keep up, and he would be lost for hours. She had even tied him to the table-leg to try to curb his energies. Another irritating development was immoderate and almost incessant laughter. He also became very mischievous and destructive, and indulged in violent fits of temper.

The case was worked out thus:

Tidy (fastidious)	Ars., Nux-v.
Mischievous	Agar., Anac., Ars., Calc., Cann-i., Cup., Hyos., Lach., Merc., Nux-v., Stram., Tarent., Verat. (with 3 other drugs in lowest type)
Laughs immoderately	Cann-i., Nat-m., Nux-m., Nux-v., Stry.
Violent anger	Ars., Anac., Calc., Nux-v., Tarent.

So he got one dose of Nux-vomica 10 M potency.

A month later, the report was "very much better. Getting back to his usual amount of intelligence, and says sensible things most of the time. Before, he seemed to be turning into an idiot. He has given up his everlasting walking: we keep an eye on him, but he has not the desire to go off now, like he had a few weeks ago. Still laughs some days, especially towards evening. To our relief, not one of those violent fits of temper for 3 and a half weeks, but is much more amiable and better tempered"; and "more intelligent".

He needed Nux again later for recurrence of ill temper, and it helped again. His mother wrote about the "walking and temper powders".

The above case shows how help can be given even where the condition is incurable, and how the drug can be found by taking into account peculiar characteristic symptoms, especially if it is a new development.

Using the cards, we can choose the peculiar and most unexpected symptom of tidiness as the eliminative rubric, but since it is too small a rubric, it is better to choose 'Mischievous' as the eliminative rubric, and we find that only Nux-v. has all the four symptoms.

Nux-v. numerically has 11/4 and Ars. and Tarent. have 6/3 values each.

See the next page for Mac Repertory graph.

CASE II

Demonstration of a Case Analysis on Kishore Cards (Kentian Method)

Case from Dr. Toman Pablo Paschero - The British Homoeopathic Journal Vol LIII No. 2, April 1964.

The case of a woman, aged 31, with three children, one of them microcephalic. She came complaining of indigestion, burning pains in stomach, weak sensation with fullness after eating, pains in right hypochondrium extending to back,

Case I **8/1/97** **Jugal Kishore, Dr**

Analysis Options: Totality, All Remedies

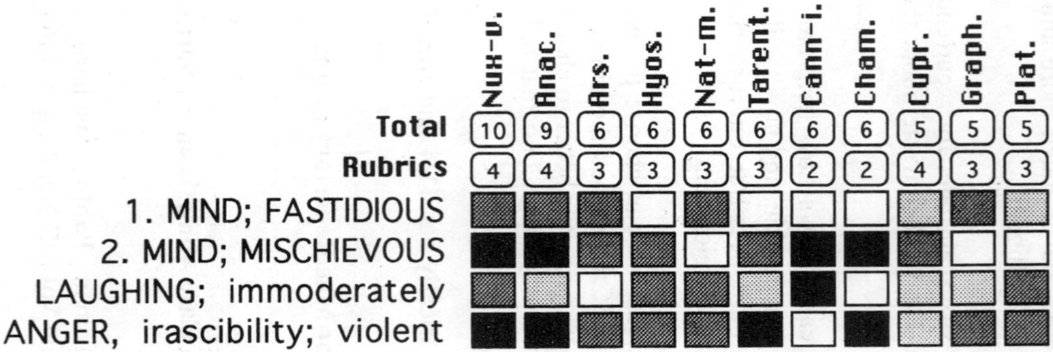

	Nux-v.	Anac.	Ars.	Hyos.	Nat-m.	Tarent.	Cann-i.	Cham.	Cupr.	Graph.	Plat.
Total	10	9	6	6	6	6	6	6	5	5	5
Rubrics	4	4	3	3	3	3	2	2	4	3	3
1. MIND; FASTIDIOUS											
2. MIND; MISCHIEVOUS											
LAUGHING; immoderately											
ANGER, irascibility; violent											

constipation alternating with diarrhoea, with physical and moral exhaustion, extreme irritability and intolerance, weeping, frigidity, vertigo and numbness in hands and legs. In her last pregnancy I and a half years ago, she had hepatitis, and a recent test showed numerous amoebae in the faeces.

Her mental state was totally referred to her mentally retarded son aged 5 who had encephalitis before he was 1 year old. She had developed a deep resentment against him; according to her, the child was aggressive, obstinate and capricious and his constant demands oppressed her.

She railed against this unjust fate and rejected all attempts at consolation. As a result of this state of intolerance, anger and despair, she developed an anxiety neurosis. A competent psycho-analyst, after 2 years, got her to recognize the abnormal emotions towards her son, reinforced by resentments and frustrations against her own parents and her husband, but he did not have any success in modifying her attitude and her general physical weakness and nervousness.

She had a deep desire for sweets, even to the extent of eating chocolates and cakes instead of lunch and dinner, which was very noticeable to her family. Moreover, her menses were of a deep brown colour, a fact often verified by her own mother. Damp aggravated all her complaints, especially the irritability, fatigue and aches round her waist. She also volunteered that spring provoked a general aggravation with twisted outlook and weariness. She felt specially weak every morning on rising, and after stool; great anxiety in the abdomen with restlessness and vague fear.

Her perspiration was profuse and offensive, breath foetid, belly painful and tympanitic; blood pressure 110/90 mm of Hg., oedema of legs and varicose veins.

The following symptoms were chosen for repertorisation both on Kishore's Cards and Kent's Repertory:

Rubrics Analysis:	**Kishore Card No.**	**Kent's Rep pg**
1. Desire, sweet	0919	486
2. Wet weather aggravates	0362	1421
3. Menses, brown	1849	725
4. Spring aggravates	0295	403
5. Abdomen, Anxiety after stool	3503	541
6. Weakness, worse morning on rising	8809	1414

The result of Kishore Cards-

I Grade- Sep.
II Grade- Bry., Carb-v.

Sepia was the only remedy which covered all the symptoms. The Materia Medica also confirmed it.

Thus, Sepia emerged clearly through repertorising and also covered the whole of the patient's picture with asthenia, laxity of parts, weariness, irritability, disgust, intolerance, unkindness and the varicose veins.

The First dose of Sepia 200 caused an aggravation with sleeplessness, increased leucorrhoea and anal itching. Then the picture remained stationary, and after two months Sepia 1M was prescribed which caused a rash on her face and neck. Forty days later, a dose of Sepia 10 M was found necessary, because her moral and physical apathy was not much modified despite general amelioration.

In only a few days after this third dose, her attitude towards her son was totally changed. She consented to his being educated in a special institution, which she had before quite refused to allow because of her feeling of tremendous aggression to this son whom she had blamed for all her misfortunes. She became tender, patient and affectionate with him, with her husband and her other two children; she also became tranquil and unselfish and never recriminated again.

This case has well-marked Mentals which can be used as Eliminative Symptoms and the case analysed.

For example, the following symptoms can be used as such-

1. Aversion to the loved ones.
2. Consolation aggravates.
3. Aversion to consolations.

The numerical evaluation has not been done. The author has, however, chosen physical generals for analysis.

See the next page for Mac Repertory graph.

CASE III

Repertorial Analysis of a Case from Dr. Harvey Farrington 'Homoeopathy and Homoeopathic Prescribing'

Mrs. W., aged 25, married, has two children, the youngest 15 months old. Since her last labour, she has had profuse, yellow leucorrhoea and violent pruritis vulvae.

She has "great bearing down of the womb," which completely incapacitates her from standing, walking, or doing her household duties such as washing or ironing.

Violent chronic headaches of a throbbing, tensive character, arising after worry or fatigue. These come on or are worse when she is constipated. Under regular treatment for headaches for two years without benefit. Sensations of heat in the vertex and as if a weight rested on top of her head. Head symptoms are more or less constant but are worse before the menses.

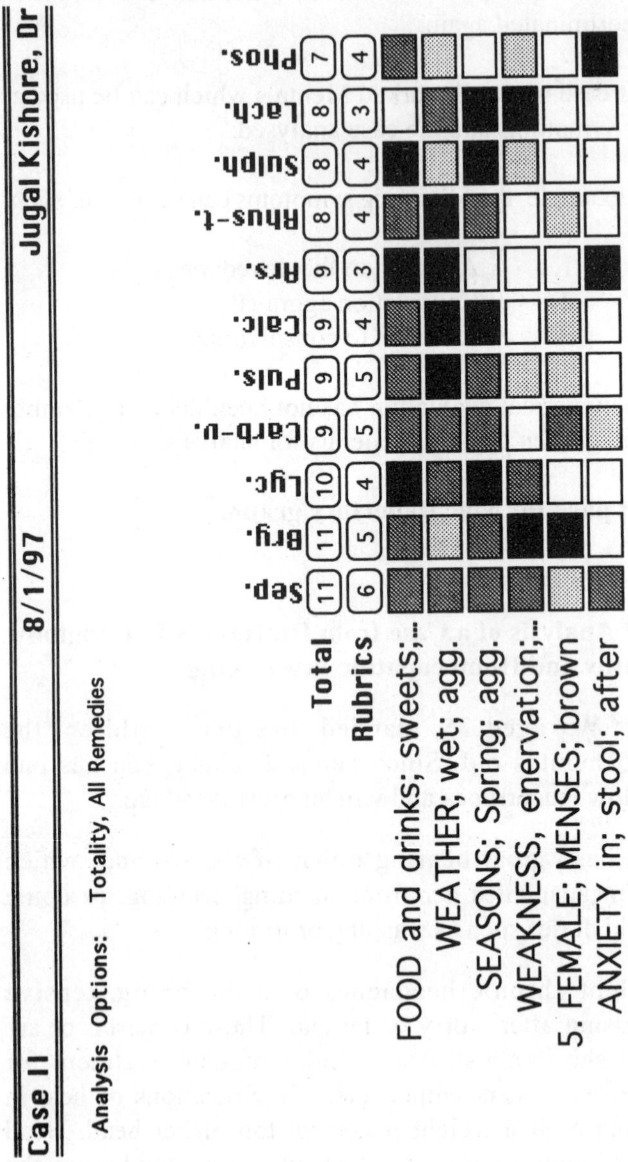

Case II **8/1/97** **Jugal Kishore, Dr**

Analysis Options: Totality, All Remedies

	Sep.	Bry.	Lyc.	Carb-v.	Puls.	Calc.	Ars.	Rhus-t.	Sulph.	Lach.	Phos.
Total	11	11	10	9	9	9	9	8	8	8	7
Rubrics	6	5	4	5	5	4	3	4	4	3	4
FOOD and drinks; sweets;...											
WEATHER; wet; agg.											
SEASONS; Spring; agg.											
WEAKNESS, enervation;...											
5. FEMALE; MENSES; brown											
ANXIETY in; stool; after											

Worried by trifles and complains that her memory is not good.

Face flushes; fainting spells while standing or without apparent cause; craving for food with an empty gone feeling in the epigastrium some time before the noon meal.

Most symptoms are worse at night, particularly the vulvar itching.

Perspiration under arms smells like garlic.

Rubric Analysis:		**Kishore Card No.**	**K-Rep pg. no.**
1.	Worse while standing	0296	1403
2.	Worse at night	0052	1342
3.	Worse From exertion	0149	1358
4.	Worse before menses	1838	1373
5.	Mind-Memory, weak	2067	64
6.	Head. pulsating	1717	223
7.	Head-Vertex, pressure on	6482	200
8.	Flushes of heat	1738	1365
9.	Ext.-Feet, cold	4995	962
10.	Female- Pain.bearing down, uterus	2780	735
11.	Female-Leucorrhoea, yellow	1820	723
12.	Female-Leucorrhoea, copious	1801	721
13.	Abdomen-Empty feeling in epig	2943	487
14.	Head-Vertex, heat of	6168	124
15.	Sweat in axillae, smelling like garlic (Sulph.)	878	

The result of Kishore Cards-

The remedies having all these symptoms i.e. I Grade (except no. 15 - Sweat in axillae, smelling like garlic) are- Calc., Graph., Nat-c. and Sulph.

Since Sulph has sweat offensive, garlic-like, it was the final choice. Sulph. was given and all the symptoms cleared up and the patient recovered complete health.

See the next page for Mac Repertory graph.

CASE IV

Demonstration of a case analysis on Kishore Cards
A Case from Dr. Toman Pablo Paschero

Case History

Some time ago, I saw a boy of 10 with bronchitis and frequent attacks of asthma. His mother stated that he had been in good health until measles at 1 & a half years. The present trouble began just after that. This categorical statement blaming measles for the onset of asthmatic bronchitis might have induced one to prescribe Morbillinum but the patient showed other symptoms. He had profuse perspiration in sleep, wetting the pillow, with a disagreeable odour. He also had the peculiarity that his skin often became "goose flesh" with little granules rendering it rough and dry. He was timid, hid from strangers, said "No" to everything and contradicted any little suggestion.

Rubrics for Repertorial analysis:		**Kishore Card No.**
1.	Goose flesh	2865
2.	Timidity	2169
3.	Disposition to contradict	1940
4.	Perspiration, foetid, scalp - (Kent p. 222- Calc, Merc, Puls, Staph)	
5.	Perspiration 'scalp during sleep	6498

On consulting the first three cards, the remedies, out of which only the similimum must be selected are:

Case III **8/1/97** **Jugal Kishore, Dr**

Analysis Options: Totality, All Remedies

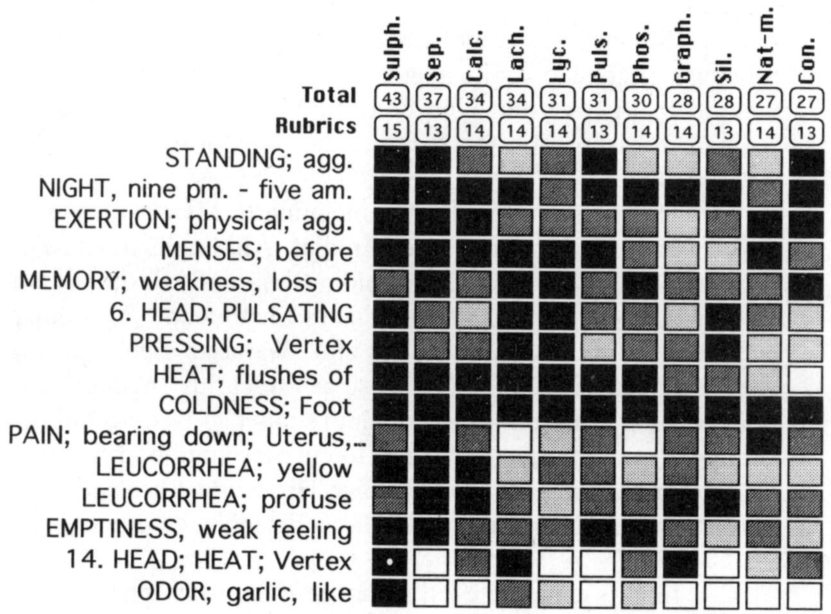

Aur-mur., Caps., Caust., Ign., Lyc., Merc., Nit-ac., Nux-v.

The last two symptoms will narrow down the selection and we have to refer to the Kent's Repertory Page 222. Mercurius is the remedy which is common to all symptoms.

(Mercurius was the remedy for this patient, with serious problems of conduct, quite aggressive and quarrelsome. He even wanted to kill anyone who contradicted him and he had a permanent disposition to contradict any proposal put to him).

The mental characteristic inclining to Merc. rather than Calc. was his disposition to contradict. Although, it was not taken into account, the other symptom 'Desire to kill the person who contradicts her' (p. 60) pertains to Merc. alone. Two other symptoms, 'Quarrelsome' (p. 70) and 'Wants to fight' (p. 48) were not necessary either. One dose of Mercurius 1M produced a dry scaling eruption on both palms similar to post-scarlatinal peeling; Profuse nasal catarrh and foetid perspiration of feet that his mother said he had when younger. His conduct became quite normal and his bronchitis and asthma disappeared completely.

In this case, the eliminative symptoms chosen are 'timidity' and 'disposition to contradict'. Here, Evaluation is not done, but straight forward elimination brings us our solution.

See the next page for Mac Repertory graph.

CASE V

(Adapted from the Homoeopathic Recorder Jan. 31)

Mrs. F. ,age 49. The symptoms are as follows- Has a constant headache which is worse lying down. The pain is in the occiput and there is a sense of pressure. Dizziness and dimness of vision. Dyspnoea on ascending stairs and when leaning backward. Recently sighs much. Sleep good but tired

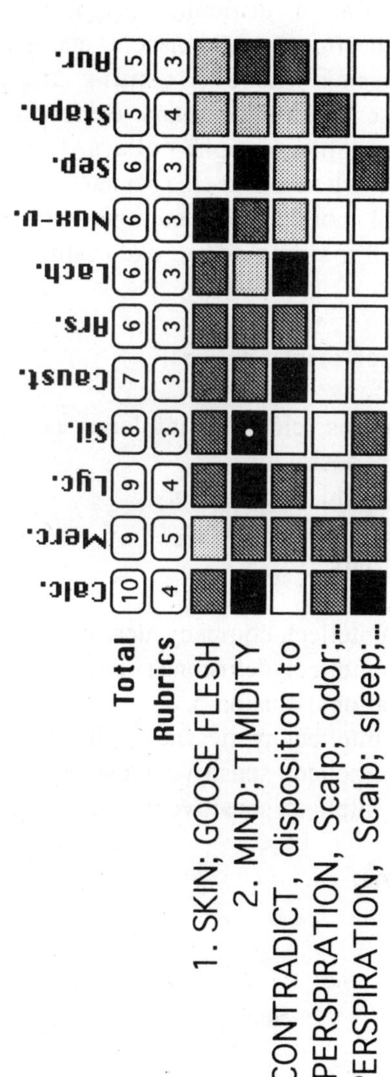
Case IU
8/1/97
Jugal Kishore, Dr
Analysis Options: Totality, All Remedies
Total
Rubrics
Calc. 10 4
Merc. 9 5
Lyc. 9 4
Sil. 8 3
Caust. 7 3
Ars. 6 3
Lach. 6 3
Nux-v. 6 3
Sep. 6 3
Staph. 5 4
Aur. 5 3
1. SKIN; GOOSE FLESH
2. MIND; TIMIDITY
CONTRADICT, disposition to
PERSPIRATION, Scalp; odor;...
PERSPIRATION, Scalp; sleep;...

in the morning. Wants to sleep all the time, worse after eating. Hungry but easily satisfied. No thirst. Considerable flatus. Very restless. Sadness from music. Memory poor. Speech stuttering recently. Concentration difficult. Imagines she sees things running across the floor, mice, insects, etc. Thinks of nothing but death. Homesick whenever visiting. Irritable and cross. Sensitive to noise. Desires company. Better in open air; must have it. Very sensible to tight collars. Urination frequent, copious, worse when on feet. Menses irregular, delayed, sometimes 2 or 3 months; flow copious; duration 3 to 4 days; discharge very dark; strong odour; excoriating during latter part of period.

Rubrics for Repertorial Analysis:		**Kishore Card No.**
1.	Aggravations, clothing, intolerance of.	0096
2.	Air, open, desire for.	0377
3.	Menses, acrid, excoriating.	1843
4.	Menses, copious, profuse.	1852
5.	Menses, dark.	1854
6.	Menses, late.	1863
7.	Mind & Intellect, company, desire for.	1933
8.	Mind & Intellect, delusions (Imaginations, hallucinations, illusions).	1956
9.	Mind & Intellect, restlessness (Nervous).	2099
10	Mind & Intellect, sensitive, music to.	2115
11.	Mind & Intellect, sensitive, noises, to.	2116

Remedy Analysis:

Ist Grade-

1.	543	Sep.	21/11

IInd Grade-

1:	191	Caust.	17/10
2.	393	Lyc.	23/10

IIIrd Grade-

1.	372	Lach.	19/9
2.	484	Phos.	16/9
3.	485	Ph-ac.	11/8
4.	506	Puls.	19/9
5.	620	Zinc.	16/9

Apparently, Lycopodium stands out even though it does not cover all the symptoms. Then also, looking back over the other symptoms, there are two very characteristic symptoms of Lyco- 'hungry but easily satisfied' and 'sleepy after eating'. After reading through the Materia Medica, Lycopodium was confirmed.

This is a balanced case, where physical generals and mentals are both present. One could use the shorter method of elimination also, by using either the mentals or the physical generals at the top.

The analysis from the Mac Repertory (Kentian approach) is given here just for interest. Here, number of symptoms covered by Puls., Sep., Sulph. and Phos. are more than the symptoms covered by Lyc.

See the next page for Mac Repertory graph.

CASE VI

(Case from Dr. Tomas Pablo Paschero - B.H.J. April 1964)

A boy, age 3 years, was brought to me with serious eczema covering almost all the body. His father, a physician, had already given him all the homoeopathic remedies usually prescribed in children's eczema- Sulph., Calc., Sep. etc.

The modalities correspond to those of Sulphur; intense itching aggravated by heat of bed, clothing, at night, walking

Case V **8/1/97** **Jugal Kishore, Dr**

Analysis Options: Totality, All Remedies

	Puls.	Sep.	Lach.	Lyc.	Sulph.	Calc.	Nux-v.	Phos.	Stram.	Ars.	Kali-c.
Total	24	24	24	24	23	22	21	20	20	19	19
Rubrics	11	11	10	10	11	10	9	11	9	9	9
CLOTHING; intolerance of											
AIR; open; desire for											
MENSES; acrid, excoriating											
4. FEMALE; MENSES; profuse											
5. FEMALE; MENSES; dark											
6. FEMALE; MENSES; late, too											
7. MIND; COMPANY; desire for											
DELUSIONS, imaginations											
RESTLESSNESS, nervousness											
SENSITIVE, oversensitive;...											
SENSITIVE, oversensitive;...											

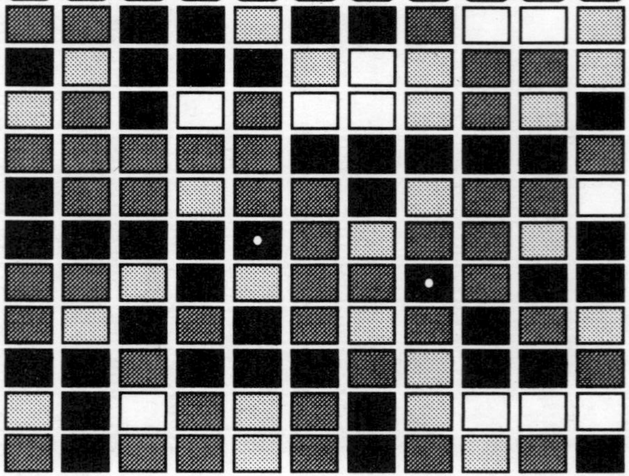

in the open air; great distress and irritability; marked thirst at meals, and intolerance of bathing. The father wondered why Sulphur did not heal his son although he had given it in different potencies.

Rubrics for Repertorial Analysis		**Kishore Card No.**
1.	Irritability in children	2046
2.	Obstinate	2086
3.	Capriciousness	1928
4.	Warm wraps aggravate	0353
5.	Warmth of bed aggravates	0349
6.	Desires cold drinks	0908

Remedy analysis:

Grade I-

1.	199	Cham.	17/6
2.	393	Lyc.	12/6

The case is more similar to Cham. than Lyco. Moreover Lyco patient usually likes warm drinks. One dose of Cham. 200 ameliorated him enormously from the first night, 25th October 1960; the eruption began to clear up three weeks later. On October 28th, 1960 another dose of Cham. 200 was prescribed and on January 19th, 1961 the boy was brought to our office quite healed of the eczema.

The last manifestation was a small plaque on the right palm, which was also the first sign of eczema two years before. The boy ceased to be irritable, obstinate and capricious and seemed in good health. But some strange features of conduct were apparent when he came to our office with his parents, who were also under treatment. They told me that the child had become quite sensitive, affectionate, loving, and remained long near his mother, kissing her and wanting constantly to caress

Case U **8/1/97** **Jugal Kishore, Dr**

Analysis Options: Totality, All Remedies

	Puls.	Sep.	Lach.	Lyc.	Sulph.	Calc.	Nux-v.	Phos.	Stram.
Total	24	24	24	24	23	22	21	20	20
Rubrics	11	11	10	10	11	10	9	11	9
CLOTHING; intolerance of									
AIR; open; desire for									
MENSES; acrid, excoriating									
4. FEMALE; MENSES; profuse									
5. FEMALE; MENSES; dark									
6. FEMALE; MENSES; late, too									
7. MIND; COMPANY; desire for									
8. MIND; DELUSIONS, imaginations									
9. MIND; RESTLESSNESS, nervousness									
SENSITIVE, oversensitive; music, to									
SENSITIVE, oversensitive; noise, to									

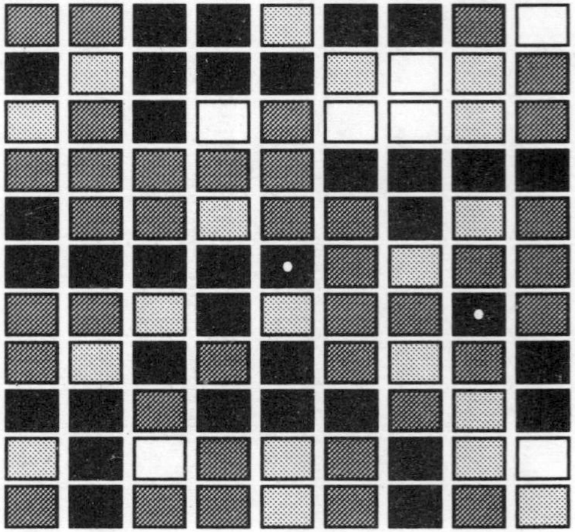

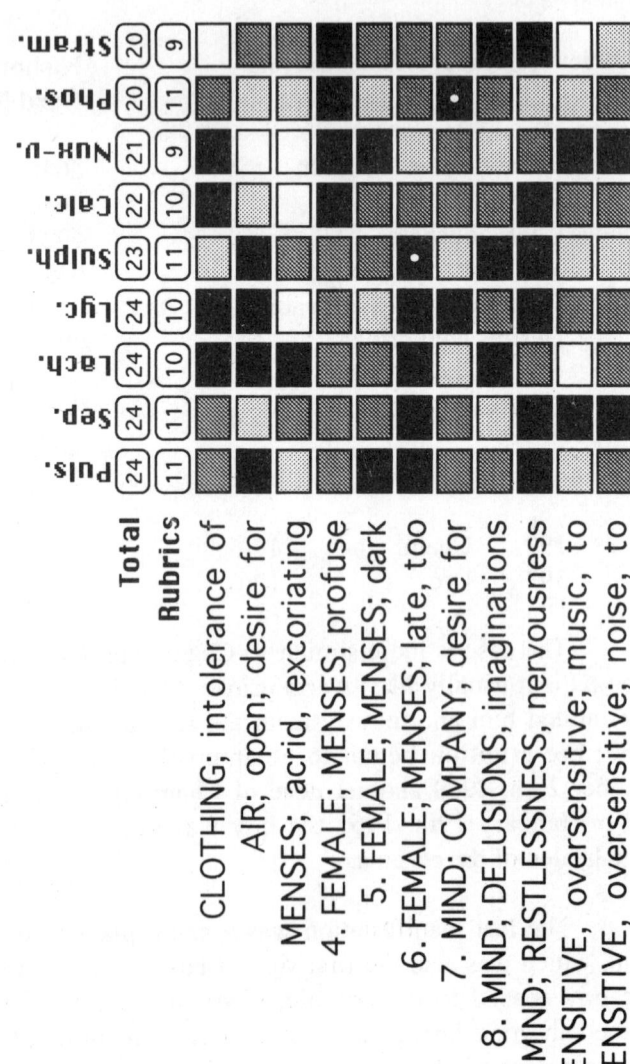

her. It was striking to hear the parents describe the soothing effect of stroking any painful part of the child's body, especially the belly. Whenever he complained of headache, the mother's hand calmed him and induced sleep.

See the next page for Mac Repertory graph.

CASE VII

Repertorial Analysis of a Case of Malarial Fever

('Homoeopathy and Homoeopathic Prescribing' by Harvey Farrington, M.D.)

The history of a young woman of twenty, who contracted malaria while traveling with her family. Massive doses of quinine stopped the chills and she was able to continue her tour.

Not long after her return home, she required a dose of Bromine, her constitutional remedy. Later, whether from the action of the Bromine or otherwise, the chills reappeared. Ars-alb was prescribed without result. The symptoms became alarming, and he gave quinine in massive doses, this time with only temporary palliative effect.

In prescribing for malarial fever homoeopathically, the exact similimum must be found if a cure is to be expected.

Since Ars-alb had been prescribed by a man of many years experience and the case presented a number of Arsenicum indications, the physician who was called at this juncture worked the case out with great care, using Kent's Repertory.

The symptoms were as follows- Chill daily at 6 or 6.30 p.m., beginning between the scapulae, as though ice water were dashed down the back; preceded by faintness and yawning; accompanied by intense thirst, great restlessness with tossing

Case VI **8/1/97** **Jugal Kishore, Dr**

Analysis Options: Totality, All Remedies

	Cham.	Bry.	Puls.	Cina	Lyc.	Sulph.	Chin.	Ip.	Merc.	Bell.	Phos.
Total	17	12	12	12	11	11	10	10	10	10	9
Rubrics	6	6	6	5	6	5	6	6	5	4	6
IRRITABILITY; children; in											
OBSTINATE, headstrong											
3. MIND; CAPRICIOUSNESS											
WARM; agg.; wraps											
WARM; agg.; bed											
FOOD and drinks; cold; drinks,...											

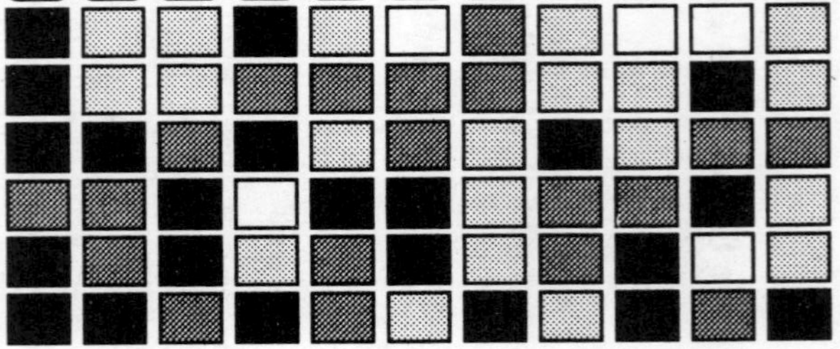

about, coldness, numbness and aching of the extremities, cold buttocks, and a sensation as though a wind blew on the feet and legs. The chill was worse from drinking cold water and from the least movement under the covers.

Fever without thirst was accompanied by throbbing headache, faintness, nausea, moaning, oppression of the chest, gasping and restlessness. The face was flushed, the skin hot and dry, and there was chilliness from lifting the covers. The temperature during the heat rose to 104.5 F.

Restlessness was the most marked mental characteristic. Therefore, it was given first place in the repertory study.

Rubrics for Repertorial Analysis	**Kishore Card No.**	**Kent's Rep pg.**
1. Mind, restlessness, tossing about	2102	73
2. Mind, restlessness, chill, during	6988	73
3. Mind, restlessness, heat, during	6991	74
4. Thirst, chill, during	3119	74
5. Chill at 6.00 p.m.	4413	1274
6. Chill, beginning in the back	0729	1263
7. Chill, worse on uncovering	4419	1275
8. Chilliness on uncovering during heat	1609	1292
9. Chill, water, as if cold water was dashed over him	4431	1276
10. Yawning, chill before	8861	1257
11. Extremities, pain, chill during	5253	1044
12. Extremities, numbness in general	5219	1035
13. Chill, wind, as if it were blowing cold upon the body	4433	1277
14. Chill, aggravated by drinking	4354	1266

Rhustox was the only remedy which was coming all through the symptoms.

By this process of elimination, Rhustox is shown to be, without doubt, the most similar remedy. The choice may be confirmed by comparing it with Arsenicum which had been selected by the former physician.

The characteristic times of onset for Arsenicum are 1:00 to 2:00 p.m., or 12:00 to 2:00 a.m. The chill is characteristically without thirst, but there is insatiable thirst during the heat for small amounts of water taken frequently. The time of appearance of the Rhustox chill ranges from 6:00 to 9:00 p.m. The absence of thirst in this case is typical of Rhustox and might introduce an element of doubt. However, the patient was actually thirsty but refrained from drinking because of its immediate chilling effect.

Numbness of the hands or any part of the extremities as a concomitant is more characteristic of Rhustox than it is of Arsenicum.

A single dose of Rhustox was given. For three days, there was no change. Then the chill was lighter and the fever not so high and there was less aching of the limbs. The next day, there was only a slight chill in the evening, and from then on, the symptoms gradually abated. The patient's general condition improved. By the sixth day, all symptoms had disappeared, and years have elapsed with no return.

Numerically also, the results indicate:

Ars.	23/11
Rhus-t.	31/14

See the next page for Mac Repertory graph.

CASE VIII

(Adapted from the Homoeopathic Recorder 1928)

Began with a cold.
It started after getting up in the morning to start the fire; not

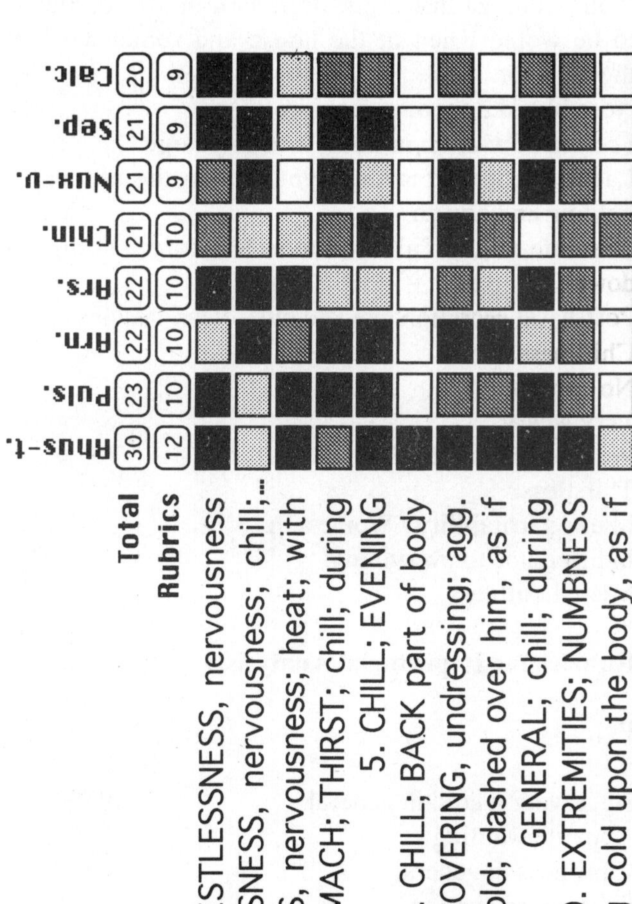

Case VII **8/1/97** **Jugal Kishore, Dr**

Analysis Options: Totality, All Remedies

	Rhus-t.	Puls.	Arn.	Ars.	Chin.	Nux-v.	Sep.	Calc.
Total	30	23	22	22	21	21	21	20
Rubrics	12	10	10	10	10	9	9	9
1. MIND; RESTLESSNESS, nervousness								
RESTLESSNESS, nervousness; chill;...								
RESTLESSNESS, nervousness; heat; with								
4. STOMACH; THIRST; chill; during								
5. CHILL; EVENING								
6. CHILL; BACK part of body								
7. CHILL; UNCOVERING, undressing; agg.								
WATER; cold; dashed over him, as if								
GENERAL; chill; during								
10. EXTREMITIES; NUMBNESS								
WIND; blowing cold upon the body, as if								
12. CHILL; DRINKING; agg.								

having a bathrobe on, became slightly chilled.
Sneezing often due to tickling in right nostril.
Watery coryza that drips, drop by drop, if not blown out. Seems to be worse when in the house and somewhat better when in the open air.
Nose blocked up on right side.
Feeling of warmth in nose, then discharge.
Lachrymation from the right eye on the second day with the tickling and coryza.
Absolute relief of all symptoms and coryza at night and on lying down.
Post-nasal secretion hawked out - clear, tasteless.
Chilliness.
No appetite.
Very weary.
Weakness in stomach.
Thirstless.
Marked irritability - Worse a.m.
Indifference to everything.
Mental dullness.

Rubrics for Repertorial Analysis **Pg.**	**Kishore Card No.**	**Kent's Rep**
Aggravation cold in general	0100	1348
Appetite wanting	0477	0479
Chilliness in general	0756	1264
Eyes, lachrymation	1386	0245
Mind and Intellect, dullness	1980	0037
Mind and Intellect, indifference(apathy)	2031	0054
Mind and Intellect, irritability	2044	0057
Nose, discharge, watery	2379	0333
Nose, itching inside	2394	0339
Nose, obstruction, one sided	2397	0341
Nose, Sneezing	2412	0350
Thirstlessness	3128	0530
Weakness (enervation)	3472	1413
Weariness	3483	1421

Remedy Analysis:

Ist Grade

1.	141	Bell.	
2.	200	Chel.	
3.	456	Nux-v.	33/15
4.	484	Phos.	33/15
5.	524	Sabad.	
6.	567	Sulph.	34/15

IInd Grade

1.	062	Agar.
2.	108	Ars.
3.	235	Con.
4.	426	Mez.
5.	444	Nat-m.
6.	450	Nit-ac.
7.	506	Puls.
8.	543	Sep.
9.	559	Staph.
10.	588	Thuj.

Nux-v. relieved the patient promptly.

See the next page for Mac Repertory graph.

CASE IX

(Adapted from the Homoeopathic Recorder 1934)

H.L., a boy seven years of age, whose maternal grandfather had died-an asthmatic sufferer, had been subjected to asthmatic attacks since eighteen months of age. There had been eczema, especially prominent on the face, when he was eight months old, which was suppressed with local applications. He has been vaccinated and 'protected' from diphtheria by the

Case VIII **8/1/97** **Jugal Kishore, Dr**

Analysis Options: Totality, All Remedies

	Sulph.	Puls.	Nux-v.	Phos.	Lyc.	Nat-m.	Sep.	Ars.	Calc.	Carb-v.	Hydrog.
Total	36	34	33	32	32	32	32	31	31	30	30
Rubrics	14	13	14	14	13	13	13	13	12	13	13
1. GENERALITIES; COLD; agg.											
2. STOMACH; APPETITE; wanting											
3. CHILL; CHILLINESS											
4. EYE; LACHRYMATION											
DULLNESS, sluggishness,...											
6. MIND; INDIFFERENCE, apathy											
7. MIND; IRRITABILITY											
8. NOSE; DISCHARGE; watery											
ITCHING, crawling and tickling;...											
OBSTRUCTION; one-sided											
11. NOSE; SNEEZING											
12. STOMACH; THIRSTLESSNESS											
WEAKNESS, enervation											
14. GENERALITIES; WEARINESS											

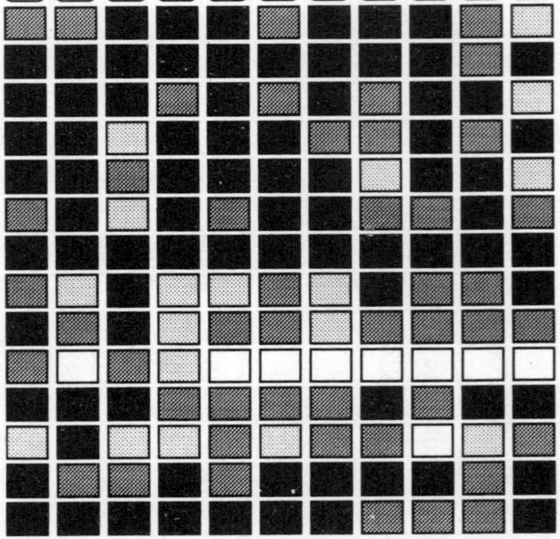

routine procedures; had received autogenous vaccine therapy for the asthma. To prove the efficacy of such treatment, he continued to grow continually worse. Then, in desperation, as a Grande finale, the tonsils and adenoids were removed. How those offending organs had escaped so long, no one seemed to know.

Every time he contracted a cold, he had an attack. Since colds were very frequent occurrences with him, one could almost always find him sneezing. With each attack, there is dry cough. Becoming overheated or bathing were frequent precipitants of cold. The asthma is worse by physical exertion, during wet weather and during cold weather. He sleeps on either side, covered lightly, occasionally trembling, jumping up or screaming during sleep; sweats freely especially about the upper parts of the body; had for over a year an ulcer on the inner surface of the left upper lid with conjunctivitis, which had been defeating constantly the efforts of a skilled ophthalmologist. The irregular teeth with notched incisors spoke of syphilis. The mother had noticed that eating tomatoes usually is followed by an outbreak of hives.

Rubrics for Repertorial Analysis:	**Kishore Card No.**	**Kent's Rep.Pg.No**
Abdomen, hypochondria.	0009	
Aggravation, air, cold.	0062	1348
Aggravation, bathing	0074	1345
Aggravation, exertion, physical	0149	1358
Aggravation, heated becoming	0184	1367
Aggravation, warm wraps	0353	1413
Aggravation, weather, wet	0362	1421
Cold, tendency to take (catching a cold easily)	0773	1349
Cough, dry	0843	0786
Eruptions, suppressed	1118	1319
Respiration, difficult	2638	0766
Sleep, restless	2910	1247
Sweat, exertion, during slightest	3033	1297
Sweat, upper parts of body	3048	1301

Remedy Analysis

Ist Grade

1.	184	Carbo-veg	27/14
2.	543	Sepia	31/14

IInd Grade

1.	156	Bryonia	30/13
2.	354	Kali-carb	30/13
3.	417	Merc-sol	22/13
4.	450	Nit-ac	25/13
5.	484	Phosphorus	25/13

IIIrd Grade

1.	393	Lycopodium	
2.	456	Nux-vomica	18/12
3.	518	Rhus-tox	24/12
4.	544	Silicea	22/12
5.	559	Staphysgaria	17/12
6.	567	Sulphur	28/12

A study of Materia Medica, pointed to Sepia as the remedy, which was given in 1M potency and repeated infrequently. The attacks of asthma stopped and the ulcer on the eyelid started disappearing.

See the next page for Mac Repertory graph.

CASE X

A case of Cancer of Soft Palate
by
Dr. J. Kishore

Mr. B.S. came to me in December, 1962 for dyspepsia.

Case IX **8/1/97** **Jugal Kishore, Dr**

Analysis Options: Totality, All Remedies

	Lyc.	Sulph.	Calc.	Kali-c.	Sep.	Bry.	Puls.	Rhus-t.	Carb-v.	Sil.	Ars.
Total	32	32	31	31	30	30	30	29	27	27	27
Rubrics	13	13	14	13	14	13	13	14	14	13	11
PAIN; general; Hypochondria											
COLD; agg.; air											
BATHING, washing; agg.											
EXERTION; physical; agg.											
HEATED, becoming											
WARM; agg.; wraps											
WEATHER; wet; agg.											
COLD; tendency to take											
9. COUGH; DRY											
ERUPTIONS; suppressed											
11. RESPIRATION; DIFFICULT											
12. SLEEP; RESTLESS											
EXERTION; slight, during											
SINGLE parts; upper part of...											

There was regurgitation of food, with lot of belching. He passed lot of flatus also. There were loud rumblings in the abdomen. The thirst was rather decreased. He loved to take more salt than others in the household. At that time, we prescribed Nat-mur which helped him for sometime. Later, Sep., Carbo-v., Nux-v., Lyc. and Nat-p. were prescribed. He was reasonably well.

In July 1965, he presented himself with a growth on the soft palate. The report of the Surgeon on 2.6.65, before the biopsy, was 'Firm swelling of the right side of the palate with ulcerating everted margins'. The biopsy had been done, and the biopsy report, dated July 1965, showed 'Pleomorphic Salivary gland Adeno-Carcinoma'.

Since the presenting symptoms were scanty and not enough for us to be any guide for selection, we took out his past history and utilized the old symptoms which were palliated but were never completely cured.

Rubrics for Repertonal Analysis:	**Kishore Card No.**	**Kent's Rep. Pg no**
1. Desire for Extra Salt	0917	0486
2. Eructations, Food (Regurgitation)	1034	0494
3. Eructations, Sour	1038	0496
4. Eructations, Eating after	4844	0491
5. Eructations, Sour, eating after	4866	0497
6. Eructations, Ineffectual & Incomplete	1031	0491
7. Indurations	1750	1367
8. Cancerous affections	0586	1346
9. Fibroid tumours	3200	1409
10. Side, right	2824	1400

Conium was the only remedy which came all-through. A reference to the Materia Medica confirmed it. He was put on Conium and the growth regressed. The cancer became silent as confirmed by the surgeons who saw him more than two years ago. There were no cervical nodes palpable. He is quite healthy, otherwise also.

In this analysis, we have utilised the peculiar combination of some particulars and some pathological generals as Boger used to do. The only uncommon general which could be used as an eliminative symptom is abnormal craving for salt.

See the next page for Mac Repertory graph.

Cases worked directly on Kent's Repertory.

Some of these cases have been reported by other workers. While repertorising, not all remedies are mentioned here but only the ones which are common to all the rubrics.

Case I

A.M., age-32.
September 30th, (An outpatient case)

Headache- vertex and eye, all his life. Getting much worse. Lasts from 3 days to 3 weeks. So severe, hardly knows what do. Worse sleep. Head very tender, can't bear being touched. Sickness last 10 hours, and vomits every 10 minutes. Always got a headache. Can't eat, therefore, very weak.

Feels well before attack. Good family history; general history also good. Burrows head in pillow. Vision good, tested lately. Tongue indented. Feels as if suffocated after eating, which greatly aggravates the headache. Averse to fats and milk.

Very sleepy at 8 p.m. Dreams exciting. Alopecia areata. < Heat; thunder; sleep. Depressed, ≤ consolation. Wants to be alone. Worse heat is used as an eliminating symptom to cut out all the cold remedies from the following lists.

Case X **8/1/97** **Jugal Kishore, Dr**

Analysis Options: Totality, All Remedies

	Phos.	Con.	Lyc.	Sil.	Nat-m.	Carb-v.	Chin.	Sulph.	Calc.	Bry.	Arg-n.
Total	25	21	19	19	19	18	18	17	17	15	15
Rubrics	10	10	9	9	8	8	8	9	8	8	7
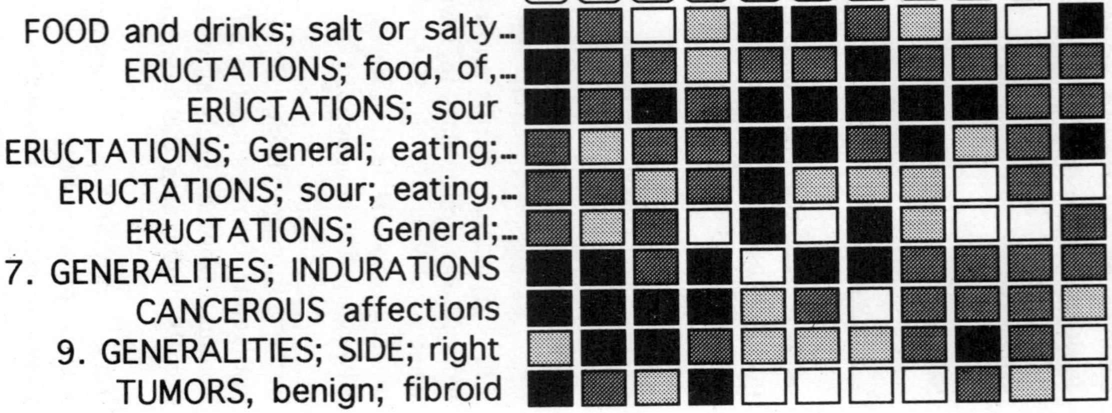 FOOD and drinks; salt or salty...											
ERUCTATIONS; food, of,...											
ERUCTATIONS; sour											
ERUCTATIONS; General; eating;...											
ERUCTATIONS; sour; eating,...											
ERUCTATIONS; General;...											
7. GENERALITIES; INDURATIONS											
CANCEROUS affections											
9. GENERALITIES; SIDE; right											
TUMORS, benign; fibroid											

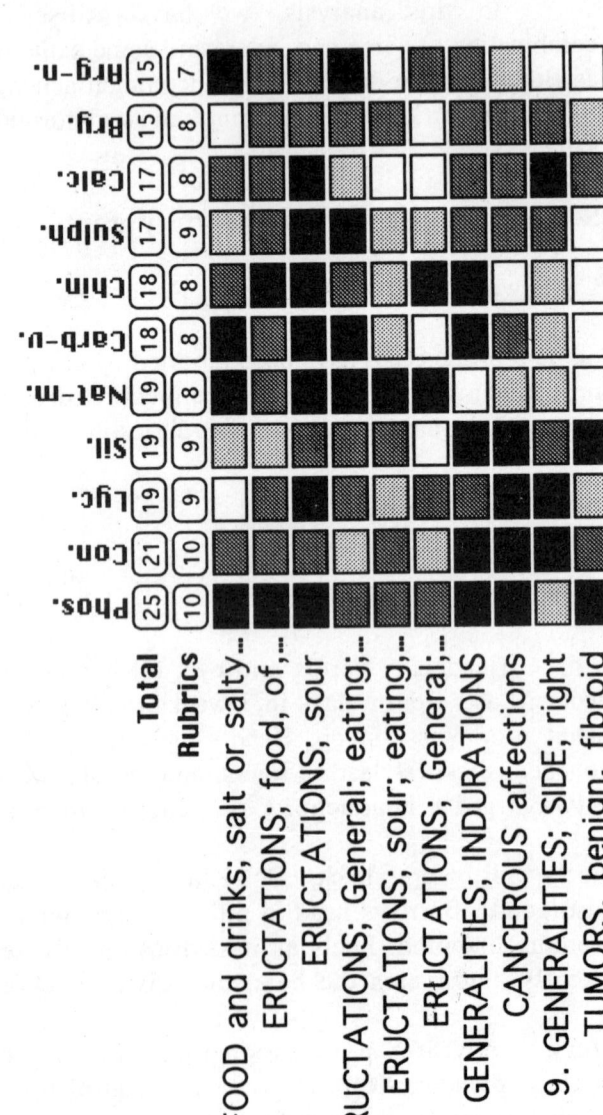

Rubric		Remedies
1. Agg. consolation (K16)	-	lyc., merc. **NAT-M.**, plat., thuj.
2. Agg. thunder, approach of (K 1403)	-	aur., bry., kali bi., lach., lyc., nat-m., puls., sulph., thuj., tub.
3. Averse to fat (K 480)	-	bry., merc., nat-m., **PTEL.**, **PULS.**, sulph.
4. Averse to milk (K 481)	-	bry., puls., sulph.
5. Headache < sleep, after (K 147)	-	arg-n., aur., bry., kali-bi., **LACH** lyc., merc., **NAT-M.**, puls., sulph., thuj.

Lach.	5/2
Lyc.	5/3
Merc.	4/3
Nat-m.	9/4
Puls.	7/4
Sulph.	7/4
Thuj.	4/3

Puls. could never come in, outruled by 'consolation' test, and by the look of patient. Leaves Nat-m. and Sulph. Aspect typical Nat-m.
Nat-m 30, 4 doses. Six hourly.

October 21st - Not been laid up with headaches for the last three weeks; and not been sick, but hardly so well in himself Has had a cold and is heavy and dull. No medicine.

November 11th - One attack threatened but passed off. If they came on before, they always laid him up for a week. He feels stronger, brighter, more heart for things. Sleep less heavy;

dreams the same. Hair the same. No medicine.

December 7th - Had bilious attack on the 3rd inst., but was not sick, only headache; same character. No medicine.

December 13th - Nat-m. 30, 6 doses 6-hourly.

Jan. 4th - Had four attacks since here, two bad. Same character. Bry. 30, six doses 3 hourly.

Remarks- It is never wise during an acute exacerbation of a chronic malady to prescribe the chronic remedy, as you are apt to increase needlessly the sufferings of your patient. Under such circumstances, one prescribes a more superficial remedy corresponding to the immediate modalities e.g. Bry. in a Nat-m. case. Bell. in a Calc. case, etc.

January 11th - Cannot eat. Though headache > Nat-m. 200, 4 doses six hourly.

February 1st - Not had an attack since here, despite heavy work, feels very well. No medicine.

March 14th - Only slight headache since here, but was able to stop at work; and right again. No medicine.

CASE 2

Miss B., aged 52. Been heavy tea drinker for 20 years; had much pain and discomfort in stomach; with flatulence immediately after eating; gradually got better till next meal; much rumbling in abdomen. Appetite poor; bowels fairly regular.

Desires - Salt, Sweets.

Averse - Fats, acids.

Flushes of heat with sweating which relieved her. She was very thin ; excitable person - a bundle of nerves. On further inquiry she was found to be very chilly.

Generals-

Very Chilly. < Spring < Before and during thunderstorm.
Irritable in morning.
Anxiety for others.
Fears. Burglars; something going to happen; crowds; being suffocated, and therefore, in tunnel.
Impatient.
Suspicious.
Very sensitive, readily offended, startled easily with least noise.

Chilly Patient - Used as Eliminating symptom; only chilly remedies are given in the following lists-

Fear, something will happen (K 45)	-	alum., ars., calc., carb-v., **CAUST**., graph., kali-ar., kali-p., mag-c., mang., nat-a., **PHOS.**
Fear, robbers (K 47)	-	alum., **ARS**., bell., con., ign., mag-c., nat-c., phos., sil., zinc.
Fear, darkness (K 43)	-	calc., camph., carb-an., carb-v., caust., rhus-t., **STRAM**., stront., valer.
Fear, suffocation (K 47)	-	carb-an., phos., stram.
Fear, crowd (K 43).	-	aloe, ars., bar-c., calc., carb-an., caust., con., ferr., graph., hep., kali-ar., kali-bi., kali-c., kali-p., nat-a., nux-v., phos., plb., rhus-t., stann
Anxiety for others (K 7)	-	ars., bar-c., cocc., phos.

Suspicious (K 85)	-	**ARS.,** aur., **BAR-C.,** bar-m., bell., bor., calc-p., carb-s., canth., **CAUST**., cham., chin., cocc., con., graph., hell., hyos., **KALI-AR.,** kali-p. mur-ac., nat-a., nat-c., nit-ac., nux-v., phos., plb., **RHUS-T.,** ruta, sep., sil., stann., staph., **STRAM.,** sul-ac., viol-t.
Offended readily (K 69).	-	agar., alum., ars., aur., bor., calc., camph., caps., calc-s., carb-v., caust., cham., chel., chin., chin-a., cocc., cycl., graph., **NUX-V**., petr., phos., ran-b., sars., sep., spig., stram., zinc.
Storm, approach of a, agg. (K 1403)	-	agar., aur., caust., hyper., kali-bi., nat-c., nit-ac., petr., phos., **PSOR., RHOD.,** rhus-t., sep., sil.
Spring, in, agg. (K1361)	-	aur., bar-m., bell., calc., carb-v., chel., colch., dulc., hep., kali-bi., nux v., rhus-t., sars., sep., sil.
Averse fats (K 480).	-	ars., bell., calc., carb-an., carb-v., **CHIN.,** chin-a., colch., cycl., hep., nat-c., **PETR.,** phos., rheum., rhus-t., sep.

Averse acids (K 480)	-	bell., cocc., ferr., ign., nux-v., ph-ac., sabad.
Desire salt. (K 486).	-	calc., calc-p., **CARB-V.**, caust., cocc., con., nit-ac., **PHOS.**, plb.
Desire Sweets. (K 488).	-	am-c., arg-m., ars., bar-c., calc., carb-v., **CHIN.**, chin-a., kali-ar., kali-c., kali-p., nat-c., nux-v., petr., plb., rheum., rhus-t. sabad., sep.

Remarks: The chief remedies running through the case are Ars., Calc., Caust, Nat-c., Nux-v., Phos., Rhus-t., Sep.

Ars.	16/8
Calc.	13/8
Caust.	14/7
Nat-c.	8/5
Nux-v.	9/6
Phos.	19/10
Rhus-t.	12/7
Sep.	11/6

The constitution of the patient suggested either Ars. or Phos.

We have thus come to these two remedies by only considering the general symptom of the patient.

The pain in stomach was > hot drinks; even wine, which suits her generally, had to be given up owing to its coldness, and as Phos. patients crave cold drinks (even ice) in gastric troubles, we are left with Ars.

Ars. 30- 3 doses at six hourly intervals.

Pain > (which had been present for years) in a few days, and in a few weeks she was almost well, being much less excitable.

This case shows the importance of Generals in their order- mental, climatic, desires and aversions in food; all of which must be markedly present to be of any value.

Case 3

Girl of 23. Ill five days. Sore (red) throat; tongue dirty; aching all over; alternatively hot and cold; heavy and tired; ill. Temp. (at 11.30 a.m.) 100°F.
Headache "thumpy". Thirsty. Desire for hot milk.
Aversion to sweet things (usually "adores sugar"). Sweet things make her feel sick.
She is worse from motion.
The case was quickly worked out, in the following way, on its peculiar features, neglecting those that belonged to "flu" and fever in general, and taking only those peculiar to this individual, sick and feverish; but novel and unusual with her.

All so marked and so new that only symptoms in black type and in italics were considered.

Aversion to sweets (K 482)	-	ars., caust., **GRAPH.,** merc., phos., sulph., zinc.,
Nausea from sweets (K 510)	-	arg-n., **GRAPH.,** ip.
Desire for hot milk (K 485)	-	calc., chel., graph., hyper.

So she got a prescription that would never have occurred to one, viz. Graphites 10M., given on the spot. In half an hour, while she was still under observation, her skin felt cooler, it had lost the feverish feel; pulse was better, and temperature had already dropped to 99.4 °F. The next day, she got two doses of Graph. 50M. And the following night she was met at a big reception, perfectly well.

The name of the disease is really of little use in prescribing - unless to a routinist - and it is a great temptation to drop into routine. It may or may not take you to a group of remedies; not even that, in this case seldom to one.

Do justice to yourself and to Homoeopathy, and in acute sickness, do not be content with palliation. Get down on it, and cure, and in order to cure (not merely palliate), one must treat not a disease-name, but the patient.

Too much trouble - in a minor illness like the above? But does not humanity demand of us that we shall take trouble? Is it not our mission in life? - and is it not what we undertook when the right to treat sickness was bestowed upon us?

Case 4

Ernest H., aged 9. Sept. 14th, 1926.

For last 5,6 years gets bilious every six weeks regularly.
Suffers with "nerves" also.
Fear of going to school, of going out to play, of the dark,
Must have a light all night.
Bad headaches - has to lie down.
Restless. Always on the fidget.
Attacks begin with nausea; then sudden vomiting of green stuff.
Lies two or three days like that, quite light-headed and feverish.
Perspires a lot during the attacks.

Always drinking water, if ill; drinks a few mouthfuls often.
Bowels act while vomiting.
Worked out on Characteristic Symptoms.

Rectum-involuntary stool during vomiting (K 622) - Arg-n., Ars.

Stomach Thirst for small quantities (K 529) - **ARS**., chin., hell., lach., **LYC.,** rhus-t., sulph.

Gen.-Periodicity (of above) (K 1390) - **ARS., CHIN.,** lyc., rhus-t., sulph.

Restless (K 72) - **ARG-N., ARS.,** chin., **LYC., RHUS-T., SULPH.**

Green vomit (K 538) - arg-n., **ARS**., lyc.

Fear dark (K 43) - lyc.

Vomiting during headache (K 533) - arg-n., ars.,

Anxiety with fear (K 6) - **ARS.** (most fearful and anxious of all drugs)

Rx Ars 200 one dose.

November1 Much Better. Sick only once, two days ago, with no headache. 'No-after-effects', soon over. No feverishness, no sweating. And this attack came on at 7th instead of 6th week, and he only vomited once. Placebo.

November 30 Much better. No attacks. Less nervy; less fear of school, and getting on better there. No headaches, no nausea, less thirst, last night asked for light to be put out, as he could not go to sleep. So much better. Placebo.

Jan No attacks at all, only that one slight one. No headaches. 'They used to be so terrible". Placebo.

He never came again. Apparently cured of these attacks of years by the one dose of Ars. 200.

Comments- Ars. in the Repertory is not one of the drugs that has caused fear in the dark; but fitting the patient, it cured that also.

Case 5

G.G., two years and nine months.

Constipated all her life. "Intussusception nine months ago, just escaped operation".

Every six or seven weeks gets attacks of sickness and prostration, goes off food and only wants to drink water.
Weak: likes to be carried. Ankles turn. Only walked very late, at two years.
Does not feel the cold.
Not fond of fuss or affection.
Better and happier out of doors; more "whining" in the house.
Fear in the dark.
Stools lienteric.

Fear dark (K 43) - acon., calc., camph., **CANN-I.**, carb-an., carb-v., cupr., lyc., med., phos., puls., **STRAM.**, stront.

Better open air (K 1344) - acon., camph., **CANN-I.**, lyc., phos., **PULS.**

Stools lienteric (K 638) - **CALC.**, lyc., **PHOS.**

Does not feel the cold is against calc., and phos.

Does not like fuss (lyc.)

We are left with Lyc.

June 21 - Lyc. 1M one dose. Plac.
July 5 Is very well. Bowels act once a day. Plac.
September 13 Going on well. Plac.
October 4 "Better every way. Bowels have been acting naturally every day except yesterday; right again today".
Appetite better. Stools not lienteric.
And she had no attacks of sickness.

Little typical cases to show how they may be worked out, and with what result.

Case 6

Nov 14
O.M, 14 yrs. Out-patient.
A year ago vomited blood (like "liver").
Nose bleeds easily and much bright red blood
Headaches 9 a.m. after rising. Shooting in forehead; better when moving about;
< 3 p.m > lying > in the dark.
Menstrual pain. Ist last week a mere spot. Pain like a knife three days before flow. Appetite good, "eats too much". Thirst for cold water.
Desires salt, fat, sweets, sugar, sours.
Worse hot weather; is never cold.
"Hysterical"; gets excited when playing.
Irritable; likes sympathy. Fear alone; in the dark.
And all the hysteria you want, gives you Arg. (Its rivals here (in desire for salt, desire for sweets), Calc., Carb-v., Plb. are chilly).

She got Arg-n. 30.

December 13 Looks better. "Dysmenorrhoea much better". Placebo.
Feb 28 "Very much better. No nose bleed or vomiting. Been at business one month. More steady; not hysterical now".

(More elaborately worked out.

Desire for sugar (K 486)	-	am-c., **ARG-N**., calc., kali-c., sec.
Desire for salt (K 486)	-	**ARG-N**., calc.
For cold drinks (K 484)	-	arg-n., calc.
Vomiting (K 531) (a huge rubric but contains)	-	**ARG-N**., calc.
Heat, sensation of (K 1366) (same applies)	-	arg-n.
Fear if alone (K 43) (same applies)	-	**ARG-N**., calc.
Excitable (K 40) (same applies)	-	**ARG-N**., calc.
Hysteria (K 52) (same applies)	-	arg-n.
Menses scanty (K 728) (same applies)	-	arg-n., calc.
Nose bleed (K 335)	-	arg-n., **CALC.**

Comments- Arg-n. does not come out in high type for nose bleed; but it not only steadied her up mentally, but cured nose bleed too.

Case 7

Mrs. E.L ., 45 came to Out Patient on March 12,1931.

Indigestion 9 or 10 years.

Pain "across waist" ; dull; lasts some hours.
Better for "hot ginger", goes in two hours.
Gets this three or four times a week. Never vomits. Costive.
Worse stews, bacon, fried foods.
Not hungry; thirst for hot drinks; worse cold drinks.
Very nervy; anticipation.
Hates sympathy; cries easily; particular; fastidious.
Fears thunder. Fear for others.
Worse cheese.
Desire oranges; lemonade; drinks it hot, etc.
Examination negative.
Worked out quickly, on the more characteristic symptoms, as below:

Fastidious (K 42)	ars., nux-v.
Anxiety for others (K 7)	ars., phos., sulph.
Stomach pain< cold drinks (K 512)	**ACON., ARS.,** calc-ar., calc-p., caust., ferr-ar., graph., iris., manc., **RHUS-T.,** sul-ac., (and a few others in lowest type, not taken)
Desire for lemonade (K 485)	**BELL.,** jatr., nit-ac., sabin., sul-i. (a few more in lowest type)
Desire warm drinks (K 486)	**ARS., BRY.,** calad., chel., hyper., **LAC-C,** lyc., sabad,, sulph.
Gen. Food, cheese, old, agg (K 1362)	ars., bry., ptel., rhus-t. (a couple more in low type)
Anxiety (K 4)	**ARS.**

The most typical characteristics of Ars. are restlessness and anxiety. So she was given Ars. 10M.

April 9 Much better. No medicine.
May "Much better, digestion improving. Appetite better. No medicine."
July 30 "Been very well; medicine did more good than anything she had ever had."
But pain recurring a little. Rx Ars. 10M.
In October she again needed repeat for "Digestion less well 4 or 5 weeks". And she got a repeat in May 1933, November 1934, Feb. 1935 and Feb. 1936 for "sleeping badly and nervy". To keep her well, she seems to have needed her Ars. repeated six times in six years.

Comments - Arsenic does not come into the rubric "worse from storms" (thunder). Had one started with that, and taken through only those drugs, one would have missed her remedy. Maybe, we should include Ars. also being aggravated by storm in our Repertory.

Case 8

A pathetic looking wee girl, of three years and eight months was brought to Hospital on April 19th 1934. Big, eyes - the note is "all eyes".

Measles last month.
Sits and cries for nothing. Likes petting.
Jealous of other children, won't play with them: won't talk to them at school. Jealous of her father, because he talks to her mother. Likes to be made a fuss of. Likes her mother to fuss over her.
Can't walk upstairs.
Not hungry; not thirsty; won't drink.
May go all day without passing urine.
"May sleep practically all day and night for two days; then all right for a fortnight."
"Sits and weeps for nothing; likes petting; jealous; shy; not

hungry and not thirsty" means pulsatilla, and nothing else.

Rx Puls. 12 t.d.s. for a few days.

May 17,1934 "Wonderful. Goes to school; they do not know what has happened to her. Walks better; eats better; plays better; a different child entirely. Everybody says 'What a difference' - completely altered."

Rx Placebo.

"Is still jealous of her father and the baby, but plays with the other children in the Square. Would not go out of the house before; now goes out and plays".

Betty is no longer "all eyes". She is laughing and playful. (We will work it out, with jealousy and desire for sympathy as the important mentals which must be there.)

Consolation amel. (K 16) - puls.

Jealousy (K 60) - apis., calc-p., calc-s., coff., **HYOS.**, ign., **LACH.**, nux-v., op., ph-ac., puls., stram.

Causeless weeping (K 93) - **APIS., PULS.**

Timidity (K 88) - nux-v., puls., stram.

Bladder, urination, seldom (K 661) - nux-v., puls., stram.

Stomach, appetite, wanting (K 479) - **NUX-V., PULS.**

Stomach, thirstless (K 530) - **PULS.**

Several other drugs have 'vomiting during stool'.

Case 9

A Mental Case [Paranoia]

She was 60 and she and her husband, who supplied much of the information were very much distressed about her condition.

First seen October, 1932.
"Bad Headaches for years" "B.P. high".
Delusions of persecution. "People spreading tales about her". "The effect of a doctor's injections": or "a friend affecting her by spiritualism".
Very miserable, cries or is violent about it.
Suspicious; "that people played a game on her";
"Very hurt that people friendly should have done her that".

"Was suspicious of husband whether he was joining in the conspiracy; is still so at times; as if he were giving her something."

"Wants revenge on those people"

There are many less important symptoms, which were neglected for the outstanding mental ones; these had to be in the picture.

Suspicious (K 85)	-	anac., bell., dros., **LACH.**, merc.
Delusions, persecuted, that he is (K 30)	-	**DROS.**.
Revengeful (K 63)	-	anac., bell., lach.
Worse windy weather(K 1422)	-	bell., lach.
Head, Pain vertex (K 171).	-	anac., bell., dros., lach., merc.
Fear, poisoned, of being (K 46)	-	lach.

Rx Lach. 12, 30, 1M on three successive days with placebo.

Nov "Brighter. Can go through her troubles better." Rx Placebo.
Dec "Feeling better. Not dwelling on her worries - no use!" No pain at root of nose now. Rx Placebo.

Jan 1933 Better, till a cold. Less depressed.
Suspicious? "Has given it up" - "It was all true, but I have put all that away". She got Pulsatilla for a stye, etc.
March Headaches again. Flushes. But better, and nerves stronger. "It comes up now and again; but she stands it better." Rx Lach. 12, 30, 1M again.
July. Not so well since the hot weather. B.P. up again. A pressing, sides of neck. Irritation and cough if anything touches throat (a peculiar lach. symptom). Flushes started again.
Repeat Lach.
August. "Better; but the hot weather! swimmy and headachy! Head feels double the size." Lach. 6, 12, 30.

1934 July (11 months later)-"A lot better and very grateful."
1935 January (when last seen) "Comes for eyes".
"Has not come for one & a half years, been so very much better". Appears quite normal; never once mentions her mental complaints. Neck feels full, and B.P. high. Repeat Lach. and Plac.

Comments- Lachesis did not come through nearly all her symptoms; probably ill-marked ones and elicited in response to questions; but it had the important mentals and it made life worth living for herself- and her husband.

Case 10

ASTHMA

Miss X., 50. Nov 19, 1928.

Asthma began last winter.

Two years ago a doctor had advised injections for frequent colds - three injections three days apart. After the second, was dreadfully ill with a high temperature. "Never asthma before this". (The patient was filling an important post, and the asthma was interfering with her work. She was sent by a nurse in one of the big hospitals, who had been cured of the same complaint.)

She had great number of very definite symptoms, chiefly qualified particulars, and this is how the remedy was arrived at.

Rubric		Remedies
Respiration, difficult, sitting, upright amel. (K 771)	-	**KALI-c.**, lach., laur., lyc., seneg., sulph., ter.
Respiration, difficult, sitting, with head bent forward on knees amel. (K 771)	-	coc-c., **KALI-C.**
Respiration, difficult, lying, while(K 769)	-	**KALI-C.**, lach., lyc., seneg., sulph.
Chest, perspiration, axillae (K 878)	-	**KALI-C.**, lach., **SULPH.**
Extremities, perspiration, feet (K 1183)	-	kali-c., **LYC.**, **SULPH.**
Extremities, perspiration, toes, between (K 1184)	-	kali-c., lyc.
Extremities, Pain, foot, heel (K 1080)	-	kali-c., lyc., sulph.

Chest, oppression (K 838)	-	**KALI-C.**, lyc., **S E N E G.**, **SULPH.**
Sleep, Dreams of the dead (K 1237)	-	kali-c., lyc., sulph.
Gen. worse from cold (K 1348)	-	**KALI-C.**, **LYC.**, sulph.
Gen. worse, air, draft of (K 1344)	-	**KALI-C.**, lach., lyc., **SULPH**
Gen. Wet feet (K 1421)	-	dulc.
Gen. bathing agg. (K 1345)	-	kali-c., lyc., **SULPH**

Rx Kali carb. 6, 12, 30, one each morning for three days followed by Placebo.

December 19- "Wonderfully better: even black fog had no effect on her". Two slight attacks only. (She was having them very frequently and much more severely). She "had two years' treatment, but never derived benefit like this". Oppression in chest gone. Can lie on either side now, not quite flat. Pain heel gone (she "had had to lie up with it"). Sweats much less. Rx Placebo.

Next heard of in December 3, 1932 (four years later). Sends another asthma patient and the message, that she "had never had an attack since coming here".

This is an interesting analysis because most of the symptoms are particular in character. There is hardly any mental symptoms to help us, but a few generals were all to help the diagnosis.

But this case could not be analysed on Boenninghausen's Repertory.

Case 11

B.S., male aged 7 and a half years.

May 31- Cough since a baby. At five months had broncho-pneumonia, and cough ever since; Cut his teeth with bronchitis.

"Any chill means bronchitis".

Practically always coughing. May go a week, or fourteen days, then a slight chill, and coughing starts again.

Coughs in sleep. Mother says, she lies awake, worrying. "When will that child get to sleep then goes in to find him fast asleep, coughing. Coughs on lying down, and generally all night."

Exam. of chest proved negative.

Likes warmth; worse for cold.

Worse cloudy weather. "Used to cry for the sun" (a strange, rare and peculiar symptom in a small boy). "He practically lived in the garden till school; then dropped".

Eats and sleeps well; likes fuss. Restless; cries easily. Jealous of the cat and dog.

The peculiar symptoms were taken-

Cough during sleep (K 804) - acon., agar., apis., arn., bell., **CHAM.**, **LACH.**, petr., rhus-t., sulph.

Gen. cloudy weather agg. (K 1348) - cham., **RHUS-T.**, sulph.

Restless at night (K 72) - apis., **RHUS-T**.,
(a huge rubric but contains) **SULPH.**

Jealous (K 60) - apis., **LACH.**

'Wants warmth and is worse for cold' is against Apis, Lach. and Sulph. Rhus-t. has 'takes cold easily'.

He got a dose of Rhus-t. CM and the cough improved.

On Sept. 26 he was brought, with a doctor's letter, 'pain in abdomen, was it perhaps appendix?'

Pain was at umbilicus; doubled him up. Coloc. 200 three doses ended that.

His mother said that, since Rhus-t. four months ago, he had never again coughed. That his neighbours asked, what has become of that boy's cough? They missed it. "It is marvelous".

It is marvelous how a few peculiar symptoms, peculiar to the patient and not common to his malady, will often provide the key to the magical remedy.

Case 12

ASTHMA

Sept 10,1929 - Mrs. C., 44 years old, came to out-patients with the complaint of Asthma for the last eight years. Gradually getting worse.

Very frequent attacks. Says she has an attack every 14 days, which keeps her in bed; then a few days free; then another attack.

Tonsils removed 2-3 months ago. "Never well since," and no improvement in asthma.

Her cough worse 3-4 a.m.
Sputum frothy - lumps of jelly - stringy phlegum.

She presented a beautiful picture of Puls.

Irritable (K 58) - **PULS.**

Mood, changeable (K 68) - **PULS.**

Weeping alternating with laughter (K 93) - puls.

Company, desire for, alone, while agg. (K 12) - puls.

Fears dark (K 43) - puls.

Fear of death (K 44) - puls.

Suspicious (K 85) - **PULS.**
("People thinking something about her")

Stomach- aversion to fat (K 480) - **PULS**.

Sleep, Dreams of cats (K 1237) - puls. (for Puls. is even one of the 10 drugs that have evoked dreams of cats).

Soon on Sept 10, 1929 she got Puls.10 M one dose and then Placebo.

In a month (October 10) "Much better. One attack only, and was able to be about". Rx Placebo.

Another month (December 12). One attack this month - after getting wet. One might have repeated? ... but she got Placebo.

January 1930. Less well. Threat of Asthma. More sputum. So Rx Puls. 10 M. Her second dose.

Seen in Feb, March, April, May, June and June, 1931, and still no Asthma. Says she is "Splendid. Was a perfect wreck when she came here." She had only needed two doses of PULS. 10 M in a couple of years.

(As seen above, this little out-patient case was typically Pulsatilla to any one who realized that remedy. It only needed to look up a couple of points, but we will work it out.

Rubric		Remedies
Suspicious (K 85)	-	**ACON**., calc-p., calc-s., **CANN-I**., **LYC.,** phos., **PULS**., **RHUS-T.,** **STRAM.**
Fear of dark (K 44)	-	acon., calc-p., calc-s., **CANN-I**., lyc., phos., puls., rhus-t., **STRAM.**
Mood changeable (K 68) (a big rubric but contains)	-	acon., calc-s., **LYC**., phos., **PULS**., stram.
Weeping causeless (K 93)	-	lyc., **PULS**.
Company, desire for. alone, while agg. (K 12)	-	calc-p., **LYC.**, **PHOS.**, puls., stram.
Fear of death (K 44)	-	**ACON**., calc-s., cann-i., lyc., **PHOS.,** puls., rhus-t., stram.
Stomach, Aversion to fat (K 480)	-	phos., **PULS**., rhus-t.
Sleep, Dreams of cats (K 1237)	-	puls.
Respiration, Asthma (K 763)	-	acon., lyc., phos., **PULS.,** **STRAM.**

Expectoration, Frothy (K 815) - acon., phos., puls., stram.

Expectoration, Viscid (K 820) - acon., calc-s., lyc., **PHOS., PULS.**, rhus-t.

The above cases illustrate not only the way in which the remedy may be determined by the help of the Repertory, but they also tend to confirm the Doctrines of Hahnemann, viz-

Covering the totality of the characteristic symptoms,
The single remedy,
The potentized remedy,
The unit dose,
Long duration of reaction, to correct the vital stimulus,
Non-interference with reaction,
Repetition only when symptoms tend to return, i.e. again demand the remedy.

Comments- Once again, in regard to the grading of symptoms, which we may call perspective in prescribing.

Dr. ERASTUS CASE. U.S.A., says in his wonderful book of 'Cases'-

"Symptoms are often conflicting, and a host in number-
peculiar to constitution of the patient,
resultant from former disease,
pathological,
sympathetic,
result of diseased conditions,
due to action of drugs,
purely imaginary."

"We are taught to give the remedy that has produced all the symptoms of the patient"

Case 13

Malaria - Arsenicum.

October 12, 1918.

Malaria in Palestine, 1918 and occasionally since; quinine sometimes. He took much quinine when out there, before he got malaria.

If tired, gets attacks. They go on with intermissions for some days. Recur whenever tired.

Gets very hot, then sweats. (No rigor)
Sleeping badly; tosses; cannot get comfortable.
Very thirsty during and after the sweats.
Had also amoebic dysentery, with blood and straining. At times this also recurs. Was sent home with a badly wounded knee.

Frontal headache, worse after malaria.
It is better lying, but he can not rest.
Walks about; Very restless; "If out, wants to be in; if in, wants to be out."

"Always wants to be doing something else".

Head splits when singing: it feels top-heavy.
Likes company. Very depressed. At times nervous when alone.
Aversion to fats. Desire for sweets.
Feels the cold lately.

Now, for the prolonged effects of malaria and quinine, a limited number of drugs have proved especially helpful. We will take these-

Fever, intermittent (K 1288) - apis., **ARS.**, **CALC.**, carb-v, **FERR.**, ferr-ar., lach., **NAT-M.**, nux-v., phos., sep., **SULPH.**

Gen, Quinine, abuse of (K 1397)	-	apis., ars., **CALC.**, **CARB-V.**, **FERR.**, ferr-ar., lach., **NAT-M.**, nux-v., phos., sep., sulph.
Fear of being alone (K 43)	-	apis, **ARS.**, calc., nux-v., **PHOS.**, sep.
Depressed ("sadness") (K 75)	-	apis, **ARS.**, **CALC.**, nux-v., phos., **SEP.**
Thirst during perspiration (K 529)	-	calc., sep.
Thirst after perspiration (K 529)	-	nux-v.
Rectum, Dysentery (K 616)	-	**ARS.**, **NUX-V.**, **PHOS.**
Stomach, Aversion to fats (K 480)	-	ars., calc., carb-v., nat-m., phos., sep., sulph.
Stomach, Desire for sweets (K 486)	-	ars., calc., carb-v., nat-m., sep., SULPH.
Hates fuss("Consolation agg")(K 16)	-	ars., calc., **SEP.**

But, without working the case out, the mentality, intense restlessness, can not lie still; if out, wants to be in; if in, wants to be out; suggests Ars. and nothing else. He got Ars. 1M one dose.

The very next night "Slept soundly and wanted to get up after six hours sleep for the first time for months. Headache gone."

He has never (1936) had any more malaria; but in 1929, tired and depressed, with a bout of restlessness, the Arsenicum was repeated, and put him right again; and once since.

What great results may follow one tiny stimulus; but it must be stimulus. Nothing else will do.

Earlier most of the cases recorded were contributed by other well known clinicians, so that the readers are given unprejudiced record of analysis of cases. Now I am giving below a few cases worked out in our own clinic, which have been given in brief but all the essential elements have been included. These are intended to show that often we are not able to prescribe the remedy without the help of the repertorial analysis and the emergence of the selected remedy could not be thought of.

CASE NO. I

A case of Neurodermatits

Miss V.L., aged 43 years , visited us in May 1983. She complained of dryness and itching of skin for the last 30 years. There was history of grief on account of her father's death. It was worse in the right elbow.

Itching was more on exposed parts. Itching was so violent that she scratched till the surface was raw. Itching was aggravated in summer; draft of air; from mental tension; .warm drinks; at night; heat of sun; hot air and better after cold bath; and covering.

She was a very chilly patient. Despite that, she had a strong desire for cold drinks and food.

She was of a tense and dominating temperament. Very irritable and indecisive. Desired to be alone

There was a past history of Filaria.

In the family, father and his brothers and sisters had Diabetes. Mother had history of Ascitis and Filaria; and her sister is suffering from Diabetes and Hypertension.

The skin on right elbow was dry and hyperpigmented.

The case was analysed on the Kishore Cards and also compared with Kentian analysis.

	Kishore Cards	Kent's Rep.
Side right	2824	1400
Agg. in sun	0306	1404
Agg. from emotional excitement	0133	0040
Agg. on uncovering	0331	1410
Agg. grief and sorrow	0136	0050
Skin Itching worse at night	7763	1327
Skin Itching, must scratch till raw	2877	1328
Irritable	2044	0057
Amel. cold bath	3817	1346

I Grade - Puls.
II Grade - Agar., Arn., Caust., Graph., Merc.

Pulsatilla 200 unit dose was given. By July 1983, she had improved to a great extent. Within this period, she was given Pulsatilla 200 unit doses 3 times.

Comments : In this, there was no single symptom which could be used as the eliminative symptom. Here the modalities were utilised for discovering the simillimum.

Here, the physical generals were much more marked and did not take the risk of imbalancing the rubrics for Repertorisation, by taking mentals regarding desire to be alone and dominating character etc., as they were not well marked symptoms.

Miss V.L.'s case could be cited under Boenninghausen concepts or Boger's Boenninghausen, as we did not take into account the mentals but depended on well-marked physical general. Very often, marked physical generals are of greater importance than so called Mentals, where one is likely to mis-interpret or elicit properly the symptoms from the patient.

The difference in grading of remedies is due to the fact that in Kishore cards, certain remedies have been known to have symptoms which were not listed in Kent. These have been later additions.

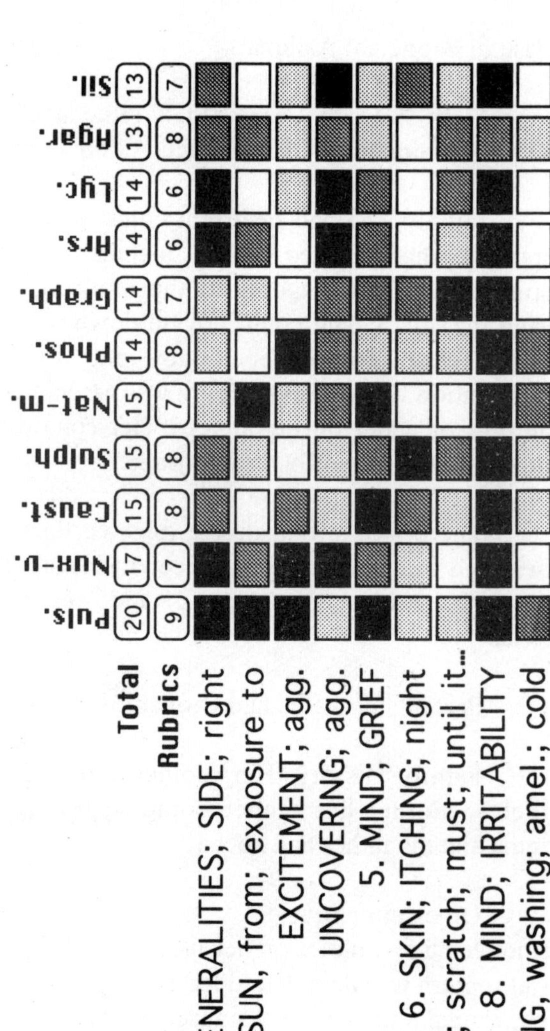
C-1
8/8/97
Jugal Kishore, Dr
Analysis Options: Totality, All Remedies
Total
Rubrics
Puls. 20 9
Nux-v. 17 7
Caust. 15 8
Sulph. 15 8
Nat-m. 15 7
Phos. 14 8
Graph. 14 7
Ars. 14 6
Lyc. 14 6
Agar. 13 8
Sil. 13 7
1. GENERALITIES; SIDE; right
SUN, from; exposure to
EXCITEMENT; agg.
UNCOVERING; agg.
5. MIND; GRIEF
6. SKIN; ITCHING; night
ITCHING; scratch; must; until it...
8. MIND; IRRITABILITY
BATHING, washing; amel.; cold

CASE NO. 2

A Case of Bronchial Asthma

Miss P.V., 21 years old, visited us first in February 1983, with complaints of Bronchial Asthma of 7 years duration.

Initialy, she had recurrent colds but during the last few years, she had started having asthmatic attacks. She had dyspnoea which was worse in the morning at about 3 A.M. During the attack, she could not lie down and felt better while sitting, better in the open air and after warm drinks. Expectoration was difficult. There was associated thirst for small quantities of water during attacks. Her condition was worse in winters and from cold foods and drinks.

There is a strong desire for sweets. She is very chilly patient and catches cold easily. Feet and hands remain cold. She is irritable and weepy, cannot stand contradiction. Fear of crowds.

Past History- She had Bronchitis at 2 years of age

Family History- Her mother's brother has asthma and diabetes, mother has diabetes and hypertension. Father had eczema and his father had kochs.

On examination-
We noticed a few moles on her face.
Nasal septum was deviated to left side.
Right frontal and maxillary sinuses were tender.
Chest auscultation showed bilateral ronchi.
X-Ray of chest showed emphysematous condition.

Treatment- She was given Silicea 200, Morning an Bedtime for 4 days. Medicine gave temporary relief. Then her case was analysed with the following symptoms,

	Kishore Cards	Kent's Rep
Irritable	2044	0057
Weeping mood	2182	0092
Contradiction, Intolerance of	1941	0016
Fear of crowd	1992	0043
Respiration difficult Agg. morning	7513	0767
Respiration difficult Agg. lying	2642	0769
Agg. winter	0372	1422
Agg. 3 A.M.	3719	1343
Agg. cold food and drinks	0164	1362
Amel. warm drinks	3825	1364
Expectoration difficult	1170	0815
Desire for sweets	0919	0486

I Grade - Nux-v.
II Grade - Ars. , Lyc.

She was prescribed Nux vomica 30, three times a day. She was kept on the same prescription till May 1983, as she reported to be much better. The chest was clear on later visits. After May, she had an attack again. On examination there were occassional ronchi in the chest. Left maxillary area was tender. She also complained of ear blockage. This time, she was given Nux Vomica 200 unit dose, followed by placebo morning & bedtime for a month. She was very soon free of the attacks. In July, her chest X-Ray was clear and sinuses were no more tender.

C-2 **8/8/97** **Jugal Kishore, Dr**

Analysis Options: Totality, All Remedies

	Lyc.	Ars.	Sulph.	Nux-v.	Puls.	Kali-c.	Sep.	Rhus-t.	Sil.	Bry.
Total	29	27	26	25	25	24	24	23	20	20
Rubrics	12	12	13	13	11	11	11	9	11	10
1. MIND; IRRITABILITY										
2. MIND; WEEPING, tearful mood										
CONTRADICTION; intolerant of										
4. MIND; FEAR; crowd; in a										
DIFFICULT; morning										
DIFFICULT; lying, while										
SEASONS; Winter; agg.										
MIDNIGHT; after; three am.										
FOOD and drinks; cold; food; agg.										
FOOD and drinks; cold; drinks,...										
FOOD and drinks; warm; drinks;...										
12. EXPECTORATION; DIFFICULT										
FOOD and drinks; sweets; desires										

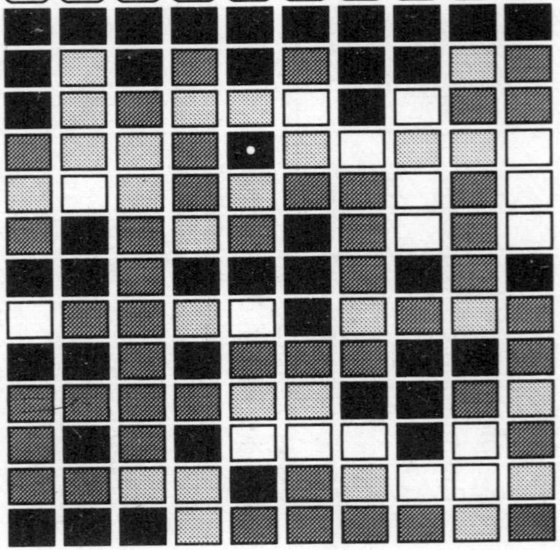

CASE NO. 3

A Case of Bronchial Asthma

Mr. A.B., 26 years old, suffered from Bronchial Asthma for the last 9 years. He first visited us in May 1983. An attack is brought on by dust, strong smell, sudden change of temperature. He is worse in winters. The attack gets worse around midnight, worse from movement. Better sitting up and in open air.

He is a chilly patient and his foot sweat is offensive. He likes to be alone and is averse to sympathy.

In the past, he has suffered from Jaundice, Chronic tonsillitis and Sinusitis.

One of his father's sister had Leukaemia and the other sister had Diabetes.

On examination there were ronchi in the chest.

The case was repertorised taking the following symptoms into account-

	Kishore Cards	Kent's Rep
Difficult Respiration - Agg. night	7516	0767
Difficult Respiration - Agg. in open air	7519	0768
Asthmatic breathing from taking cold	7503	0764
Difficult Respiration - Agg. from dust	7527	0769
Difficult Respiration - Amel. sitting	7551	0771
Agg. change of weather	0355	1347
Agg. change of temperature	0091	1347
Agg. winter	0372	1422
Agg. consolation	0108	0016
Indisposed to talk	2155	0086
Chilliness	0756	1264

I Grade- Nux-v. II Grade- Ars. III Grade- Graph.

After a week of Nux Vomica 30 repeatedly, she was much better. There were hardly any ronchi in the chest. In July and August, he again had mild attacks of asthma which were relieved after Kali-p and Mag-p in 3X. Later Nux-v 200, a single dose, followed by placebo, held the case for a long time. Then again, another unit dose of Nux-v 200 was given. The patient never had any attacks after this.

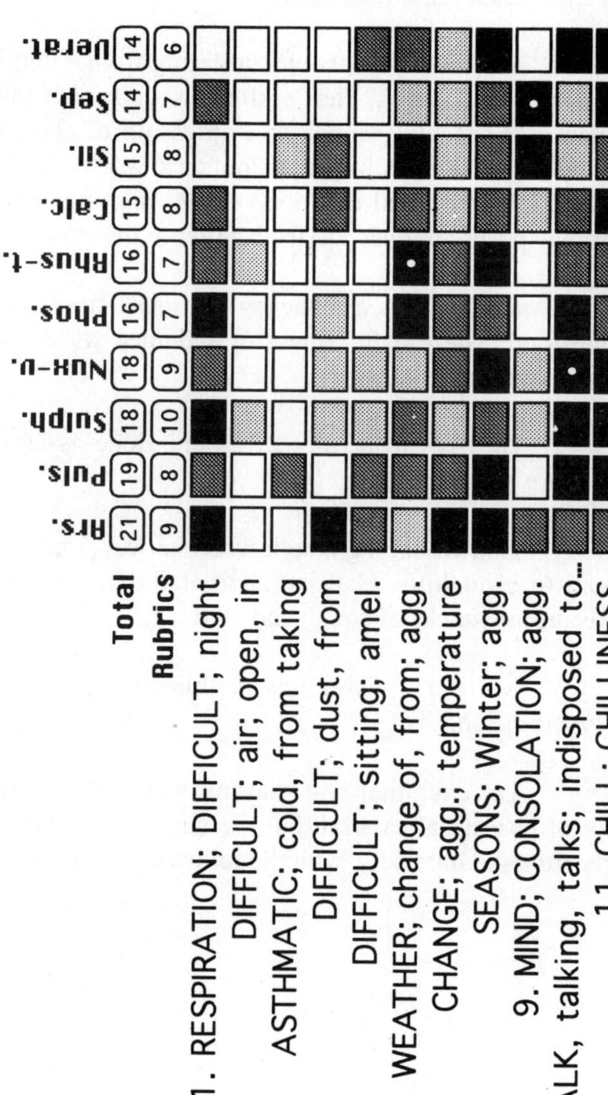
C-3
8/8/97
Jugal Kishore, Dr
Analysis Options: Totality, All Remedies
Ars. 21 9
Puls. 19 8
Sulph. 18 10
Nux-v. 18 9
Phos. 16 7
Rhus-t. 16 7
Calc. 15 8
Sil. 15 8
Sep. 14 7
Verat. 14 6
Total
Rubrics
1. RESPIRATION; DIFFICULT; night
DIFFICULT; air; open, in
ASTHMATIC; cold, from taking
DIFFICULT; dust, from
DIFFICULT; sitting; amel.
WEATHER; change of, from; agg.
CHANGE; agg.; temperature
SEASONS; Winter; agg.
9. MIND; CONSOLATION; agg.
TALK, talking, talks; indisposed to...
11. CHILL; CHILLINESS

CASE N0.4

A Case of Allergic Bronchitis

Mr. I.R., 27 years old, suffering from Allergic Bronchitis for the last 2 years, first visited us in June 1983. Recurrent attacks of sneezing, cough and opression of chest are his main symptoms. He feels his complaints are worse in air-conditioned room, after physical exertion, in the morning, lying down and from exposure to dust. He feels better in the evening.

He also has a tendency for loose stools after fried and rich food. There is heaviness of abdomen which is ameliorated after stools and flatus.

He likes to be alone. Suffers alone as he does not like to share his troubles.

Had whooping cough when he was 6 months old, which lead to bronchitis. Had jaundice at the age of 19 years. Also Recurrent attacks of cough and cold.

Mother's sister has Asthma and both parents have Hypertension.

On examination- Pharynx was congested, there was a lot of post-nasal catarrah but the chest was clear. The case was repertorised hurriedly, with the following symptoms.

	Kishore Cards	Kent Rep
Chest opression while lying	4164	1371
Agg. in the morning	0051	1341
Agg. physical exertion	0149	1358
Amel. when alone	6752	0012
Amel. after stool	0443	-----
Amel. Flatulance	0405	0617
Anxiety about health	1920	0007
Abdomen heavines	3533	0551
Abdomen fullness after eating	3527	0549
Chest opression agg. morning	4155	0839

I Grade - Sep.
II Grade - Phos., Sulph.

He was given a unit dose of Sepia 1M on 15 June.
On 12 July he was comparatively better. Another dose of Sepia 1M was repeated. He showed steady improvement and Sepia 1M was repeated two more times in the next 2 months.

C-4 **8/8/97** **Jugal Kishore, Dr**

Analysis Options: Totality, All Remedies

	Sep.	Sulph.	Nux-v.	Lyc.	Phos.	Puls.	Bry.	Carb-v.	Nat-m.	Alum.
Total	22	18	18	17	15	14	13	13	13	12
Rubrics	9	10	8	8	8	7	6	6	6	8
1. CHEST; OPPRESSION; lying, while										
MORNING, five am. - nine am.										
EXERTION; physical; agg.										
COMPANY; aversion to, agg.; alone;...										
STOOL; amel.; after										
FLATUS passing; amel.										
7. MIND; ANXIETY; health, about										
HEAVINESS as from a load or...										
FULLNESS, sensation of; eating;...										
10. CHEST; OPPRESSION; morning										

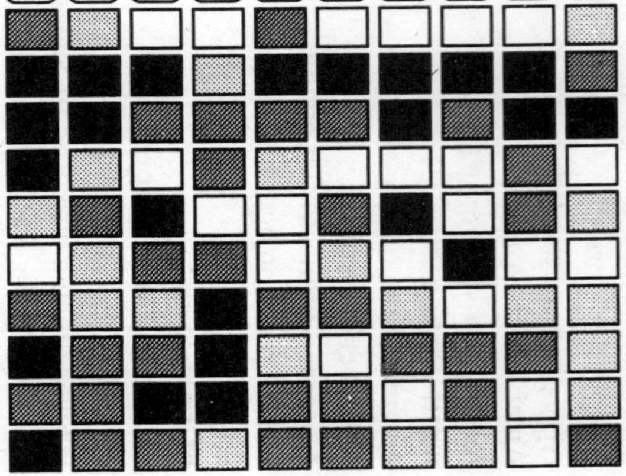

CASE N0.5

A Case of Rheumatoid Arthritis

Mrs. S.T. 35 years old, suffering from Rheumatoid Arthritis, came to us in October 1982. She had pain in the joints for 5 years. It started with the joints of left hand and later other joints were involved. The following modalities were noted down. Aggravation morning, before menses, in cold air, hot fomentation and better by continued movements.

Desire for juices, salty food. She is a hot patient. Liking for winter but cold weather aggravates her complaints. Sensation of heat in the soles. She cannot stand tight clothings around neck. Menses were regular.

Introvert, weeping nature. Worse from excitement and contradiction.

There was ulnar deviation of left hand. She was underweight, just 36.5 kg.

She was given Symphytum 10 M with temporary relief. After this, pains increased with swelling of joints. Symphytum 50M did not give any relief. The pains remained unchanged. At this stage, the case needed repertorisation.

	Kishore Cards	Kent's Rep
Extremities, Joints; complaints in general	4944	No such rubric
Extremities Heat soles	1278	1013
Extremities Pain joints	1300	1047
Gen. intolerance of clothing	0096	1348
Agg. rest	0259	1374
Agg. winter	0372	1422
Agg. before menses	1838	1373
Agg. cold air	0062	1348
Agg. warmth in general	0346	1349
Amel. continued motion	0428	1375
Desire for liquid food	4665	0485
Contradiction, is intolerant of	0134	0016

I Grade- Bry., Ferr.
II Grade- Lyc., Merc.

Bryonia 200, QID was given in March 1983. In April, her weight was 37.5 kg. We repeated Bryonia 200. On 23 April, her pains were better. Weight improved to 39.30 kg. She complained her menses were delayed and scanty but protracted for 10 days. This time, Bryonia 1M was prescribed and she started showing improvement steadily. The unit dose was repeated a few more times.

C-5 **8/8/97** **Jugal Kishore, Dr**

Analysis Options: Totality, All Remedies

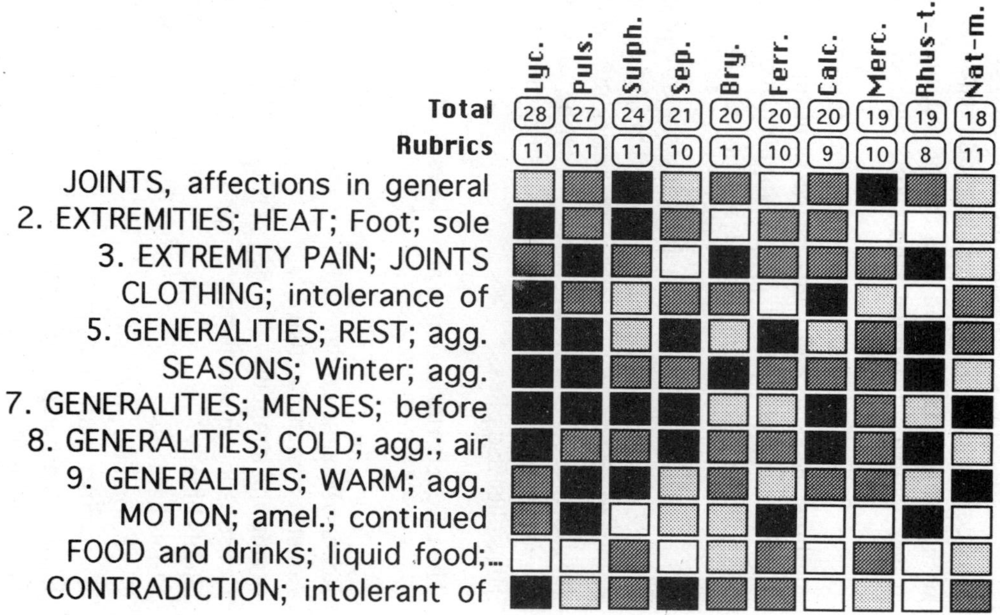

	Lyc.	Puls.	Sulph.	Sep.	Bry.	Ferr.	Calc.	Merc.	Rhus-t.	Nat-m.
Total	28	27	24	21	20	20	20	19	19	18
Rubrics	11	11	11	10	11	10	9	10	8	11
JOINTS, affections in general										
2. EXTREMITIES; HEAT; Foot; sole										
3. EXTREMITY PAIN; JOINTS										
CLOTHING; intolerance of										
5. GENERALITIES; REST; agg.										
SEASONS; Winter; agg.										
7. GENERALITIES; MENSES; before										
8. GENERALITIES; COLD; agg.; air										
9. GENERALITIES; WARM; agg.										
MOTION; amel.; continued										
FOOD and drinks; liquid food;...										
CONTRADICTION; intolerant of										

CASE N0. 6

A Case of Bleeding Haemmorhoids

Mr. N.K.G, 43 years old, complained of bleeding piles with constipation. Stools were hard and required lot of straining with cutting pain. Blood was bright red, and after the stools. It was worse in winter, after taking alcohol and spicy food.

There was also thick, greenish expectoration in the morning. He also had pains in the right hip. It was aggravated in winter, on physical exertion, slightest movement, turning in bed and he felt better while lying down still and by pressure.

Desires Sweets. There is history of extra salt. Now, he has reduced as a precaution for piles. As a person, he likes company and is quite social. Can easily mix with new people. He likes to go out in open air. Sweating of soles in summer. Sweat on face. No significant past history of illnesses.
His father had piles.

The case repertorisation is as follows-

	Kishore Cards	Kent's Rep
Rectum haemorrhoids	2576	0619
Constipation ineffectual urging and straining	0790	0606
Constipation unsatisfactory stools	0791	0607
Stools bloody	2966	0635
Stools hard	2977	0638
Expectoration greenish	1177	0816
Extremities pain right hip	5375	1067
Extremities perspiration soles	5491	1184
Face perspiration	3059	0390

I Grade- Kali-c.

II Grade- Arn., Ars., Calc., Carb-an., Kali-bi., Merc., Nat-m., Petr., Plb., Sep., Sil., Sulph.

Kali Carb 30 repeatedly, and later 200 unit dose, helped this case.

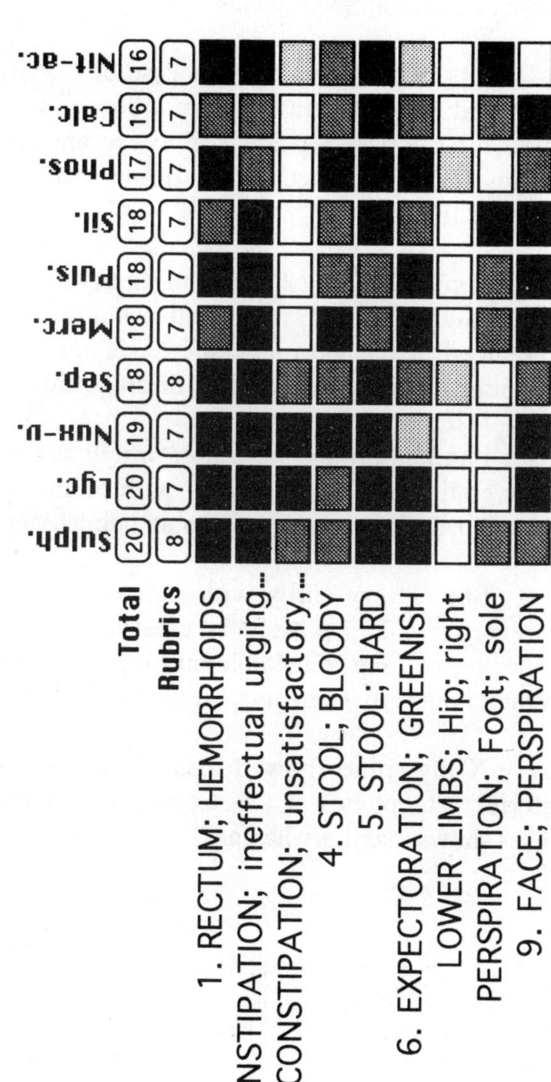
C-6
8/8/97
Jugal Kishore, Dr
Analysis Options: Totality, All Remedies
Sulph.
Lyc.
Nux-v.
Sep.
Merc.
Puls.
Sil.
Phos.
Calc.
Nit-ac.
Total
20
20
19
18
18
18
18
17
16
16
Rubrics
8
7
7
8
7
7
7
7
7
7
1. RECTUM; HEMORRHOIDS
CONSTIPATION; ineffectual urging...
CONSTIPATION; unsatisfactory,...
4. STOOL; BLOODY
5. STOOL; HARD
6. EXPECTORATION; GREENISH
LOWER LIMBS; Hip; right
PERSPIRATION; Foot; sole
9. FACE; PERSPIRATION

CASE N0.7

A Case of Cervical Spondylosis

Mrs. S.L., 38 years old, a case of Cervical Spondylosis, first visited the clinic in January 1984. She complained of vertigo for the past 1 year. It is worse on standing. There is heaviness in nape of neck with stiffness which is acute in the morning.

She has a long history of flatulant dyspepsia for 20 years, which gets aggravated after heavy food and is more pronounced in the morning. She has flatus, sour eructations, water brash, sense of fullness. No desire to eat.

She had an abortion after which she has weakness of the lower limbs. It is associated with numbness and is worse before and during menses and on standing. Menses are regular.

She is very chilly with icy coldness of feet, difficult to warm up. The patient is clairvoyant and is afraid of thunderstorms. She is irritable and loses her temper from least contradiction. Hypersensitive, weeps easily.

X-ray spine showed loss of normal curve. There are posterior osteophytes at C5, C6 and C7. X-ray of Para nasal sinuses shows maxillary haziness.

	Kishore Cards	Kent's Rep.
Flatulence	1617	Flatus- 0617 Eructations-0489
Stomach eructations sour	0496	0496
Abdomen fullness	3526	0549
Stomach eructations waterbrash	1039	0497
Vertigo agg. standing	8669	0104
Gen. lack of vital heat	1741	1366
Extremities coldness feet	4995	0962
Weeping	2182	0092
Sensitive	2114	0078
Clairvoyance	6751	0011

I Grade - Calc., Lach. and Phos.
II Grade- Acon., Arn., Cocc., Kali-bi., Lyc., Nat-m., Nux-m., Rhus-t., Sil., Stann. and Sulph.

The treatment was started on 13 January. Calcarea carb 200, 1M, 10M in unit doses gave her instant relief. Only placebo was repeated on 27 January. She soon found herself cured of her ailment.

C-7 **8/8/97** **Jugal Kishore, Dr**

Analysis Options: Totality, All Remedies

	Phos.	Sulph.	Calc.	Lyc.	Puls.	Caust.	Nux-v.	Sil.	Graph.	Kali-c.
Total	23	22	21	21	20	19	19	18	18	18
Rubrics	9	8	9	8	8	8	7	9	8	8
1. STOMACH; ERUCTATIONS; sour										
FULLNESS, sensation of										
ERUCTATIONS; waterbrash										
4. VERTIGO; STANDING, while										
HEAT; vital, lack of										
6. EXTREMITIES; COLDNESS; Foot										
7. MIND; WEEPING, tearful mood										
8. MIND; SENSITIVE, oversensitive										
9. MIND; CLAIRVOYANT										

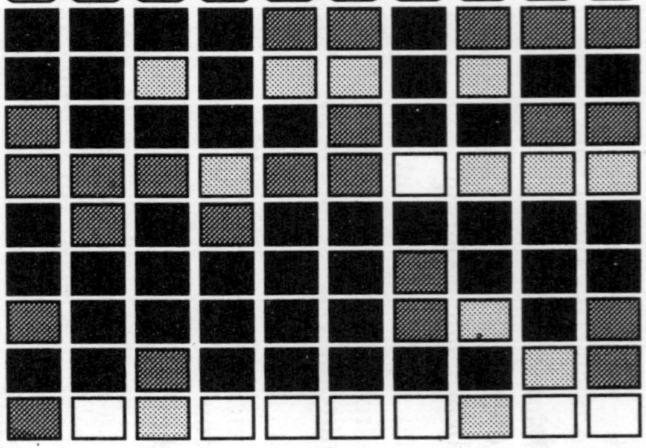

CASE NO. 8

A Case of Osteo-Arthritis

Mrs. H.B., aged 70 years, was suffering from arthritis of the knee joints - Pain and swelling, more in the right knee. It gets worse on walking and there is some relief with warm application.

She also had severe constipation with hard stools. Required lot of straining. Unsatisfactory stools and misses a day.

Head sensitive to cold air. She suffers cramps of hands. Itching of palms in winters. Desires salty food and salts her food extra. Patient was quite irritable.

	Kishore Cards	Kent's Rep
Extremities pain knees.walking on	5392	1073
Extremities pain joints, walking after	5278	1048
Extremities pain joints, amel. warmth	5281	1048
Extremities swelling knee	5538	1200
Extremities cramps hands	4636	0972
Extremities itching palms	5180	1023
Constipation-difficult stool on acount of hard faeces	0784	0607
Stools hard	2977	0638
Head sensitive to, cold air	6108	0109
Desires salty food	0917	0486
Irritable	2044	0057

II Grade - Nat-m.

On 14 Oct. 1983 she was given Nat-mur 30 three times a day. Two weeks later she felt better. Nat-mur 10M unit dose was given. She came back on 26 November and was much better. This time placebo was given for the next two months. After this, another unit dose of Nat-mur 10M was repeated.

C-8 **8/8/97** **Jugal Kishore, Dr**

Analysis Options: Totality, All Remedies

	Nat-m.	Sulph.	Nux-v.	Sil.	Hep.	Caust.	Kali-c.	Lyc.	Bry.	Calc.
Total	21	19	19	19	18	17	17	17	17	17
Rubrics	10	9	8	8	7	9	8	8	7	7
LOWER LIMBS; Knee; walking; on										
JOINTS; walking; after										
JOINTS; warmth; amel.										
4. EXTREMITIES; SWELLING; Knee										
5. EXTREMITIES; CRAMPS; Hand										
ITCHING; Hand; Palm										
CONSTIPATION; difficult stool										
8. STOOL; HARD										
9. HEAD; COLD air, sensitive to										
FOOD and drinks; salt or salty...										
11. MIND; IRRITABILITY										

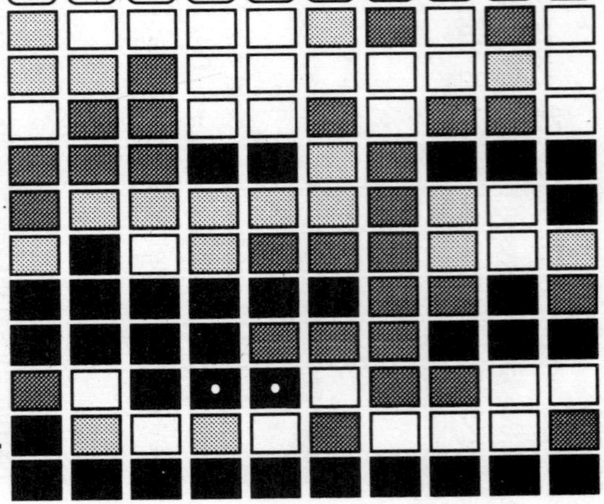

CASE NO. 9

A Case of Anxiety Neurosis

Mr. H.B., 25 years old, appeared to be suffering from Anxiety Neurosis. The patient gets attacks of nervousness, anxiety with fear, palpitation, anticipatory tension with irritability, fear of disease. There was history of shock, tension and grief when his father died after a heart attack 2 years ago.

He also complains of dull headache in the temples and forehead region which is worse on waking in the mornings. He felt great burning in stomach with flatulence. This got worse whenever he was emotionaly tense. His temperament is mild and he is prone to worry and broods on trifles.

In the family, his father's mother had Anxiety neurosis after her brother's death. Father also had nervous breakdown after excessive drinking. He was diabetic and he died of M.I. Father's father also had M.I. Mother and sister Thalassaemia Minor.

	Kishore cards	Kent's Rep
Anxiety with fear	1917	0006
Averse to being spoken to	2138	0082
Desire for salty things	0917	0486
Irritable	2044	0057
Fear of impending disease	1995	0044
Anxiety	1914	0004
Indisposed to talk	2155	0086
Agg. due to grief	0136	0051
Head pain agg. morning on waking	6198	0133
Head pain agg. after sleep	6318	0147

I Grade- Nat-rn.

II Grade- Calc., Ign., Kali-p., Nit-ac., Nux-v., Phos., Sep., Staph., Sulph. and Tarent

From November to February of the next year he was prescribed Nat-mur 200, 1M, 10M unit doses followed by placebo. Only 3 such courses, lasting 6 weeks each, were needed to set his mind to rest.

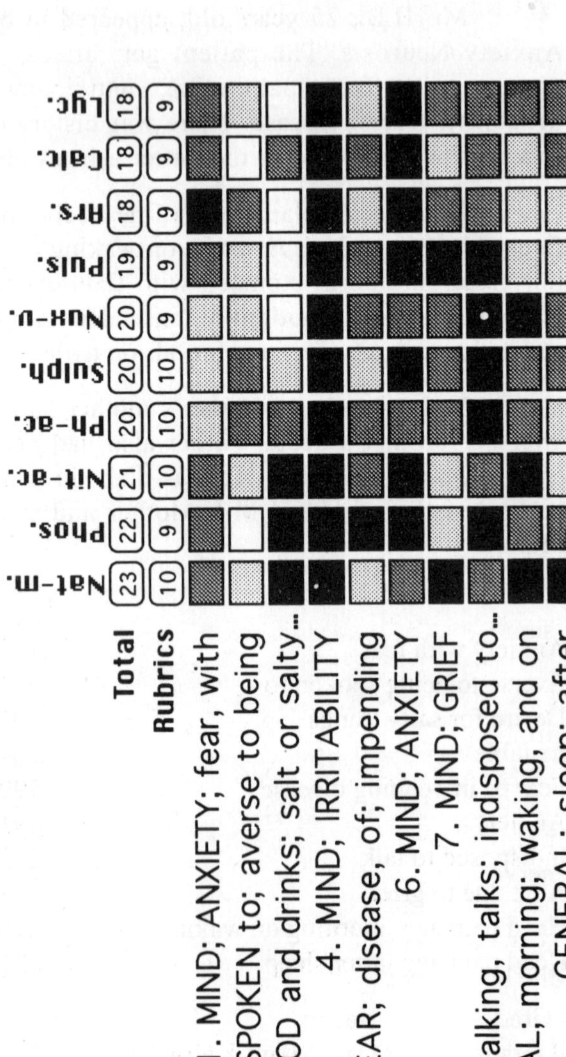
C-9
8/8/97
Jugal Kishore, Dr
Analysis Options: Totality, All Remedies
Nat-m. 23 10
Phos. 22 9
Nit-ac. 21 10
Ph-ac. 20 10
Sulph. 20 10
Nux-v. 20 9
Puls. 19 9
Ars. 18 9
Calc. 18 9
Lyc. 18 9
Total
Rubrics
1. MIND; ANXIETY; fear, with
SPOKEN to; averse to being
FOOD and drinks; salt or salty...
4. MIND; IRRITABILITY
FEAR; disease, of; impending
6. MIND; ANXIETY
7. MIND; GRIEF
TALK, talking, talks; indisposed to...
GENERAL; morning; waking, and on
GENERAL; sleep; after

CASE NO. 10

A Case of Neuralgia

Mr. L.H. aged 26 years complained of pain tip of coccyx for one month. Four years ago he fell down on the road, falling on the right side of body but with no apparent injury at that time. He cannot sit without feeling acute pain. His movements are restricted.

Pain is worse from sneezing, coughing or any jarring movement and by bending forward; and better by lying on back, warmth and pressure.The pain radiates to thighs and legs. Pain in the legs at times on waking in the morning.

He complained also of hyperacidity, burning pain in epigastrium after eating. Better when stomach is empty. Appetite is reduced.

Ringworms in the groins. Worse in rainy season and summer.

Headache in the heat of sun; from tension; and better from pressure.

He is a hot patient. Gets chillblains in winters and also pain in the knee joints in cold weather. He experiences nervousness in anticipation.

The following rubrics were selected for analysis from the Kishore Card Repertory.

	Kishore's Cards	Kent's Rep
Back pain coccyx	4022	912
Back pain coccyx agg. sitting	4024	912
Abdomen pain after eating	3557	558
Perspiration odor offensive	3037	1298
Extremities chillblains fingers	4304	955
Agg. winter	372	1422

I Grade- Petr.
II Grade- Bell., Carb-an., Rhus-t. and Sulph..

Petroleum in 1M and 10M potency has not only removed the Coccalgia but removed his hyperacidity and other complaints also.

C-10 **8/8/97** **Jugal Kishore, Dr**

Analysis Options: Totality, All Remedies

	Petr.	Rhus-t.	Sulph.	Nux-v.	Puls.	Carb-an.	Lyc.	Verat.	Carb-v.	Graph.
Total	13	10	10	10	10	9	9	9	8	8
Rubrics	6	5	5	4	4	5	4	4	4	4
1. BACK; PAIN; general; Coccyx										
PAIN; general; Coccyx; sitting;...										
PAIN; general; eating; after										
4. PERSPIRATION; ODOR; offensive										
CHILBLAINS; Fingers										
SEASONS; Winter; agg.										

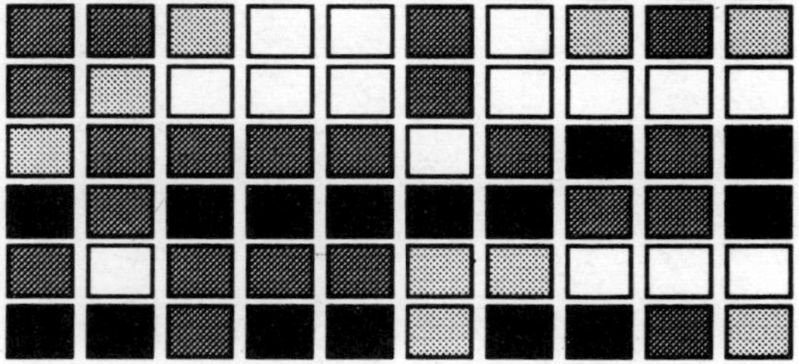

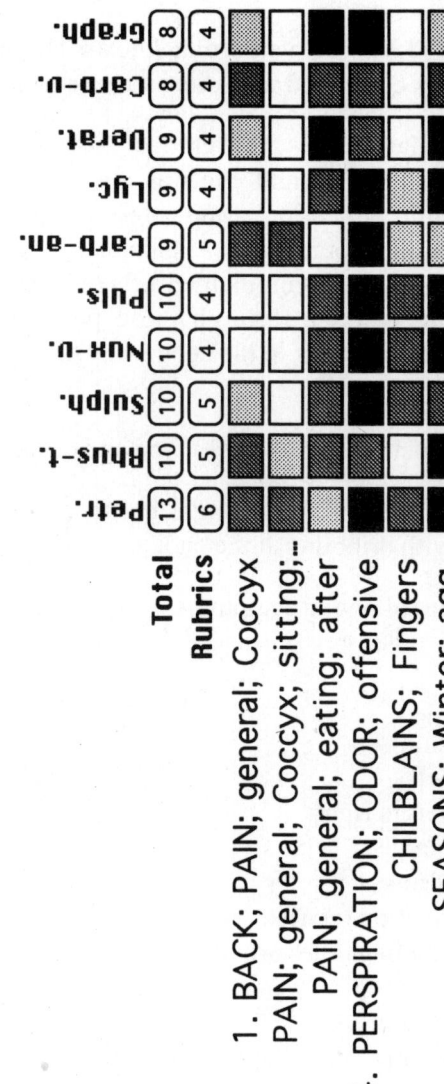

CASE NO. 11

A Case of Diabetic Retinopathy

Mr. J.V.P. 52 years old, known Diabetic for 5 years. Diabetes was controlled with diet and exercises.

In March 1984 had gradual loss of vision in the left eye. In May 84, the right eye was also affected. He had been given Insulin injections and steroid therapy. Slit Lamp examination and Flourescence Angiography indicated 'Geographic Choroiditis.' Patient complained of grey patches in vision. In bright light, can see through these patches. Also sees two crimson coloured rings in the centre of vision. Steroids had been stopped.

Throat sensitive to cold food and drinks.

Enlarged prostate. Slight hesitency in the beginning of urination with dribbling at the end.

The following symptoms were selected for case analysis.

	Kishore Cards	Kent's Rep
Loss of vision	3422	0281
Gen. side left	2822	1401
Gen. side left to right	2823	1401
Prostate enlarged	3283	0667
Agg. cold drinks	0165	1362
Bladder urination retarted	3332	0660
Bladder dribbling, after urination	3318	0656

I Grade - Arg-n.
II Grade- Clem., Sil,, Staph. and Thuj.

The only remedy which came through was Arg-nit. So Arg-nit 1M and later 10 M were given. After four months, we found that vision was definitely better, patches had disappeared and urinary symptoms were much better.

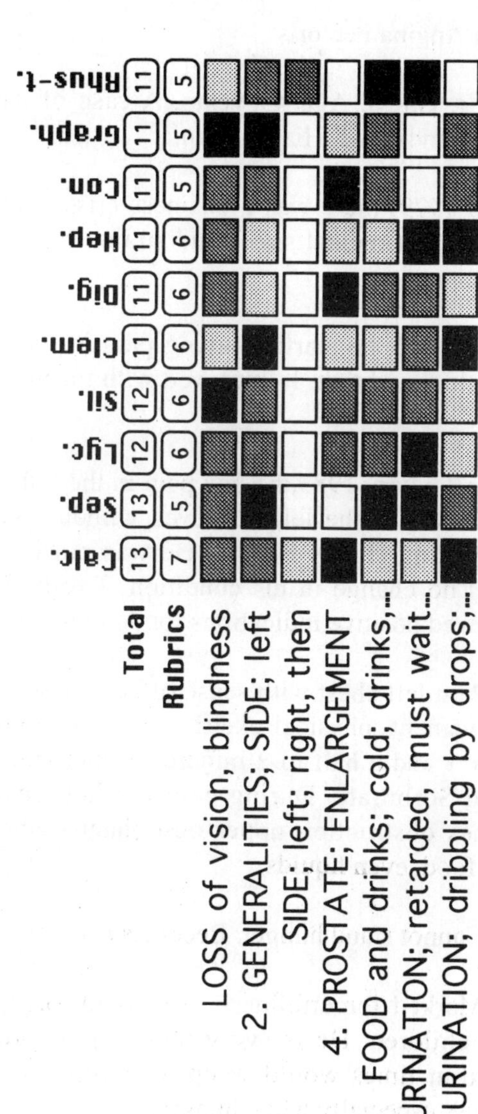
C-11
8/8/97
Jugal Kishore, Dr
Analysis Options: Totality, All Remedies
Calc.
Sep.
Lyc.
Sil.
Clem.
Dig.
Hep.
Con.
Graph.
Rhus-t.
Total
13
13
12
12
11
11
11
11
11
11
Rubrics
7
5
6
6
6
6
6
5
5
5
LOSS of vision, blindness
2. GENERALITIES; SIDE; left
SIDE; left; right, then
4. PROSTATE; ENLARGEMENT
FOOD and drinks; cold; drinks,...
URINATION; retarded, must wait...
URINATION; dribbling by drops;...

CASE NO. 12

A Case of Angina Pectoris

Mr. G.R.S. Age 49 years. A case of Angina Pectoris, Cervical Spondylosis, Hiatus Hernia

In 1979, there was a business crisis and for 3 years he was under great mental stress and strain. Since then he has not been well.

In 1982, he started having pain in the cervical region, right shoulder and arm. It improved with traction, diathermy and exercises.

In January 1983, he had pain in the left side of the chest with heaviness in the left arm even without exercise. Ba Meal showed sliding Hiatus Hernia. He was put on Cemitidine but there was no change in his condition. Treadmill's Test in June 1984 showed positive indications for Angina Pectoris.

Pain left chest with sense of heaviness which was worse from movement, physical exertion and emotional tension. Pain lasted for 1 and a half to 2 minutes. Better from rest and better on taking Sorbitrate. During pain felt hot, anxious and dizzy. Sometimes obstruction upper oesophagus when he started to swallow food, even liquids.

Cannot stand hunger. Becomes restless.

Marked forgetfullness. He would forget names of even his own children. He is very tense and depressed. Desire to weep and at times would weep without cause. He is irritable and restless especially when hungry.

Two elder brothers suffer from Angina Pectoris

	Kishore Cards	Kent's Rep
Agg. hunger	0188	1367
Sadness	2106	0075
Forgetfulness	2005	0048
Weeping, causeless	2186	0093
Angina Pectoris	0619	0822
Heart pain or its affections with pain in the left arm or hand	4199	1049 & 850
Desires sweets	0919	0486

The remedies that emerged were Lycopodium and Rhustox in the first grade and Ars-alb, Kali-carb and Nux-v in the second grade.

Lycopodium was prescribed and the results have been gratifying. He was treated with Lycopodium for a few months and continued to be better.

Comments-

In 'Aggravation from hunger', Kent's Repertory does not give Lycopodium, although in our annotated copy of Kent, it has been added. In 'Aggravation from fasting' Lycopodium has been included in Kent.

In Heart pain, Kishore Card Repertory has a combined rubric, where as in Kent, we have to seek two places and use them as combined rubric.

In popular parlance, it has been suggested that grades of the individual remedies should be added together and the totality of the value should finally decide the choice. In our experience, this is not always correct. Many of the remedies have not had sufficiently large provings or confirmation especially for some particular symptoms or complaints.

We have to keep an open mind and the final decision

should be left to the study of Materia-Medica and the patient's picture of sickness as a whole. This way we can add to the Materia-Medica and enlarge the therapeutic horizon of the remedies, which otherwise would have been left unexplained.

These cases have been analysed in a fairly busy clinic and the point here stressed is that it pays to do a repertorial analysis. Otherwise, one goes on to 'hit or miss' spree.

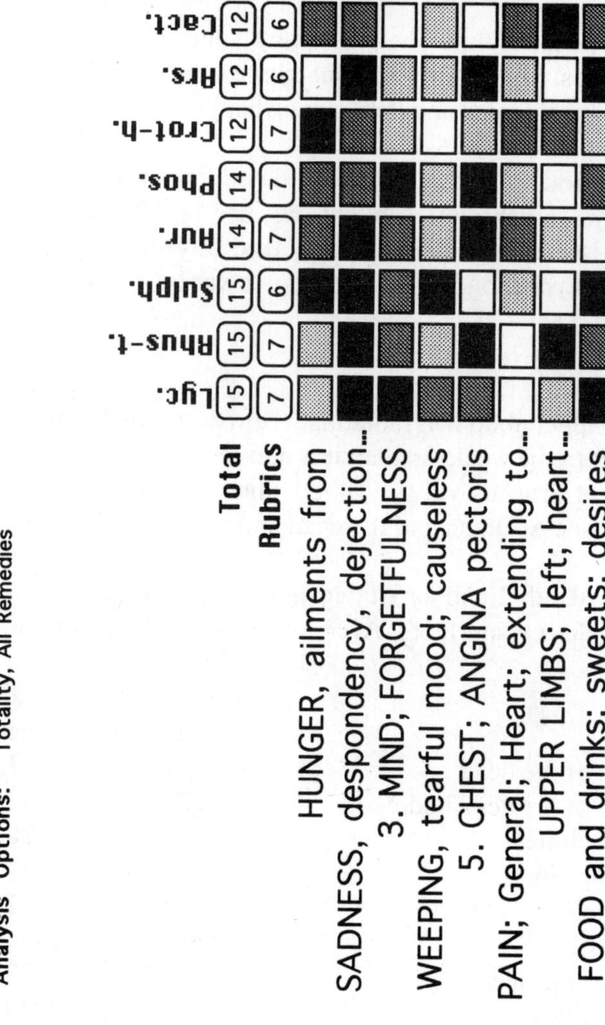
C-12
8/8/97
Jugal Kishore, Dr
Analysis Options: Totality, All Remedies
Lyc.
Rhus-t.
Sulph.
Aur.
Phos.
Crot-h.
Ars.
Cact.
Acon.
Kali-c.
Total
15 15 15 14 14 12 12 12 11 11
Rubrics
7 7 6 7 7 7 6 6 6 6
HUNGER, ailments from
SADNESS, despondency, dejection...
3. MIND; FORGETFULNESS
WEEPING, tearful mood; causeless
5. CHEST; ANGINA pectoris
PAIN; General; Heart; extending to...
UPPER LIMBS; left; heart...
FOOD and drinks; sweets; desires

CASE NO. 13

A Case of Menorrhagia

Mrs. N.D., 49 years of age, compalined of Menorrhagia for the past 7 to 8 months.

Onset- While she was doing some religious ceremony, her clothes caught fire and she got extensive burns and later developed insomnia and then menorrhagia.

Menses- every 20 to 25 days, very profuse, lasting 6 to 7 days. Thick clotted blood. For the last 3 months she was having labour like pains on the first day of menses. Pain in back and hypochondria radiating downwards.

Concomitants-

Pain in upper abdomen radiating to throat usually at night during sleep. Extreme weakness, anxiety and restlessness.
Recurrent Pruritus vulvae. Blood sugar at random was 280 mg.
Sleeplessness. Dreams of the dead and of dead bodies.

Mind- Easily irritated and wants her way. Forgetful. Forgets names and faces. Aversion to noises. Wants to be alone.

	Kishore Cards	Kent's Repertory
Dreams of the dead	0944	1237
Dreams of the dead bodies	4736	1237
Menses clotted	1850	0725
Menses profuse	1852	0725
Restlessness	2099	0072
Agg. fasting	0153	1361
Agg. during sleep	0289	1402
Agg. fright	0135	0049

The result according to Kishore Cards was-

I Grade- Am-c.,. Calc., Nit-ac.

She was given Am-carb 200, 1M, 10M in December 1983. Patient had no menses after 27 December 1983. Treatment was continued, but her blood sugar was still high. For this, she was given Syzygium Jambolinum mother tincture. Post parandial blood sugar dropped down to 149 mg. The last prescription was in April 1984 and her blood sugar was normal. She had undergone menopause without any further problems.

C-13 8/8/97 Jugal Kishore, Dr

Analysis Options: Totality, All Remedies

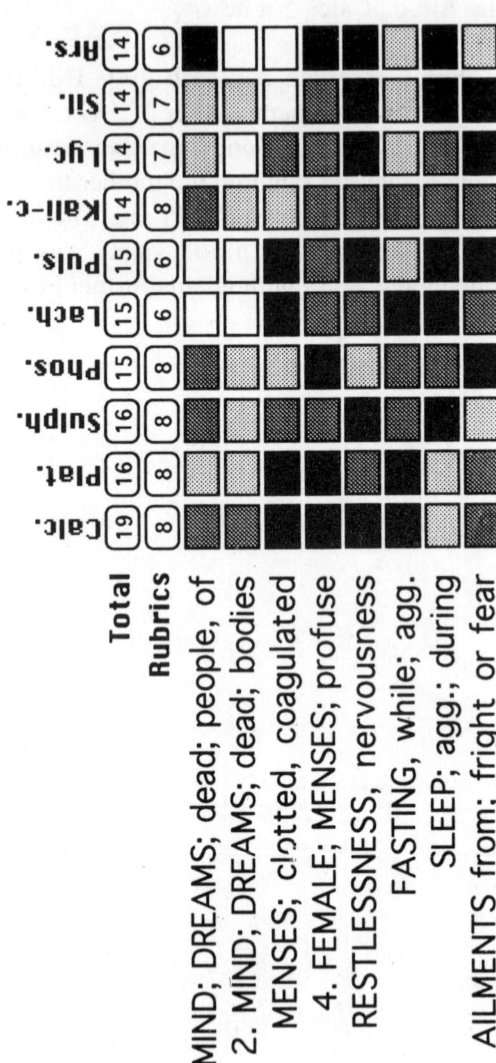

CASE NO. 14

A Case of Eczema

Mrs. P.K., 60 years of age, first visited the clinic on 6 March 1985. She had various Complaints-

1. Flatulance for the last 20 years. No relation to meals. There is loud belching at frequent intervals. Upper abdomen feels bloated which got worse after fried food. It is better by passing flatus.

2. Attacks of palpitation and breathing difficulty. Palpitation from loud talking and from watching TV, worse from ascending stairs, physical exertion and better by rest.

3. For the past few months she is becoming very forgetful. Forgets her way to different places. Aversion to work and to talking. Feeling of helplessness. Weeps easily without any cause.

4. Eczema for the past one year and a half. Eruptions with cracks on palms and soles, worse from washing with cold water.

There is lack of vital heat. She must cover her head in winters.
20 years ago, was operated for severe otitis media.
There is history of moist eczema on the occiput.
7 years ago, lost her speech which was relieved by 50 injections of vit. Bl, B6 and B12.

The Family History was not significant.

She has been on homoeopathic treatment.

Pulse and Respiration were normal. There is slight dark pigmentation on forearms

On 8 March 1985, she was given Silicea 1M. On 22 March 1985, there was not much change in her condition. Repertorisation was done taking the following symptoms-

	Kishore Cards	Kent's Rep
Rectum sudden urging	7491	0634
Skin dryness	2857	1307
Mouth taste bitter	2260	0422
Extremities cracks hands	1271	0970
Skin cracks in general	2839	1305
Stomach empty eructations	1033	0493
Forgetfulness	2005	0048
Aversion to company	1931	0012
Weeping on trifles	7052	0094

I Grade- Petr.
II Grade- Bar-c., Calc., Graph., Lach., Nat-c., Nat-m., Puls., Rhus-t, Sep., Sulph. and Zinc.

Petroleum 1M was prescribed on 22 March and on 8 April she reported to be much better in every respect. Behaviour improved. She was now cheerful whereas she used to cry when asked about her complaints. Her appetite improved, less of gases. Eruptions on hands are 70 % better. Following this, only placebo was given.

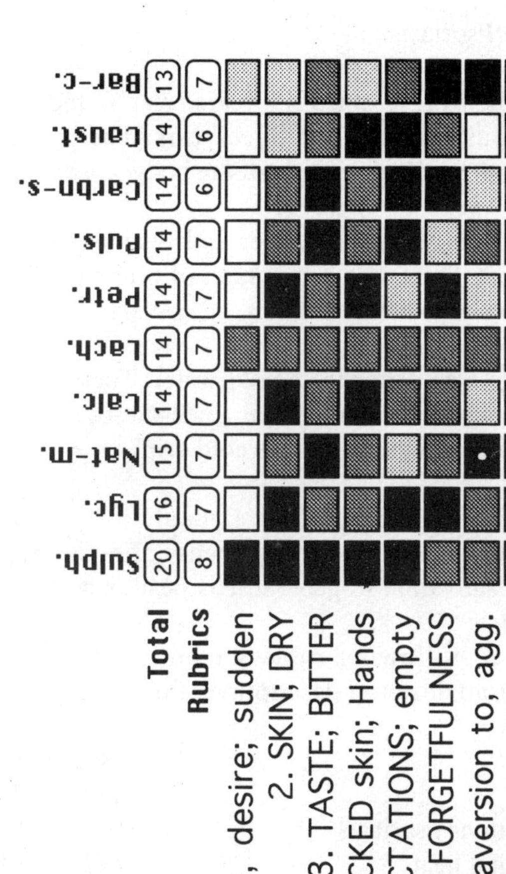
C-14
8/8/97
Jugal Kishore, Dr
Analysis Options: Totality, All Remedies
Total
Rubrics
Sulph. 20 8
Lyc. 16 7
Nat-m. 15 7
Calc. 14 7
Lach. 14 7
Petr. 14 7
Puls. 14 7
Carbn-s. 14 6
Caust. 14 6
Bar-c. 13 7
URGING, desire; sudden
2. SKIN; DRY
3. TASTE; BITTER
CRACKED skin; Hands
5. STOMACH; ERUCTATIONS; empty
6. MIND; FORGETFULNESS
COMPANY; aversion to, agg.
WEEPING, tearful mood; trifles, at

CASE NO. 15

A Case of Psoriasis

Mr. M.L.K. aged 45 years, was found to be suffering from psoriasis for the last three years. The psoriatic eruptions covered practically the whole of the body.

It was worse in winter and responded to Graphites to some extent There was a sensation of pricking all over the body when exposed to the winter sun.

He was better from cold water. There was tendency for tonsillitis which is worse from acids or sour food and pickles. During such attacks, he desires cold drinks.

There is lack of vital heat, but there is copious perspiration and he is generally better after sweat. There is also increased salivation in general. His head is sensitive to cold air.

The following rubrics could be made available for analysis from this brief description of the case-

	Kishore Card	Kent's Rep
Skin eruptions psoriasis	1098	1316
Lack of vital heat	1741	1366
Head sensitive to cold air	6108	0109
Agg. in winter	0372	1422
Agg. from sour food	0175	1364
Agg. from sour drinks	0174	1364
Amel. during perspiration	0447	1391
Amel. after perspiration	0448	1391
Desire for cold drinks	0908	0484
Mouth salivation increased	2245	0417

I Grade- Ars., Nat-m.

II Grade- Calc., Lyc. and Rhus-t.

The remedies which appeared to have all the symptoms are Ars-alb and Nat-mur.

Since January 1984, he was kept on Nat-mur 200 and later 1M and has continued to improve.

In this case, the concomitant symptoms of salivation and sweating with its modalities, tilted the grading of symptoms in favour of Nat-mur. He lacked the characteristics of either Ars or Rhustox. Psoriasis is a very difficult disease to cure. In this case, follow up later also indicated that there was no return of symptoms.

C-15 8/8/97 Jugal Kishore, Dr

Analysis Options: Totality, All Remedies

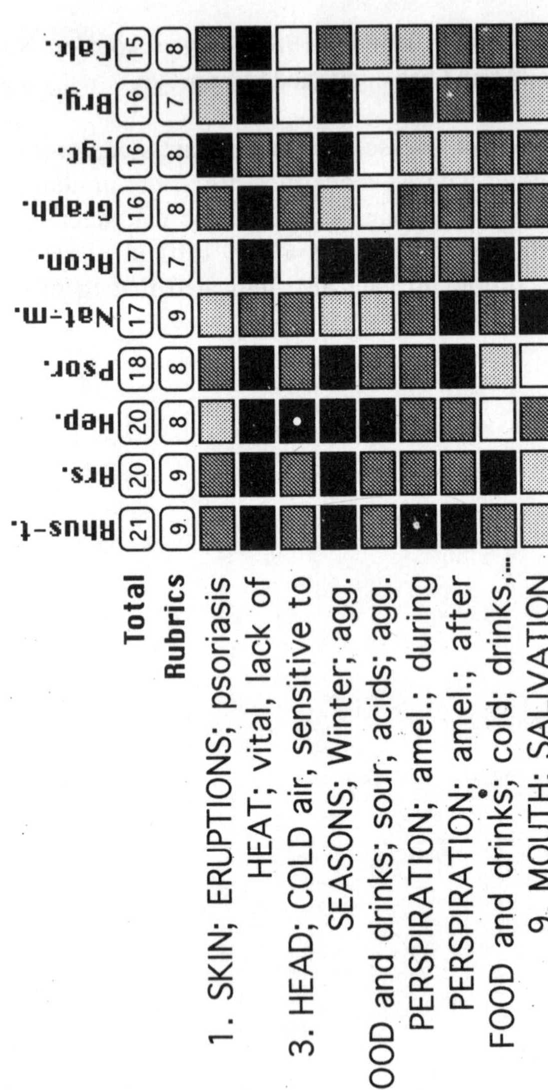

Total
Rubrics
Rhus-t. 21 9
Ars. 20 9
Hep. 20 8
Psor. 18 8
Nat-m. 17 9
Acon. 17 7
Graph. 16 8
Lyc. 16 8
Bry. 16 7
Calc. 15 8
1. SKIN; ERUPTIONS; psoriasis
HEAT; vital, lack of
3. HEAD; COLD air, sensitive to
SEASONS; Winter; agg.
FOOD and drinks; sour, acids; agg.
PERSPIRATION; amel.; during
PERSPIRATION; amel.; after
FOOD and drinks; cold; drinks,...
9. MOUTH; SALIVATION

CASE NO. 16

A Case of Neurological Demyelotrophy.
Example of a rarer remedy coming through the analysis.

Dr. R.B. aged 35 years, has been diagnosed as a case of 'Neurological Demyelotrophy' by the neuro-surgeons. He himself is a medical doctor. He has severe pain in the shoulders, upper arms. There is increasing weakness of upper and lower extremities.

Pain is worse in winter, from lying on sides, lying on back and in the morning at 4 or 5 a.m. He is ameliorated by movements, warmth and heat of the sun.

Fasting or work-stress gives him a headache. There is dizziness at times.

He desires sweets very much.

Investigations-

EMG indicated Neuro-demyelotrophy.
X-ray spine- NAD
ENT checkup- NAD
Myelogram- NAD
ESR- 8 mm 1st hour.

The following rubrics were utilised for repertorisation-

	Kishore Cards	Kent's Rep.
Agg. in winter	0372	1422
Agg. in morning	0051	1341
Amel. continued motion	0428	1375
Amel. external warmth	0456	1413
Agg. from rest	0259	1374
Agg. lying on sides	0220	1372
Amel. by motion of affected part	0429	1375
Headache from fasting	6248	0140
Desire for sweets	0919	0486

I Grade- Kali-c. and Sabad.
II Grade- Ferr., Lyc., Rhus-t., Sep., Sil. and Sulph.

The remedies that had all the symptoms were Kali-carb and Sabadilla.

Sabadilla was prescribed in 30th potency. Later, 200 unit dose in a week and later in 1M potency. Gradually, his pain and muscle tone improved to a great extent. Six months later, he was practically cured. The last report was on 20.4.85 and since then there has been no recurrence.

Comments- The question that props up here is why was Kali-c not given, when it has 4-5 a.m. aggravation. There are certain imponderables which cannot be searched in the Repertory and which influence the judgement of any experienced prescriber. Here we found that the patient, a medico, had certain amount of obscessiveness which was evident in the narration of his complaints and was also very chilly. Sabadilla hit the bull's eye.

C-16 **8/8/97** **Jugal Kishore, Dr**

Analysis Options: Totality, All Remedies

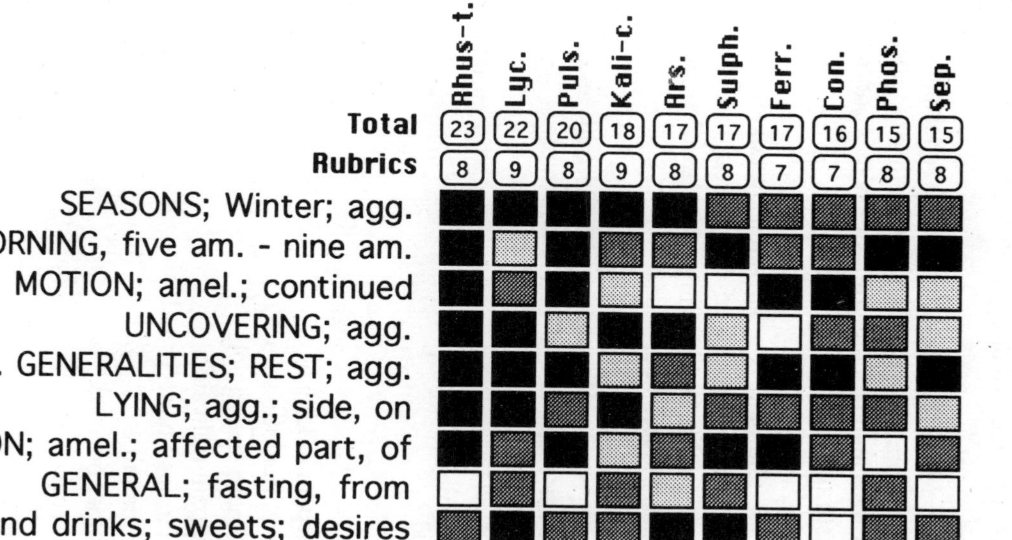

	Rhus-t.	Lyc.	Puls.	Kali-c.	Ars.	Sulph.	Ferr.	Con.	Phos.	Sep.
Total	23	22	20	18	17	17	17	16	15	15
Rubrics	8	9	8	9	8	8	7	7	8	8

SEASONS; Winter; agg.
MORNING, five am. - nine am.
MOTION; amel.; continued
UNCOVERING; agg.
5. GENERALITIES; REST; agg.
LYING; agg.; side, on
MOTION; amel.; affected part, of
GENERAL; fasting, from
FOOD and drinks; sweets; desires

CASH NO. 17

A case of Facial Neuralgia

Mr. R.S., aged 37 years, reported in October 1982 of severe vibrating pain starting from right jaw extending to the right temple. The pain comes in waves and starts in the morning on getting up.

The pain is aggravated by talking, eating, every motion of the jaw or jarring of body; coughing; spitting or blowing of nose; worse on thinking of it; better when occupied; bending head on the left side.

He is subject to gastric upsets and flatulance. Desires more salt in food. Indolent and irritable.

History of eczema 18 years ago, suppressed by local applications.

	Kishore's Cards	Kent's Rep
Face pain talking agg.	5914	0383
Face pain motion agg.	5904	0382
Face pain eating agg.	5900	0381
Face pain right side	5888	0380
Pain in face-paroxysmal	5908	0382
Desires salt	0917	0486
Occupation amel.	0430	0069
Indolence	2306	0055

II Grade- Mez.

The only remedy that emerged was Mezerium.
Mezerium in 30, 1M and later 10M at intervals relieved the pain to a great extent. Earlier remedies like Phos, Verat, Rad-br, Passiflora etc. had not made any impression.

Comments- In this case, without the help of a Repertory, we could not have solved the case. A number of remedies were already given on the basis of the diagnosis of Neuralgia, coupled with a modality here and there by thumbing up the pages of Repertory or on one's so called experience. The analysis humbles us and points to the need for a proper systematic analysis of the case.

C-17 **8/8/97** **Jugal Kishore, Dr**

Analysis Options: Totality, All Remedies

	Spig.	Bell.	Nux-v.	Mez.	Phos.	Sep.
Total	12	11	11	10	10	10
Rubrics	7	5	5	6	6	5
PAIN; General, aching, prosopalgia; talking;...						
PAIN; General, aching, prosopalgia; motion;...						
PAIN; General, aching, prosopalgia; eating;...						
PAIN; General, aching, prosopalgia; right						
PAIN; General, aching, prosopalgia;...						
FOOD and drinks; salt or salty food; desires						
7. MIND; OCCUPATION, diversion; amel.						
8. MIND; INDOLENCE, aversion to work						

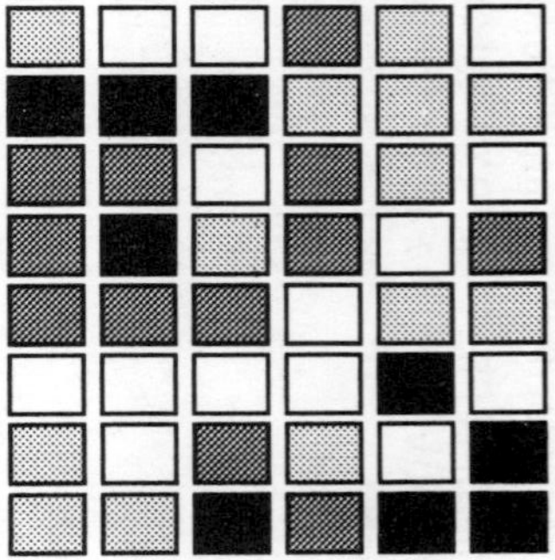

CASE NO. 18

A Case of Dysmenorrhoea

Here is another case which required repertorial analysis second time when the indicated remedy improved the patient, but later due to a relapse and appearance of a few new symptoms necessiated the need for a review and a further analysis.

Miss V.B., aged 37 years, was seen in March 1982. She complained of severe dysmennorhoea on the first two days of menses, better slightly by lying on the abdomen and by pressure. Menses scanty, blackish, clotted with frequent urging for stool.

She had gastric distention with belching, worse at night and in summer. Desires warm food. Premature grey hair. There is a cyst in the inner canthus of right eye. Dark rings around eyes. Backache before menses.

	Kishore Cards	Kent's Rep
Back complaints in general before menses	6629	0896
Menses painful	1966	0727
Menses clotted	1850	0725
Menses scanty	1871	0728
Menses black	1846	0724
Head hair premature grey	1660	0120

II Grade- Lyc., Puls. and Sulph.

She was kept on Lyc. till January 1983, and later on, 1M till September 1983. The cyst had disappeared, and the dark rings around the eyes became much less. Dysmenorrhoea had disappeared and menses became normal.

On 24 November, she developed fever. Her menses became very painful. She had diarrhoea, vomiting and great weakness. There was a recent history of mental tension. The following symptoms were elicited and a second analysis was made-

	Kishore Cards	Kent's Rep
Menses clotted	1850	0725
Menses dark clots	1851	0725
Menses offensive	1865	0727
Menses black	1846	0724
Menses protracted	1868	0728
Menses tenacious	1874	0729
Menses dark	1854	0726
Anxiety with fear	1917	0006
Menses Painful	1966	0727

It is quite apparent that almost all the symptoms here are centered around the character of menstrual discharge and pain connected with it. We did not have any other reliable data to fall back on excepting her anxiety with fear.

I Grade- Plat., Puls. and Sec.
II Grade- Bell., Croc., Ign. and Lach.

She was placed on Sec-cor off and on and reported by June 1983 to be much better.

Comments- In this case, in the absence of any other important general or mental symptoms, we had to depend upon the menstrual discharge and other associated symptoms, as these were the only complaints dominating the patient's economy. In the analysis done in the first time, Lycopodium held the ground for sometime, but later on giving way to Sec-cor, which seemed to put an end to the complaints. Here we could make a note in our books that Sec-cor follows Lycopodium. This is in consonance with recordings as given in Hering's Guiding symptoms.

C-18 8/8/97 Jugal Kishore, Dr

Analysis Options: Totality, All Remedies

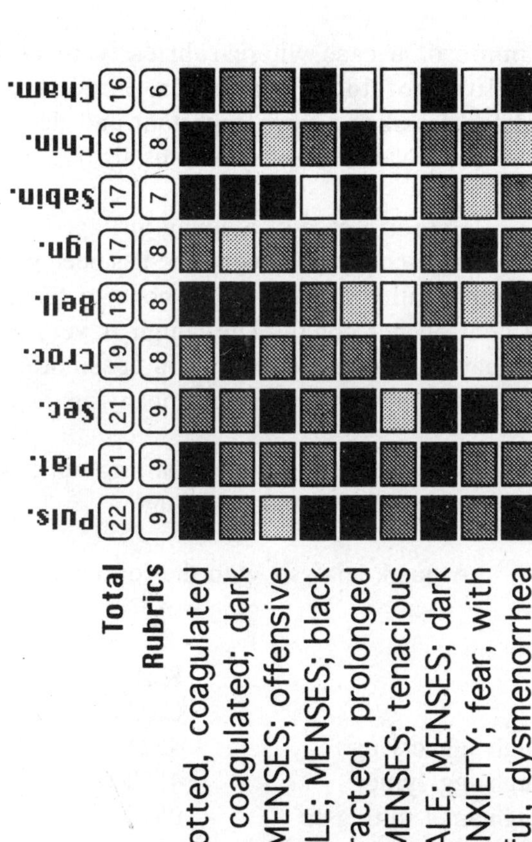

CASE NO. 19

A Case of Allergic coughs and colds

Example of a case where rubrics were collected from the modalities of local symptoms. Peculiar combination of modalities makes a very important and decisive factor in the evaluation (Evaluation of symptoms also).

Here is a case of a young girl aged 3 years who suffers from allergic colds and cough. She has been prescribed a number of homoeopathic medicines but none of them seemed to make any dent on her cough. The cough is very loud and resonant like that of Spongia cough. It is spasmodic and continuous. There is at times, wheezing accompanying the cough.

The cough is better by sitting up, and by eating. It is worse on lying down; and on crying.

A quick analysis with the following rubrics gave us the clue.

	Kishore's Cards	Kent's Rep.
Cough agg. crying	4521	0785
Cough agg. lying	4557	0796
Cough amel. sitting up	0876	0803
Cough amel. eating	**4538**	**0790**
Cough spasmodic	0877	0804

I Grade- Ferr
II Grade- Ars., Hep. and Phos.

Ferrum-met has all these symptoms, whereas Ars-alb, Hep-sulph and Phos were runners up.

She responded to Ferr-met 30 beautifully. It has always helped her whenever she had any episode of cold and cough. Last report was in December 1984.

In this case, we could include in Ferr-met as one of the remedies for croupy type of cough and for deep cough. Spongia etc. had not helped here. We could welcome any other confirmation.

This simple case illustrates the value of Repertorisation and no amount of hit or miss method or key-note prescriptions could have helped us.

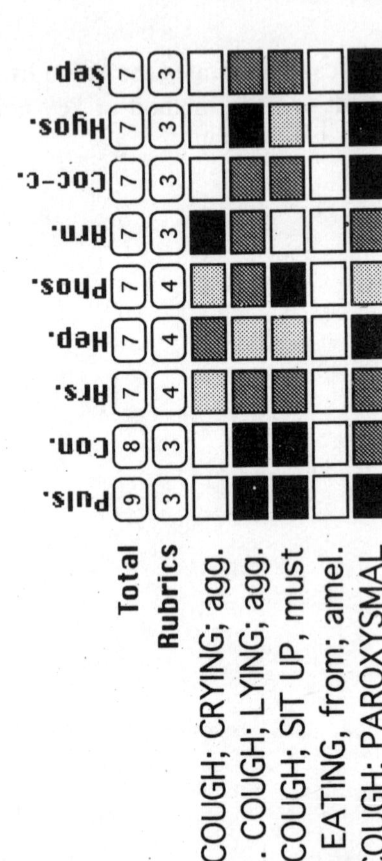
C-19
8/8/97
Jugal Kishore, Dr
Analysis Options: Totality, All Remedies
Total
Rubrics
Puls. 9 3
Con. 8 3
Ars. 7 4
Hep. 7 4
Phos. 7 4
Arn. 7 3
Coc-c. 7 3
Hyos. 7 3
Sep. 7 3
1. COUGH; CRYING; agg.
2. COUGH; LYING; agg.
3. COUGH; SIT UP, must
4. COUGH; EATING, from; amel.
5. COUGH; PAROXYSMAL

CASE N0.20

A Case of Bleeding Haemorrhoids

Mr. N.B., 34 years of age consulted us on 16 January, '87 for bleeding haemorrhoids. He was, otherwise, a very healthy person but due to irregular food habits, he developed piles. The bleeding would occur after spicy food or alcohol. There is prolapse of piles from least straining. The stools are unsatisfactory and incomplete. There is desire for sweets and fruits.

With this data, our first impulse was to give Nux-vomica because of his food habits, intake of alcohol and the nature of stools. It seemed to be too obvious. But we decided to use the Kishore Cards for intellectual curiosity. We put through the data whichever was available to us. The following rubrics were utilised-

	Kishore Cards	Kent's Rep
1. Rectum haemorrhoids	2576	0619
2. Rectum constipation unsatisfactory stools	0791	0607
3. Gen agg. from alcoholic stimulants	0120	1344
4. Desire for sweets	0919	0486
5. Desire for fruits	0911	0485

I Grade- Ars., Carb-v., Chin. and Nat-m.

Carbo-veg 30 3 times a day was started on 16.1.87. He reported to be much better on his next visit.

On 2.3.87, he reported that he was practically cured. No further medication was given.

The lesson we learnt from this case is that one should not have pre-conceived notions or prejudices on examining any new case. Each new case is a unique entity and has to be evaluated as such. It is only then one gets Kentian cures. In the above case, I could not think of Carbo-veg, at least not in the first few instances.

C-20 8/8/97 Jugal Kishore, Dr

Analysis Options: Totality, All Remedies

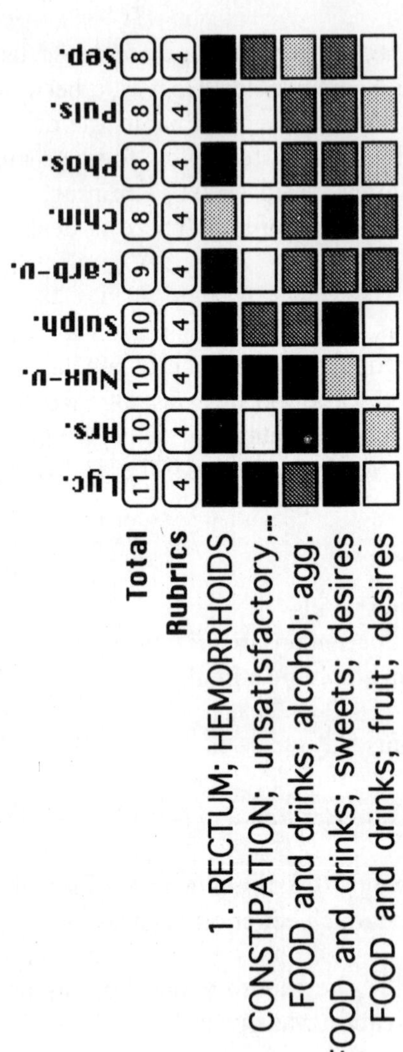

	Lyc.	Ars.	Nux-v.	Sulph.	Carb-v.	Chin.	Phos.	Puls.	Sep.
Total	11	10	10	10	9	8	8	8	8
Rubrics	4	4	4	4	4	4	4	4	4

1. RECTUM; HEMORRHOIDS
CONSTIPATION; unsatisfactory,...
FOOD and drinks; alcohol; agg.
FOOD and drinks; sweets; desires
FOOD and drinks; fruit; desires

CASE N0.21

A Case of Rectal polyp

This is a case of a young man, C.K., 12 years of age, who was having a rectal mass which prolapsed while passing stools. He was having it for the last one year. There was often bleeding from rectum during stools. He had to push the mass manually after stools. The surgeon had diagnosed it as rectal polypus and had advised immediate operation.

He had also developed dark circles around eyes. He had blepharitis and itching around the eyes. There is dryness of lips with rough, scruffy skin around the lips. He is an irritable child, obstinate and quarrels frequently with his younger brother.

He is fond of sweets, cold drinks and eggs. He is fond of cold in general. His mother suffers from Migraine and has had asthma. We did a rapid going through the Kishore Cards with the following data-

Kent's	Kishore Cards	Rep
1. Rectum polyp	2524	0631
2. Agg. warmth in gen. (hot patient)	3808	1412
3. Mind irritability	2044	0057
4. Mind obstinate	2086	0069
5. Desire for sweets	0919	0486
6. Face dryness lips	1487	0364
7. Mouth discoloration tongue white	2281	0402
8. Face discoloration (color) bluish, eyes around	1453	0358

II Grade- Calc., Lyc., Nux-v. and Sulph.

It was easier now to select the remedy for the patient. His obstinacy and desire for eggs with polypoidal growth in the rectum throws greater weight for Calc-carb even without the repertorisation, but this exercise gives one great confidence in the prescription.

Calc-carb 30 and later 10M potency cured the patient of all his complaints including a very obstinate blepharitis.

Discussion- Why did I jump suddenly from 30 potency to 10M? The answer is that when I am sure of a remedy especially in children's complaints like this, I give higher potency of Calc-carb. It does cut short the duration of the curative reaction. Calc-carb 30 gave some relief but it seemed to be a rather slow process. This case reminded me of two other cases of rectal polypus and they too responded to only Calc-carb. I would recommend raising its grade in Kent's Repertory to highest grade in 'Rectum-Polypi', where only Phos has been given in highest grade.

In this case, it was not only the polypus which disappeared, but the skin and eye symptoms also vanished and the boy was less irritable and more cooperative.

I am firmly convinced that physicians would do good to younger generations if they prescribe only Homoeopathic medicines from infancy to adulthood. These remedies can, not only modify most of the genetically inherited tendencies but also restore balance, thus enabling them to pursue higher purposes in life as Hahnemann put it.

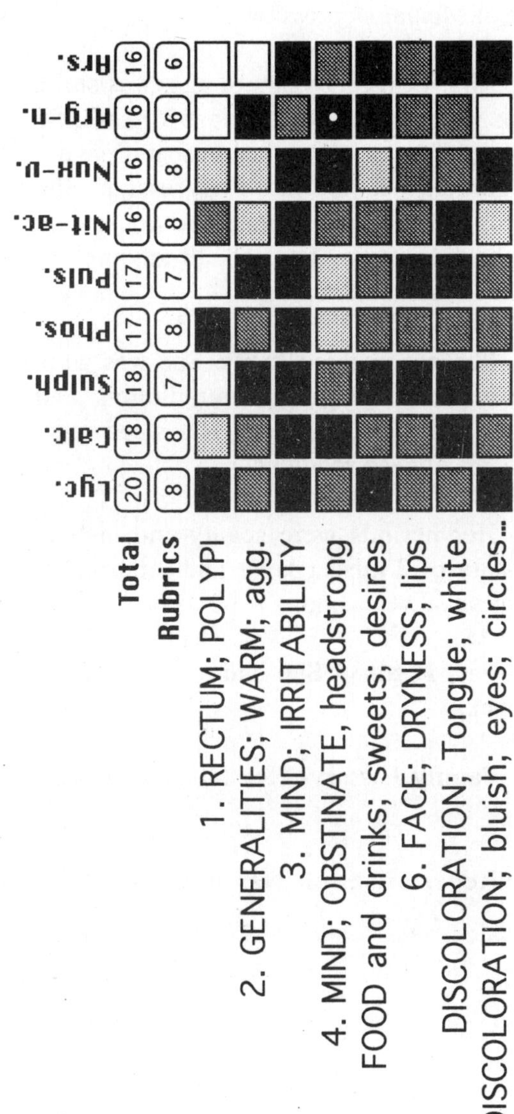
C-21
8/8/97
Jugal Kishore, Dr
Analysis Options: Totality, All Remedies
Total
Rubrics
Lyc. 20 8
Calc. 18 8
Sulph. 18 7
Phos. 17 8
Puls. 17 7
Nit-ac. 16 8
Nux-v. 16 8
Arg-n. 16 6
Ars. 16 6
1. RECTUM; POLYPI
2. GENERALITIES; WARM; agg.
3. MIND; IRRITABILITY
4. MIND; OBSTINATE, headstrong
FOOD and drinks; sweets; desires
6. FACE; DRYNESS; lips
DISCOLORATION; Tongue; white
DISCOLORATION; bluish; eyes; circles...

CASE N0.22

A Case of Mental Depression

Mrs. U.M., 39 years of age, was suffering from psycho-neurosis, depression for the last 3 years. She suffered from a lot of complexes. After her husband gave up his job 3 years back, she had become more aggressive. She was listless and even stopped working around the house. She could not weep or laugh, did not want to talk to anyone. There was loathing of life and suicidal thoughts.

She got irritated easily. She was worse in general after physical exertion; from contradiction and ameliorated in company and when occupied. Her sleep was disturbed and she had dreams of dead relations.

Her periods were scanty and lasted only 2 days. She had history of 2 miscarriages and 2 normal deliveries. Her last delivery was 8 years ago.

Past History- She had similar attacks of depression 2 years back.

Family History- Her father and brother suffered from M.I.

Repertorisation was done with the following data-

	Kishore Cards	Kent' Rep
Mortification	2083	0068
Company amel.	0107	0012
Occupation amel.	0430	0069
Contradiction intolerant of	1941	0016
Irritable	6692	0057
Suicidal thoughts	2152	0085
Dreams of dead	0944	1237

I Grade- Aur.
II Grade- Ign., Lyc.

Aur-met 30, 200, 1M in unit doses reduced the depression and suicidal thoughts. The same course was repeated again. Later Sepia had to be given due to indifference of the patient to herself and her children.

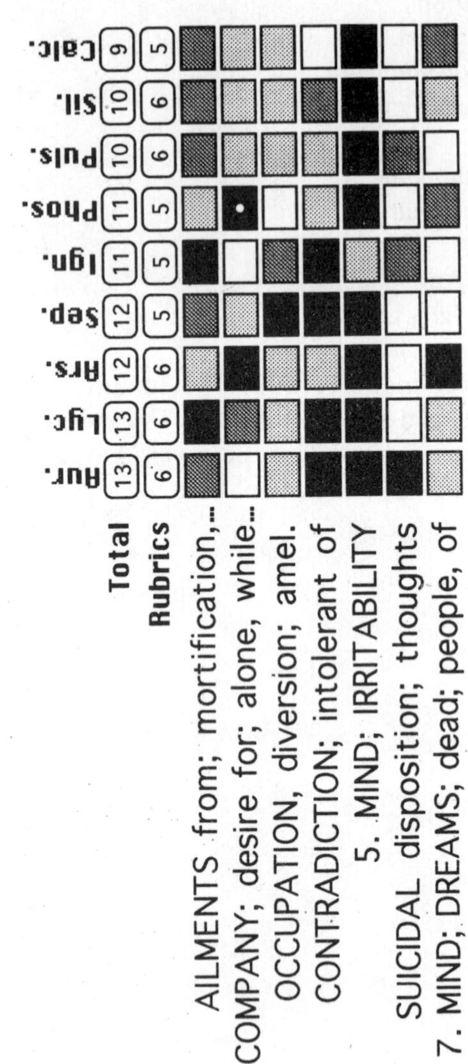
C-22
8/8/97
Jugal Kishore, Dr
Analysis Options: Totality, All Remedies
Aur. Lyc. Ars. Sep. Ign. Phos. Puls. Sil. Calc.
Total 13 13 12 12 11 11 10 10 9
Rubrics 6 6 6 5 5 5 6 6 5
AILMENTS from; mortification,...
COMPANY; desire for; alone, while...
OCCUPATION, diversion; amel.
CONTRADICTION; intolerant of
5. MIND; IRRITABILITY
SUICIDAL disposition; thoughts
7. MIND; DREAMS; dead; people, of

CASE N0.23

A Case of Persistent Backache

Mr. R.G. 28 years old, suffering from lumbar backache ever since he hurt his back 2 years ago. Pain is aggravated on bending; standing; sitting and from exposure to cold air. It is relieved by lying on the back and hot fomentation.

There is lot of hair falling and dandruff. He also has lot of flatulence and pain in abdomen after eating, which is relieved after passing flatus. He has dreams of quarrels and fights.

On examination his blood pressure is 150/100.

In the Family History his father has asthma.

Repertorisation was done taking the following symptoms-

	Kishore Cards	Kent's Rep
1. Dreams of fights	4746	1239
2. Head hair, falling of	1658	0120
3. Back Pain lumbar region	3982	0905
4. Back Pain - when stooping	3947	0898
5. Gen. agg. cold air	0062	1348
6. Gen. agg. sitting	0283	1401
7. Gen. agg. standing	0296	1403
8. Gen. amel. lying on back	0419	1372
9. Gen. amel. external warmth (Uncovering agg.)	0456	1410

I Grade- Con.

II Grade- numerous

Conium-mac 30 was prescribed after trying Bryonia. There was a great response after Conium. The same prescription was repeated several times till the patient was finally free of his backache.

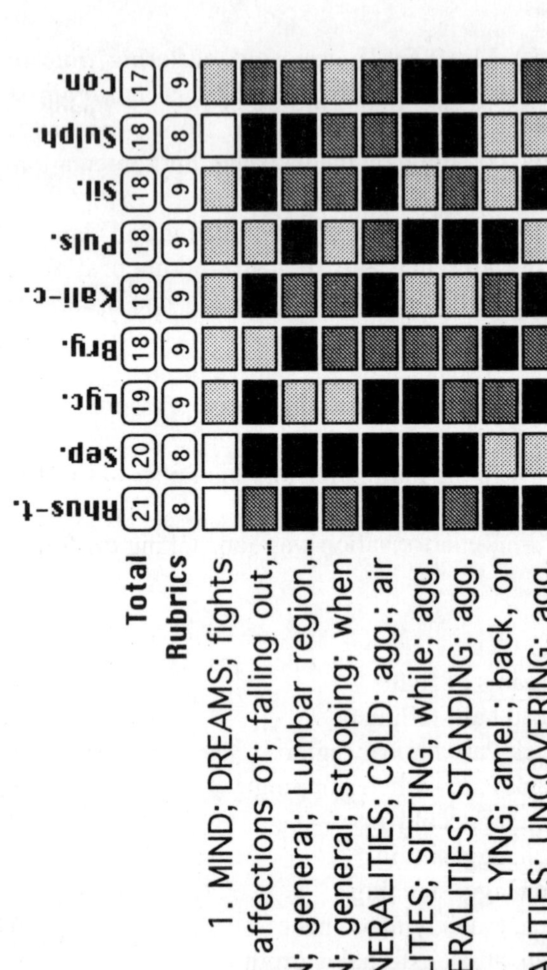
C-23
8/8/97
Jugal Kishore, Dr
Analysis Options: Totality, All Remedies
Rhus-t.
Sep.
Lyc.
Bry.
Kali-c.
Puls.
Sil.
Sulph.
Con.
Total
21
20
19
18
18
18
18
18
17
Rubrics
8
8
9
9
9
9
9
8
9
1. MIND; DREAMS; fights
HAIR, affections of; falling out,...
PAIN; general; Lumbar region,...
PAIN; general; stooping; when
5. GENERALITIES; COLD; agg.; air
6. GENERALITIES; SITTING, while; agg.
7. GENERALITIES; STANDING; agg.
LYING; amel.; back, on
9. GENERALITIES; UNCOVERING; agg.

CASE NO. 24

A Case of Warts

Mr. M.K., 24 years old, had warts on dorsum of hands for the last one year. Onset was from left hand. Later right hand also. There were about seven warts on the left hand and three on the right and there was no pain or itching associated.

On interrogation, we came to know that he has also been suffering from allergic rhinits for the last 10 years, which was worse in change of season. Thin nasal discharge in the morning, nasal obstruction. Tongue indented. Increased saliva.

He had already taken Thuja and had applied some medicine locally.

We took the following rubrics for analysis-

	Kishore Cards	Kent's Rep
1. Gen. side left	2822	1401
2. Gen. side left to right	2823	1401
3. Ext. warts hands	1322	1223
4. Warts hard	8792	1339
5. Warts flat	8791	1339
6. Mouth salivation increased	2245	0417
7. Gen. tendency to take a cold	0773	1349

I Grade- Dulc.
II Grade- Calc., Caust., Lach. and Sep.

On 10.6.86, Dulc. 1M was given. There was no change after a month and Caust 1M was tried. Warts became smaller and flatter but were still persisting after repeating Caust 1M. In October, Lach 1M was prescribed. There was no change in the warts, but her thirst and perspiration on palms increased even though it was winter. Thirst for large quantities of water.

Tendency to catch colds was much better. Dulcamara was again given on 18 October. In November, warts had disappeared. She had dark circles around eyes for 6 months. It was more noticable in the morning. Itching in the eyes and sweating of the soles. When he returned next time on 22 January 1987, there was no problem and he needed no further medication.

Comments- In this case, repertorial analysis helped us in the selection of the indicated remedies and their relationship in the clinical progress. Dulcamara, though, having all the symptoms did not make any impression in the beginning but was able to finish the curative process in the end. Causticum as a deep anti-sycotic remedy modified the patient's response so that ultimately Dulcamara finally cured the case.

C-24 **8/8/97** **Jugal Kishore, Dr**

Analysis Options: Totality, All Remedies

	Dulc.	Calc.	Sep.	Lach.	Sulph.	Caust.	Thuj.	Nit-ac.	Ant-c.
Total	15	14	14	13	12	11	11	11	10
Rubrics	7	7	6	7	5	6	6	4	6

1. GENERALITIES; SIDE; left
SIDE; left; right, then
3. EXTREMITIES; WARTS; Hand
4. SKIN; WARTS; hard
5. SKIN; WARTS; flat
6. MOUTH; SALIVATION
COLD; tendency to take

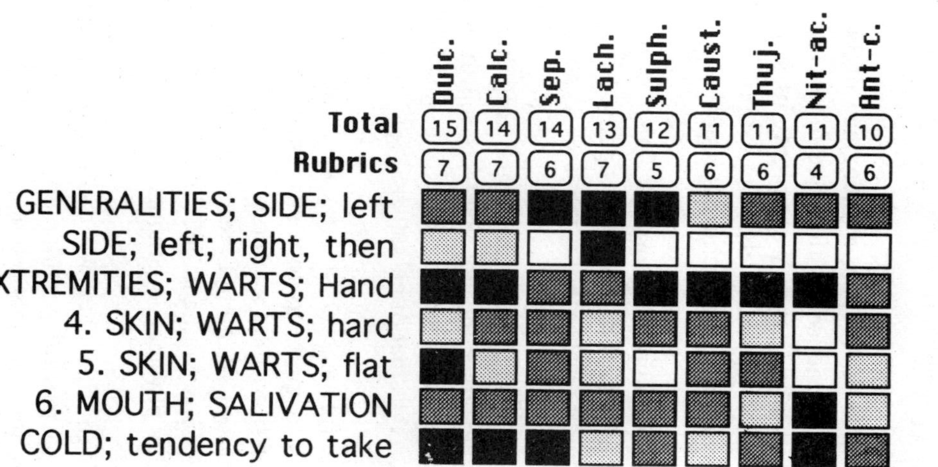

Case No. 25

A Case of Acne

On 11 June 1986, a youngman of 18 years of age, Mr. A.G. presented himself with a face full of acne, mostly pustular and very painful. There were plenty of scar marks. He had a greasy skin. It appeared that the eruptions were more on the right side and there was itching at times.

In the family history his father also had Acne Rosacea in his younger days. He accompanied his son and his face showed pock marks as the relics of the violence of the acne.

Both father and son were very anxious, naturally so because the father did not want his son to go through what he had suffered, and the son was afraid that he might have a face as disfigured as that of his father.

Unfortunately, there were no other characteristic symptoms to guide us to a similimum. The patient, however, is fond of fried food and cold drinks, likes company. There is some amount of mental tension due to the eruptions, but otherwise he is calm and does not show any mental abberations or any other physical complaints.

With this data, we could think of Hep or Lyco; Hep because of painful pustular eruptions, and Lyco because the eruptions were concentrated more on the right side of face.

We decided, however, to work out the case on the Kishore Cards to make a satisfactory prescription. A little extra work - yes, but the results usually are worth the trouble. I chose to work with the following data-

	Kishore Cards	Kent's Rep
1. Desires cold drinks	0908	0484
2. Desires fats	4660	0485
3. Gen. side right	2824	1400
4. Face eruptions acne	1502	0366
5. Face eruptions pustules	5839	0371
6. Mind desire for company	1933	0012

I Grade- Ars., Mez.

On 12.6.86, we prescribed Mez 200, a unit dose which was repeated every 15 days for two months. He responded very well.

On 18.8.86, Mez 1M was given, as the effect of the last dose of Mez 200 was short lived and a few pustular eruptions had appeared. About 2 months later i.e. 28.10.86, he needed another dose of Mez 1M. He was practically cured. Subsequent enquiries elicited no relapse. We need not mention that placebo, Hahnemann's second prescription, was utilised regularly.

Comments- Kent's Repertory does not show Mez in the rubric 'Desire for fats' and 'Face- eruptions, acne' whereas in Kishore's cards, we had made certain additions.

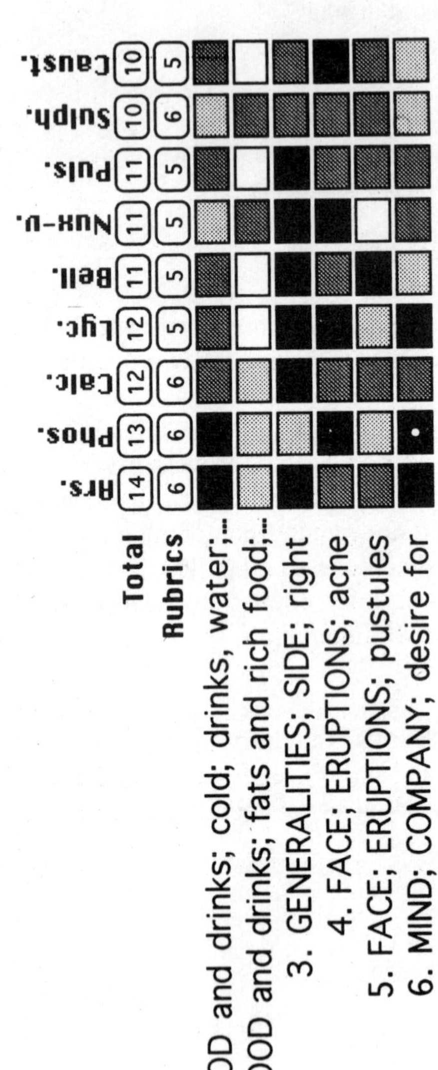
C-25
8/8/97
Jugal Kishore, Dr
Analysis Options: Totality, All Remedies
Ars. Phos. Calc. Lyc. Bell. Nux-v. Puls. Sulph. Caust.
Total 14 13 12 12 11 11 11 10 10
Rubrics 6 6 6 5 5 5 5 6 5
FOOD and drinks; cold; drinks, water;...
FOOD and drinks; fats and rich food;...
3. GENERALITIES; SIDE; right
4. FACE; ERUPTIONS; acne
5. FACE; ERUPTIONS; pustules
6. MIND; COMPANY; desire for

Case No.26

A Case of Warts

Mr. A.K.S., 25 years of age, suffering from warts on face for last six months. Onset was from left side of forehead and warts were more on left side of face. Flat warts. No itching.

Concomitant- Diarrhoea from rich, fried food; flatulance and distention from fatty food. His appetite is poor, prefers sweets and fried food, which, however, disagrees.

Worrying type; tense and short tempered. Reserved nature, broods about his feelings.

On examination liver left lobe is palpable and tender. Colon and Ileocaecal region is also tender.

Cauterisation was done twice, but there was recurrence. Homoeopathic treatment for 3 to 4 months. Thuj., Sil. and Calc. were given.

Rapid repertorisation on Kishore Cards with the following rubrics-

	Kishore Cards	Kent's Rep
1. Desires sweets	0919	0486
2. Desires fats	4660	0485
3. Skin warts flat	8791	1339
4. Gen. Agg. from rich food	3761	1363

I Grade- Nat-m.
II Grade- Sep.

On 4.8.87, Sepia 30 was given twice daily for sometime but there was no improvement. Later, he was given Nat-mur 30, but it did not help. The warts were increasing in size and in number. Dulcamara was prescribed without any effect on the warts, though his appetite improved. On 19.10.87 Nat-mur 200, 1M and 10M were given on three successive days with sac-lac to follow. Warts started shrinking after this. The same course was repeated and he was cured by the end of the year.

Comments- In Kents Repertory, Sepia is mentioned as a remedy for warts on face but not Nat-mur. The prescription was made on generals with the help of Kishore cards. Nat-m 30 did not help but higher potencies did help the case. Was the stock of 30th potency defective? We discover new things with every case we treat.

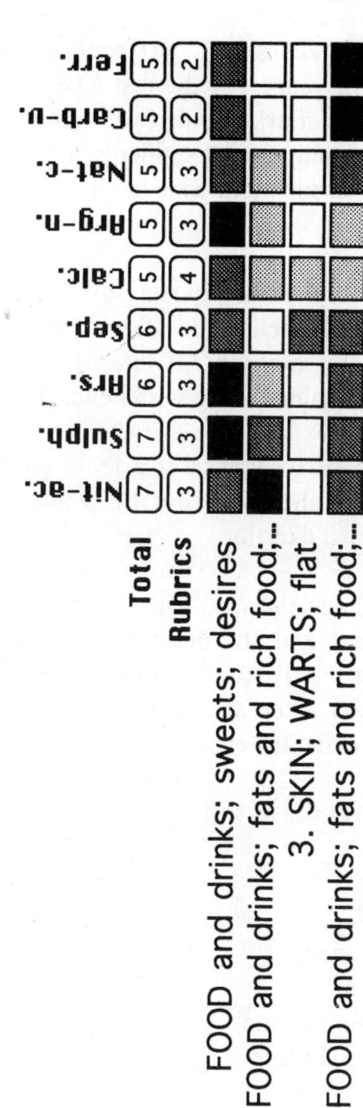
C-26
8/8/97
Jugal Kishore, Dr
Analysis Options: Totality, All Remedies
Total
Rubrics
Nit-ac. 7 3
Sulph. 7 3
Ars. 6 3
Sep. 6 3
Calc. 5 4
Arg-n. 5 3
Nat-c. 5 3
Carb-v. 5 2
Ferr. 5 2
FOOD and drinks; sweets; desires
FOOD and drinks; fats and rich food;...
3. SKIN; WARTS; flat
FOOD and drinks; fats and rich food;...

CASE NO. 27

A Case of Migraine

Mrs. H.S., 35 years old, suffered from attacks of Migraine for the last 12 years. For the last 4 years, the headache was of severe intensity. Earlier pain was generalised, now it is one sided. Pulsating pain comes suddenly and goes gradually. Lot of vomitings are associated. She has nausea especially in the morning.

Headache is worse from exposure to sun; mental tension; before menses, and it is ameliorated after sleep; from pressure; after vomiting and after menses. Of late, there is stiffness of one side of neck and shoulder along with headache.

She has a lot of weakness and feels giddy often. Her face is oedamatous and she has palpitations after vomiting and after any sort of physical exertion.

As a person, she is very sensitive to heat of the sun. Her appetite is normal and she desires sour things and extra salt in her food. She has frequent thirst. She is irritable and weeps easily, especailly when she faces contradiction. She likes to be consoled and is offended easily.

The case analysis is as follows-

	Kishore Cards	Kents Rep
Head pain one sided	6420	0166
Head pain amel. after sleep	6319	0148
Head pain amel. pressure	0630	0145
Head pain agg. exposure to sun	6333	0149
Head pain agg. menses, before	6274	0142
Generalities agg. sun	0306	0149
Mind offended easily	2087	0069
Weeping	2182	0092
Stomach desires salt	0917	0486

II Grade- Calc., Carb-v., Nat-m., Sulph.

The treatment was started with Nat mur 30 three times a day. After 5 weeks of this treatment her headaches improved. She was generally worse before menses. Appetite was somewhat poor. This time she was given Nat-mur 1M, followed by placebo for 2 weeks.

After 2 weeks, we were disappointed to note that her headaches were back with the same intensity. She had left sided pain. She was averse to milk and had frequent nausea aggravated by strong odors. This time the other first grade remedy i.e. Sulph was given to her in 6 potency morning and bedtime. For the next 2 months, she remained free of migraine. Then it got worse again. There was lot of distention in the abdomen and gases. Lycopodium 30 was the next choice. This remedy has given her so much relief. For the last 2 years, she has visited us only thrice, and each time Lycopodium has helped immediately.

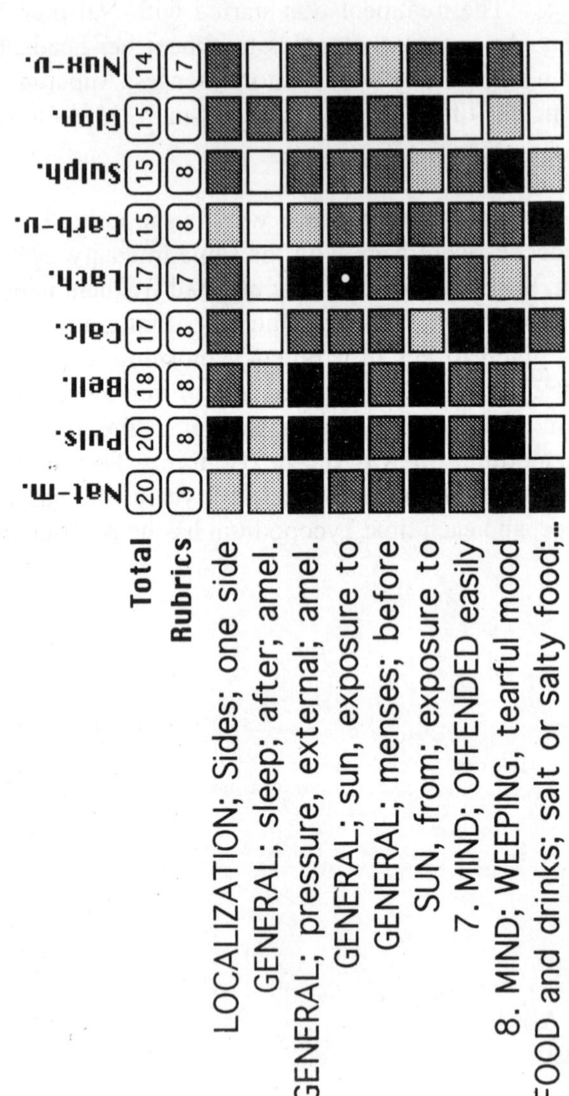
C-27
8/8/97
Jugal Kishore, Dr
Analysis Options: Totality, All Remedies
Nat-m.
Puls.
Bell.
Calc.
Lach.
Carb-v.
Sulph.
Glon.
Nux-v.
Total
20
20
18
17
17
15
15
15
14
Rubrics
9
8
8
8
7
8
8
7
7
LOCALIZATION; Sides; one side
GENERAL; sleep; after; amel.
GENERAL; pressure, external; amel.
GENERAL; sun, exposure to
GENERAL; menses; before
SUN, from; exposure to
7. MIND; OFFENDED easily
8. MIND; WEEPING, tearful mood
FOOD and drinks; salt or salty food;...

CASE NO. 28

A Case of Fibroid Uterus

Mrs. S.M., aged 45 years, had profuse menses, dark bleeding with dark clots which left stains. The flow lasted for 10 days. She had a period every 2 months. During menses she had backache, pain in legs and nausea and anorexia. Irritability before and during menses

She also suffered from pain in knees on standing; squatting; on initial movement; cold weather. She felt relief on rest.

There was headache and giddiness. General weakness. Pain in the legs. Desire to rest.

She had Grade II toxic Goitre. She was given Iodine 131.

She had 4 normal deliveries and 2 abortions.
Thirst- Increased for large quantities
Desires spicy and sour food. Takes 4-5 cups of tea.
Perspiration- excessive on scalp
Stools- hard, difficult, painful
Urine- Bladder control poor. Incontinence sometimes.

Irritable due to disease. Suppresses anger. Offended easily.

The following investigations had been done-

US Abdomen- Ut. is enlarged. Shows an anechoic area measuring 3 cm X 3 cm suggestive of a fibroid.

Urine exam.- Albumin traces, WBC-2-4/hpf, RBC- 8-10/hpf, Ca oxalate crystals.

Serum cholesterol 183. Hb- 10 gms %, TLC- 11,700, DLC P70 L20 E7 M3
B.P.- 120/80

The case was analysed with the following rubrics-

	Kishore Cards	Kent's Rep
Mind Irritable before menses	6929	0059
Mind Irritable during menses	6930	0059
Menses dark	1854	0726
Menses profuse	1852	0725
Female genitalia, tumor, uterus fibroid	3200	0745
Urination involuntary	3325	0659
Head perspiration scalp	3061	0221
Perspiration profuse	3042	1299
Desires sour food	0918	0486
Nausea during menses	7234	0508

I Grade- Calc.
II Grade- Cham., Nat-m., Sep.

On 3 Dec. 1988, she was given Calc-carb 30 repeatedly for a month.

On 31 Dec 1988, she reported to be much better. The same treatment was continued.

In May 1989, there was pain and stiffness in the knees, especially right knee. Sensation as if menses will start. This time she was prescribed Tuberculinum 1M unit dose followed next day by Lyco 30 morning and bedtime for a month.

Patient came back in September 1989. She had menopausal amenorrhoea. The latest US Abdomen showed that there was no mass or fibroid in the uterus.

C-28 **8/8/97** **Jugal Kishore, Dr**

Analysis Options: Totality, All Remedies

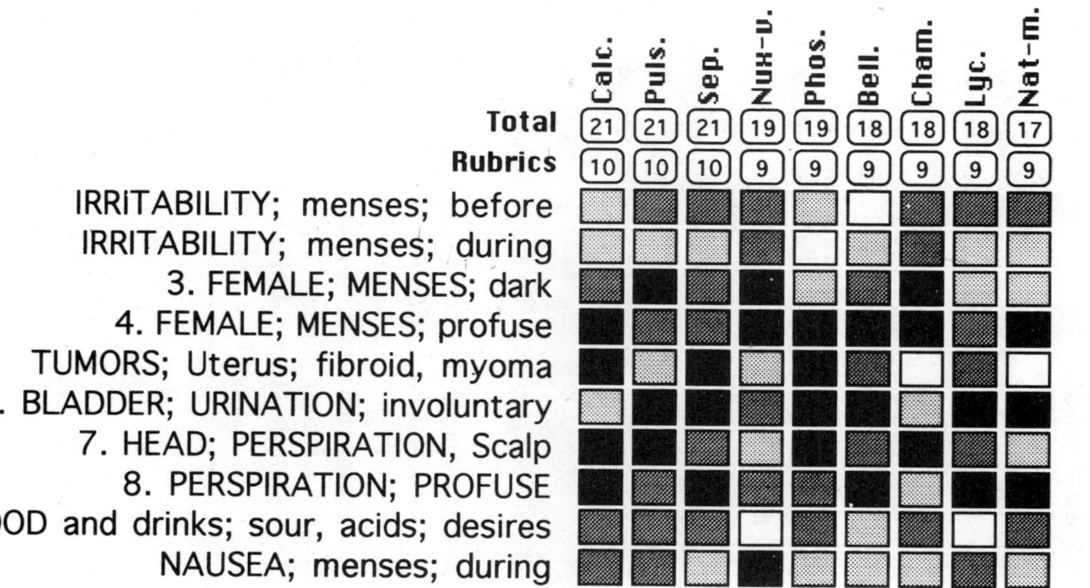

CASE NO. 29

A Case of Seizures

It is the story of a lady(Mrs. C.O.), aged 40 years, who one day suddenly developed numbness and stiffness of the left arm while washing clothes. It was the month of July 1981. Since then she started having frequent attacks of stiffness and seizures involving the right arm with dizziness. There was associated anxiety with coldness of extremities and a sense of dispropotion of limbs of the body as if they are distorted and there was a feeling of weightlessness.

On investigation, her ECG was found to be within normal limits. CT scan was also normal. She was put on Gardenal for three years. Convulsions became better but feeling of anxiety has persisted.

The present picture of her sickness is as follows-

1. Attacks of internal coldness in waves. Numbness and formication of the head.
2. Weakness of both the extremities.
3. Internal trembling of the limbs.
4. Stiffness of neck.
5. Urine is turbid and there is frequent urination. There is associated nausea. When urine becomes clearer, the attacks improve.

During this period (1981 - 1984), while she was having these attacks, she had delusions of weightlessness, with a feeling that she might fly away.

There was also a feeling as if different parts of the body have become distorted or abnormal. For example, once she complained that nose and ears have become smaller.

She is now averse to tight clothes. Gets startled by sudden

noises. There is a sensation of burning of the limbs. She starts weeping at times which seems to give her relief.

There is aversion to relatives but wants the company of her husband and children. She has been married for 22 years and has three children.

Menses were eariier rather early and profuse. But now they are normal and last only 4 days. There is pre-menstrual. tenderness of breasts and a state of anxiety. She feels abnormal weakness after menses.

Her appetite is normal but cannot stand hunger. She must eat something every 2 to 3 hours. She prefers warm food and drinks. Her thirst is normal. Iced water gives her internal coldness in the stomach. She gets a sore throat when she takes something sour.

She is rather a chilly patient, gets easily tired and exhausted by manual exertion like washing clothes or kneading dough. Sleeps poorly during sickness. Sometime back, she used to have dreams of snakes.

During sickness, she becomes very irritable and is averse to talking. She likes company of her family only, and is worse when alone.

Family history- Father has asthma.

Face is marked with cholasma. Tongue is indented but clean. Heart, Lungs NAD. EEG was normal in 1981.

Past treatment- was on Phenobarbitone and Gardenal for 3 years. She was also under treatment of a Psychiatrist. Now she takes it only when she is not well.

	Kishore Cards	Kent's Rep
1. Lack of vital heat	1941	1367
2. Gen. Agg. cold	0100	1348
3. Gen. Agg. fasting	0153	1361
4. Convulsions	0807	1351
5. Weakness after menses	8828	1418
6. Desire for company	1933	0012
7. Desire for company, alone, while agg.	6756	0012
8. Sensitive to noises	2116	0079
9. Delusions of personal identity	1963	0027

I Grade - Phos.
II Grade - Calc., Kali c., Sep.

On 30.3.91 Phos 30 was given 3 times a day

On 4.5.91 Pain chest was gone. General condition is better. Medicine was repeated for 3 weeks.

On 5.6.91 General condition continues to improve. At times vertigo with darkness in front of eyes. Menses normal. Very slight internal trembling. No dreams. Can now sit alone in the house.

On 17.8.91 Better. Numbness, anxiety and trembling before and after menses. Repeated the medicine. The patient has not reported after that.

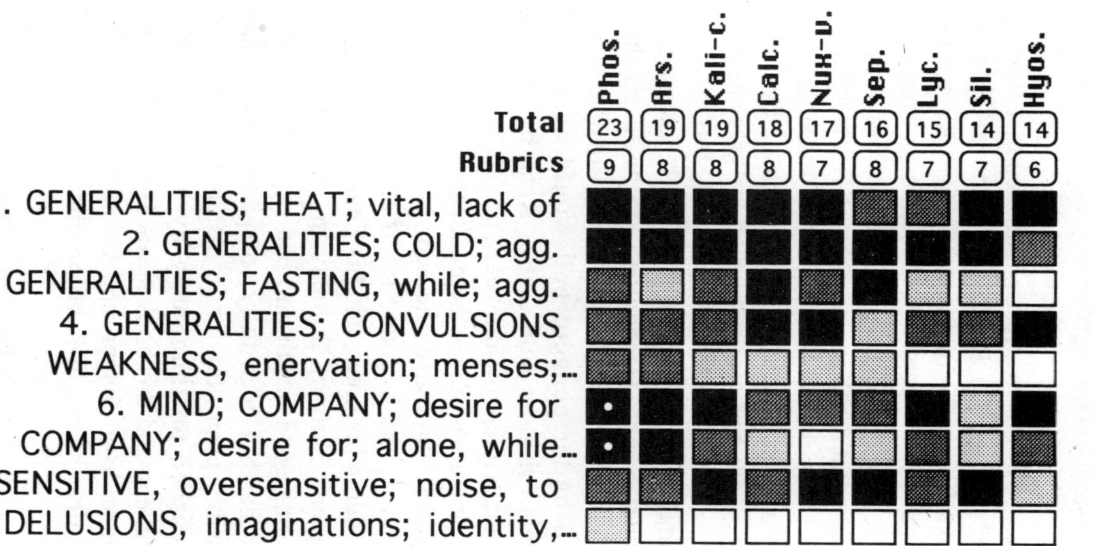

C-29 **8/8/97** **Jugal Kishore, Dr**

Analysis Options: Totality, All Remedies

	Phos.	Ars.	Kali-c.	Calc.	Nux-v.	Sep.	Lyc.	Sil.	Hyos.
Total	23	19	19	18	17	16	15	14	14
Rubrics	9	8	8	8	7	8	7	7	6
1. GENERALITIES; HEAT; vital, lack of									
2. GENERALITIES; COLD; agg.									
3. GENERALITIES; FASTING, while; agg.									
4. GENERALITIES; CONVULSIONS									
WEAKNESS, enervation; menses;...									
6. MIND; COMPANY; desire for									
COMPANY; desire for; alone, while...									
SENSITIVE, oversensitive; noise, to									
DELUSIONS, imaginations; identity,...									

BOGER'S BOENNINGHAUSEN REPERTORY

Philosophical background

As I have already indicated that Boger took up the work of Planning of a Repertory based on Boenninghausen's first book 'Repertory of the Antipsoric Remedies' but there were naturally many gaps and the number of remedies was very much limited. Boger was not only a great intuitive prescriber because of his great depth in the study of Homoeopathic Materia Medica as well as the original works of the older masters, but he had also a great logical mind like that of Boenninghausen. By this time, Kent had also published his great Repertory. Boger could see certain drawbacks in that, but he could also see the limitations of Boenninghausen Repertory called "Therapeutic Pocket Book'. He decided to build up the structure of his Repertory on the earlier works of Boenninghausen, as that would be a better concept and would combine the wisdom of Boenninghausen with that of Kent, by integrating the concepts of both without the drawback or deficiencies of both the masters. His first attempt was the publication of the integrated Repertory in 1905. Naturally, the rubrics were not complete regarding remedies, and he found lot of scope for improvement. He went on adding his notes, and his final work was published by Mssrs. Roy and Sons of Bombay in 1932, but by then, he was not keeping good health and had expired. Unfortunately, this book also has not been fully completed and contains errors, either possibly in printing or in manuscripts. Possibly this book was published posthumously by his wife. Yet, the concept is excellent, and this book needs to be updated and edited properly. Had he lived longer, and given more time from his very busy practice, he might have produced the most perfect Repertory.

In his book, he incorporated the concepts and rubrics from Boenninghausen's work, as mentioned earlier. Repertory of the Antipsoric; Sides of the Body; Repertory of Intermittent Fevers; and Whooping Cough and also the Therapeutic Pocket Book. Apart from these sources, be incorporated Kentian rubrics also, at suitable places. He added numerous clinical additions which had been verified time and again. In this final work, Boger avoided the extreme generalization of Boenninghausen's Therapeutic Book and extreme particularisation of Kent. He took the best part of both.

Let us, for example, take up the symptoms irritability, anger and sadness before menses. In Kent, there are only very few remedies listed in the rubric Irritability before menses', where as, in clinical practice, we find a fairly large number of cases where females have these symptoms, and none of the remedies found in Kent's Repertory seem to be indicated in a number of cases. Here Boger has taken up Boenninghausen's concept, by introducing a rubric 'Aggravation of mental symptoms before menses'. This larger rubric has a better chance of covering a larger number of cases, which means, whether irritability or anger or depression, they will have to be looked in this generalised rubric for Repertoric analysis.

These are many such instances where similar generalization has been done.

Since Boenninghausen was severely criticised by a number of well-known authorities of Homoeopathic Medicine especially Kent, for his unqualified modalities of Aggravation and Amelioration in local symptoms which had opposite modalities to the general symptoms, Boger included modalities of local or particular symptoms also in the relevant sections.

With regard to concomitant symptoms (the 'unassociated attendants' or so called unrelated symptoms) which are not diagnostically connected with the main symptoms or complaints, Boger has given them under each section and given a better defined place.

Structure of the Boger's Boenninghausen

This work is structured, as already written, on

Boenninghausean concept in his earlier Repertories.

He has divided the book into following chapters, along with relevant locations, modalities and concomitants.

(1) Mind
(2) Sensorium
(3) Vertigo
(4) Head; Internal; External
(5) Eyes; Vision
(6) Ears
(7) Nose; Coryza
(8) Face; Lip; Lower jaw and maxillary joints; Chin
(9) Teeth
(10) Mouth; Palate; Throat and gullet; Saliva; Tongue
(11) Appetite
(12) Thirst
(13) Taste
(14) Eructations
(15) Waterbrash and Heartburn
(16) Hiccough
(17) Nausea and Vomiting
(18) Stomach
(19) Epigastrium
(20) Hypochondria
(21) Abdomen
(22) External abdomen
(23) Inguinal and pubic region
(24) Flatulence
(25) Stools
(26) Anus and Rectum
(27) Perineum
(28) Prostate Gland
(29) Urine; Micturition
(30) Urinary organs; Kidney; Bladder; Urethra
(31) Genitalia, Male and Female
(32) Sexual Impulse
(33) Menstruation; Leucorrhoea
(34) Respiration

(35) Cough and Expectoration
(36) Larynx and Trachea
(37) Voice and Speech
(38) Neck and External throat; Nape of neck
(39) Chest, inner and external; Axillae; Mammae; Heart; Region of heart
(40) Back, Scapular, Dorsal and Lumbar region; Sacrum and Coccyx; Spinal column and vertebrae
(41) Upper extremities
(42) Lower extremities
(43) Sensations and Complaints in General
(44) Glands
(45) Bones
(46) Skin and Exterior of Body
(47) Sleep
(48) Dreams
(49) Pathological types
(50) Blood
(51) Circulation; Palpitation; Heart beat and Pulse
(52) Chill
(53) Heat and Fever in general
(54) Sweat
(55) Compound fevers
(56) Conditions of aggravation and amelioration in general, of time, situations, positions, circumstances.
(57) Concordances

The main divisions could be divided into seven chapters, as given in Boenninghausen Therapeutic Pocket Book as follows-

(1) Mind, Intellect; Sensorium and Vertigo
(2) Locations of complaints etc. in different anatomical parts
(3) Sensations in general; Glands, Bones, Skin
(4) Sleep and Dreams
(5) Fever, Blood, Circulation, Chill, Heat, Perspiration
(6) Conditions of Aggravation and Amelioration in general
(7) Relationships of remedies (Concordances)

It may be noted here that Kent in his Repertory, kept in one chapter, both General sensations and General modalities, where as Boenninghausen and later Boger kept them in different distinct chapters.

In the anatomical divisions also, Boger has followed the division from above downwards and front to back. For example, nape of neck i.e. cervical region of back, is given after the frontal part of neck, that is External throat.

Similarly, Back dorsal, lumbar etc. are given after the frontal portion of the body like Chest

Regarding Mental symptoms - Boger, like Boenninghausen, kept broad general mental symptoms for reasons already given in the description of Boenninghausen Repertory, yet, he has mental concomitants, as well as mentally related with other rubrics.

Unlike in Boenninghausen's Therapeutic Pocket Book, Boger in his Repertory, has given sensations etc. of the particular region or area along with their locations. The former follows the locations. These are followed by the modalities of the local organs or area, but here he has done some generalisations unlike in Kent For example, in Kent Repertory, on the section of Pain in general, under Head, the modalities are extensively given, and in practice, we rather utilise these modalities to even when we take up other locational rubrics of head and different kinds of pains or sensations. Boger has given only generalised modalities of the Head. Of course, the patients modalities attending different organs covered by the same modalities are given, as already pointed out, in the main chapters on Aggravation and Amelioration. This is practically the same as given by Boenninghausen in his Therapeutic Pocket Book. Kent, too, has followed more or less the same in his chapter on Generalities.

Although Kent has given concomitants or associated

symptoms spread all over the book wherever a particular sensation or location has been refered- For example, coughing associated with pain in chest is different from coughing associated with pain in head or coughing associated with involuntary urination, Boger, however, followed the logic of Boenninghausen, and remedies given under Concomitants of coughing are all put together in a generalised way i.e. whatever be the area or location, cough producing associated sensation or pains has been included under one bead.

Of course, he has, now and then, given them also in local modalities. He has specially mentioned the concomitant groups of remedies in the following sections, and this is apart from modalities mentioned in the relevant chapters.

For example, under 'Mind' the rubric Aggravations (of mental symptoms) from approach of persons, the remedies are Con, Ign, Lyc, Stry. Aggravations on ascending(steps), the remedies given are Ars, Iod, Nit-ac. These might be considered peculiar concomitants and listed like what Kent has given in some places. Boger has generalised here, as we do not know what particular(mental) symptom is aggravated by ascending. Is it anger or anxiety or fear of death? Of course, at the end of this chapter, he kept concomitants in general (pg 229). These are the mental concomitants.

Mind
Vertigo
Head(Under Head, he has not given any generalised group of concomitants, but under Aggravation, he mentioned here and there peculiar concomitants of headache. For example,
"Headache, after tearing pains in limbs", "Headache, torticollis, with", or "Headache, toothache, with".)
Nausea and Vomiting
Stomach
Stool- before; during; after
Urinating, before; during; close of; after
Concomitants after coition

Concomitants after pollutions
Menses before; at start of; during; after
Leucorrhoea
Respiration
Cough
Fever (chill)
Heat and fever in general

Of course, no concomitants have been given by Kent and Boger in their chapter on Sensation in general and Modalities respectively.

One of the most useful contributions made by Boger was in giving cross-references towards the end of every chapter. His cross-references in the chapter on Mind are the most valuable, as it is in this area that the patient may not be able to express his feelings well enough, or clear enough, so that we could translate his symptoms in the terms of rubrics in the Repertory. Even on the part of the physician, it may be difficult to assess the mental make up of the patient, and he may not be able to pen down the rubric.

Regarding Boger's chapter on Concordances, one has to refer back to Boenninghausen's Therapeutic Pocket Book.

Many of the so called concomitants are actually the causative symptoms or rubrics based on causation, specially where mental and emotional upsets or shocks are associated with physical ailments. Some of these symptoms or rubrics are of the utmost importance.

I would like to quote here Dr. Bhanu D. Desai's comments on concomitants. He has said that a concomitant having the same aggravation or amelioration as the general symptoms, represents a highly characteristic feature of the remedy and is of great importance. In other words, a modality which is common to the chief complaint, as well as a concomitant complaint, is all important For example, if the eruption on the head and whitish stools, which is a concomitant, are both aggravated by milk, this common modality would leave no doubt regarding Calc-carb being the curative remedy.

Similarly, mental concomitants in physical ailments, and physical concomitant in mental ailments, are an unfailing guide to the similimum. For example, cutting, cramping pain in the abdomen after indignation, if relieved by doubling up, would call for Colocynth, but without the amelioration from doubling up would indicate Staphysgaria.

As I have already mentioned. Dr. H.A.Roberts has summed up that the concomitant symptom is to the totality what the condition of aggravation or amelioration is to the single symptom. It is the differentiating factor.

I am giving a number of cases worked out on Boger's Boenninghausen. As I have mentioned earlier that Dr. B.D. Desai has made a singular contribution to the relevance and usage of this Repertory in analysing the case records. I am quoting the following cases worked by him on the Repertory. Detailed histories of the cases have not been given, but the complaints or the relevant symptoms have been indicated by the rubrics taken.

Case 1

Mr. R.S.T. age 48 years- Ankylosis of spine (dorsal)- **Lyco**
Ref: Dr. Bhanu.D.Desai

Rubrics-	B-B Rep Page No.
1. Agg. sitting erect	1141
2. Agg. rest	1137
3. Agg. lying down	1128
4. Agg. 4 a.m.	(Page 19 of Boger's Synoptic Key)
5. Spine dorsal	788
6. Stiffness	792
7. Memory weak	211

	1	2	3	4	5	6	7	Total
Carbo-v	2	2	2	-	3	4	3	16/6
Cham	2	3	4	-	2	-	x	
Coloc	3	3	2	1	1	-	-	
Con	3	4	4	3	2	-	4	20/6
Lyco	3	4	4	3	4	1	4	23/7
Sabad	2	4	3	-	2	-	x	

Comments- The most striking modalities were first taken up and remedies common to the first two noted as the eliminative group. Lyco 30 for a week, and then 200, at infrequent intervals, cured the patient in two months.

Case 2

Mr. Rao, age 42 years - Unsteady gait for the last two months which other systems had failed to cure- **Agar**
Ref : Dr. B.D.D.

Rubrics -	B-B Rep Page No.
1. Stumbling, uncertain gait	868
2. Uncertain, unsteady gait	855
3. Mind intoxicated, as if	208
4. Reeling staggering gait	916
5. Agg. after motion	1132
6. Vertigo	239
7. Hips- Lower ext.	842
8. Weakness	873

	1	2	3	4	5	6	7	8	Total
Agar	3	2	2	4	4	2	4	2	23/8
Arg-n	3	1	-	-	x	x	x	x	
Bar-c	3	2	-	-	x	x	x	x	
Cocc	1	2	1	4	2	2	2	-	14/7
Sec	1	2	-	3	-	2	x	x	
Stann	1	1	-	-	4	1	3	3	13/6

Comments-As there are four different rubrics on the chief complaint, it was thought advisable to take common remedies from the first. A modality and three concomitants gave a massive vote for Agaricus which effected a smooth and speedy cure.

Case 3

This is a case, given by Elizabeth W.Hubbard (Homoeopathic Herald, Octobe 1977), of cracks and fissures on face. The remedy mentioned by her, **Nitric acid** has been worked out by us here, with the help of Boger Boenninghausen's Repertory.

Rubrics-	B-B Rep Page No.
1. Face cracked, fissured	405
2. Anus- fissure of	611
3. Urine ammoniacal	621
4. Thirsty	480
5. Desires fat	476
6. Averse to milk	474

	1	2	3	4	5	6	Total
Ars	4	-	-	4	1	1	
Carb-v	4	-	2	3	-	2	
China	4	-	-	3	-	1	
Ign	4	-	-	3	-	4	
Merc	4	-	-	4	-	1	
Nat-m	4	3	-	4	-	1	
Nit-ac	4	4	3	3	2	1	17/6
Verat	4	-	-	4	-	-	

Comments- As there are a number of drugs in the highest grade in the first rubric, only those were taken in the 'eliminative' group.

Case 4

A case of cardiac disorder (Endocarditis) Rheumatism treated by Dr. J.T.Kent (Indian Journal of Homoeopathic Medicine, 12/1-1978)- **Aurum**

Rubrics B-B Rep Page No.

1.Rheumatic metastasis to heart 775
2. Agg. rest(Amel. by motion) 1137
3. Amel. open air 1105
4. Desires meat 476
5. Hungry, very 478

	1	2	3	4	5	Total
Acon	3	1	2	-	2	
Ars	1	2	1	-	2	
Aur	1	4	2	2	2	11/5
Bry	2	1	2	1	3	
Caust	3	1	2	-	2	
Kalm	2	-	-	-	-	
Lach	4	2	3	-	4	
Puls	2	4	4	-	4	
Spig	2	1	1	-	2	

Comments- All the remedies in Rubric 1 were taken to begin with. Note how Kent, a master prescriber, selected only 5 rubrics to get to the remedy. Note also, how the same remedy of Kent was arrived at, from the Boger-Boenninghausen's Repertory. Note further, how remedies with even 3 or 4 marks in the first rubric were thrown out, and Aurum with only 1 mark came through as it has all the five selected symptoms - a point stresses the need for selecting the characteristic general symptoms which pertain to the patient and touch him in his depths.

Case 5

Peritonitis- **Ars**
Ref: Dr. Edward P.Van Tine, M.D. (Homoeopathic Herald, Sept. 1978, Page 170)

Dr. Tine discussed these symptoms in an article while pointing out how to differentiate one drug from another. In this particular case, he was pointing out that though many of the symptoms are common to Ars and Sec, the symptom better by warmth would point to Ars, while worse by heat would lead to Secale. The symptoms are repertorised here with Boger-Boenninghausen's Repertory to show once again, how this Repertory can be a wonderful guide even in serious and complicated cases.

Rubrics-	B-B Rep Page No.
1. Abdomen inflated(distended)	551
2. Vomiting bloody	502
3. Rectum bleeding	610
4. Desires hot food and drinks	477
5. Agg. from cold in general	1110
6. Restlessness, mental	214
7. Burning internal	886
8. Thirst	480
9. Tongue dry	464
10. Tongue red	467

	1	2	3	4	5	6	7	8	9	10	Total
Arn	3	4	-	-	2	3	3	1	3	-	
Ars	4	4	1	3	4	4	3	4	4	3	34/10
Bell	4	4	-	-	3	3	4	4	4	3	
Carb-v	4	3	3	-	2	2	4	3	4	-	
Chin	4	3	-	-	-	x	x	x	x	x	
Nux-v	4	4	2	-	4	4	4	4	2	1	29/9
Phos	4	4	4	-	2	2	4	4	4	1	29/9
Sec	4	3	1	-	-	2	3	3	1	x	
Calc	4	4	2	-	1	2	3	3	4	-	

Comments- As there are a large number of remedies in the highest grade in the first two rubrics, only those remedies which together made at least 7 marks in the two rubrics, were selected for eliminative purposes, to save time and labour.

Case 6

Melancholia, twisted outlook. This is a case reported by the famous Dr. Tomas Pablo Paschero in the British Hom. Journal, Vol LIII, No. 2, 1964, and which Dr. Jugal Kishore has used to demonstrate a case analysis with Kishore Cards. It relates to a woman, aged 31 years, suffering from exhaustion, extreme irritability and intolerance, weeping, frigidity, etc. This condition developed on account of her mentally retarted son aged 5, who had encephalitis when a year old. The first dose of Sepia 200 caused an aggravation. Sepia 1M after two months caused a rash on the face. Sepia 10M given forty days later modified her apathy, and her attitude towards her son was totally changed. She became tender, affectionate with him, with her husband and her other two children, and she herself became tranquil.

Rubrics-	B/B Rep Page No.
1. Wet, drenched etc. agg.	1152
2. Spring agg.	1142
3. Desires sweets	477
4. Anxiety(after stool) in abdomen	545
5. Weakness, exhaustion	935
6. Agg. morning	1103
7. Agg. on rising	1137
8. Aversion to loved ones	193
9. Agg. from consolation	1112

	1	2	3	4	5	6	7	8	9	Total
Calc	4	3	-	1	4	4	3	1	-	
Lach	3	4	-	-	1	3	4	x	x	
Lyc	3	3	-	1	4	2	3	1	-	21/8
Nat-m	2	2	1	-	4	4	3	-	-	
Rhus-t	4	3	2	1	4	4	3	-	-	
Sep	4	2	1	2	4	3	2	3	2	23/9
Sil	3	2	-	-	3	2	3	x	x	
Sulph	3	3	2	3	3	3	3	-	1	

Case 7

This case illustration is taken from Dr. Harvey Farrington's 'Homoeopathy Prescribing'. At page 245 he says- 'This method of repertorising employs the physical general characterisitics and is usually chosen when mental symptoms are not characterisitc, or are lacking. The mental symptoms, if any, are considered second in order, and the particular symptom last. To illustrate by a case from actual practice- The symptoms given, have been chosen because of their value in Repertory work. Irrelevant symptoms have been omitted. The diagnosis was 'pruritus vulvae' due to toxic acidosis. Mrs. W. aged 25, married, has two children. Since her last labour, she has had profuse, yellow leucorrhoea and violent pruritus vulvae. The case analysed with Kent's Repertory brought out Sulphur as covering all the symptoms.Working with Boger-Boenninghausen's Repertory also, gives Sulphur the highest rank. The order of symptoms taken by Farrington is adhered to, in the following working, except for Rubric 1, which is taken first (instead of its original 10th place), in order to reduce the work involved, with remedies with only 4 marks in it being taken for eliminative purpose. It will be noted that Sulphur scores 3 or 4 marks against all rubrics, except for only two. This evidences its highest rank in this case.

Rubrics-	B/B	Bell	Nat-c	Sep	Sul
1. Female Genitalia-pressure down	663	4	4	4	4
2. Agg. standing, while	1143	1	2	3	3
3. Agg. night	1104	3	2	2	3
4. Agg. physical exertion	1117	-	2	2	4
5. Agg. before menses	678	1	1	2	4
6. Memory weak	211	3	3	3	4
7. Head throbbing	277	4	-	4	4
8. Vertex, pressure on	270	2	1	2	2
9. Flushes of heat	1048	3	3	4	4
10. Feet cold	1027	3	4	4	4
11. Leucorrhoea	687	1	3	4	3
12. Leucorrhoea yellow	689	1	2	4	2
13. Stomach empty feeling	517	1	2	3	3
14. Vertex heat	1050	-	2	-	4
15. Sweat axillae	1082	-	-	4	4
16. Sweat odorous	1078	3	-	4	3

This is yet another case taken from the above mentioned book of Dr. Harvey Farrington, M.D. illustrating his method 1, viz, Starting with the mental symptoms; then taking the physical generals, followed by the particular symptoms of the case.

This is a case of malaria, treated first with massive doses of quinine, then with Ars, by an experienced homoeopath. The temperature during the heat rose to 104.5° F. "In prescribing for malarial patients homoeopathically, the exact similimum must be found, if a cure is to be expected." Hence, after taking detailed symptoms and consulting Kent's Repertory, Rhus-tox was found to be the similimum. A single dose of Rhustox (obviously a high potency) was given. For three days, there was no change. From the fourth day, the symptoms gradually abated, and by the sixth day, all the symptoms had disappeared. Years have elapsed with no return of symptoms.

All the symptoms, in the order given by Farrington, were referred to the Boger-Boenninghausen's Repertory, and the analysis is given below.

Rubrics-	B/B Rep Page No.
1. Restlessness	917
2. Restless during chill	1037
3. Restless during heat	1064
4. Thirst during chill	1041
5. Chill at 7 p.m.	1032
6. Back chill	1026
7. Back chill scapulae	1029
8. Intolerance of uncovering	1075
9. Sensation as if dashed with cold water	1021
10. Yawning with chilliness	981
11. Ext. upper, pain during chill	1044
12. Ext lower, pain during chill	1045
13. Ext. numbness in general	883

	1	2	3	4	5	6	7	8	9	10	11	12	13
Anac	4	1	-	-	-	-	-	-	x	x	x	x	x
Bell	4	4	4	1	-	-	-	-	x	x	x	x	
Hyos	4	-	-	-	x	x	x	x	x	x			
Merc	4	1	1	-	-	-	x	x					
Rhus	4	3	4	2	2	3	3	3	4	1	2	3	3
Sep	4	4	1	4	-	-	-	x	x	x	x	x	x
Staph	4	x	1	1	x	x	x						
Stram	4	-	1	-	-	-	x	x					

Comments- To arrive at the first eliminative group of remedies, only the remedies in the highest rank in Rubric 1 were taken, in view of the extreme restlessness and tossing about, and because of which also, it was selected as the first rubric for repertorial analysis. When any remedy drew a blank more than twice, it was eliminated from the contest.

Case 8

Child, aged 1 and a half years. Rickets, Calc, Ref- Dr. B.D.D.

Pathetic case of a male child of a mill-worker, born in the sick country-side, from infancy, now brought to the city for treatment. Calc-carb was obviously the curative remedy, as would have been obvious to any Homoeopathic practitioner. However, the recorded symptoms are repertorised here with Boger Boenninghausen's Repertory, which puts Calc-carb as the similimum beyond question. Truly enough, the child responded to Calc 30 from the beginning, and as improvement progressed, raised potencies at infrequent intervals were enough to take the child to full, vigorous health.

	Rubrics-	B/B Rep. Page No.
1.	Obstinate	203
2.	Walk, learns with difficulty	934
3.	Irritable	212
4.	Head enlarged	300
5.	Abdomen large	552
6.	Head fontenelles open	903
7.	Emaciation	895
8.	Hungry	478
9.	Aversion to milk	474
10.	Desires earth, chalk	476
11.	Desires egg	476
12.	Constipation	583
13.	Teething delayed	903
14.	Face wrinkled	403

	1	2	3	4	5	6	7	8	9	10	11	12	13	14	Total
Bell	4	3	2	-	1	-	-	3	2	-	-	-	3	3	21/8
Calc	4	4	4	4	3	4	3	3	2	1	4	4	4	4	47/14
Sil	3	4	1	3	2	3	3	3	3	2	-	4	-	-	31/11
Sulph	2	3	4	2	3	2	4	4	2	1	-	4	4	-	35/12

Case 9

Mrs. Lakshmi, aged 38 years, with two children. Since child-birth 1 and a half years ago, has never been well. Pale, anaemic, exhausted. Fer-met steered her to health in a couple of months. (Ref. Dr. J.K. Clinics)

Rubrics-		B/B Rep. Page No.
1.	Weakness, exhaustion	935
2.	Excitable	200
3.	Flushes of heat to face and head	396
4.	Vomiting, while eating	507
5.	Anaemia	1009
6.	Eggs agg.	1120
7.	Lips pale	407
8.	Walking amel.	1149
9.	Throbbing occiputal headache	278
10.	Menses, too late	675
11.	Menses too scanty	676

	1	2	3	4	5	6	7	8	9	10	11	Total
Ars	4	3	-	1	4	-	-	2	-	1	-	
Asar	3	3	-	-	-	-	-	x	x			
Bell	3	4	3	1	-							
Calc	4	2	-	1	-							
Camph	3	3	-	-	-							
Cann	3	3	-	1	-							
Cham	3	4	-	-	-							
Coff	2	4	-	-								
Ferr	4	3	4	3	4	2	2	4	3	3	3	11/3
Gels	3	3	4	-	-							
Iod	4	3	-	-	-							
Lyc	4	2	-	-	3	-						
Merc	3	3	-	-	-	-						
Nat-m	4	2	3	-	-	-						
Nit-ac	2	4	2	-	-	-						
Nux-v	4	4	3	1	4	-						
Phos	4	2	3	x	3	-						

Chapter Five
THE CONCLUDING CHAPTER

Regular growth of Repertory, like that of Materia Medica, is the true index of the progress and richness of the Homoeopathic system of medicine. Their growth, therefore, is most vital for the very existence of the system and its contribution for the health and welfare of the society.

The changing pattern of sickness, the tremendous atmospheric and environmental changes, and use and abuse of potentially toxic drugs (crude) have created challenges today which were not known in Hahnemann's time. It is, therefore, tragic if our instruments are not geared up to these challenges. The Materia Medica and its field of application and repertorial indices have to grow rapidly and made up to date. The background of our earlier workers in these areas should inspire us to do such things more extensively and with much greater speed, because of tremendous technological advances that modern world has seen. These problems should be taken up more seriously at the International meets.

Even in our daily clinical practice, there are cases with paucity or absence of mentals or generals and we have to depend upon the local or particulars that are available. This is often seen in cases of ordinary acute coughs and colds, where we depend upon only the regional modalities. If there are more of common (generals) and regional symptoms, then Boenninghausen's approach has to be seriously considered for repertorial analysis and evaluation.

It may again be emphasised that Homoeopathic Materia Medica has been basically built up on the provings of medicines.

Some medicines have been overproved or have been used and confirmed much more frequently than others. Therefore, they have a large data of clinical provings and application. So, in the process of developments of Homoeopathic Repertories and their usage in the analysis of remedies, there is overwhelming dominance of such remedies, with the result that the lesser known remedies, which would be the right similimum in a particular case, are not brought to the surface and are missed. To overcome such difficulties, Boenninghausen conceived the idea of completing symptoms of a remedy by analogy, and thus enlarging the capacity or scope of even lesser known remedies or of remedies with inadequate proving for more extensive application. This has tended to repair this deficiency, but even then it makes only a small dent in the dominance of the bigger remedies. Here it is desirable to integrate both the Kentian and Boenninghausen's concepts for use in the application, and might help us in many situations.

It may be mentioned here that numerical totality will pay great dividends on working with Boenninghausen or Boger's Boenninghausen Repertory than with Kentian methods. In the Kentian method, the dependence on numerical summation can often be misleading. Here, we have to make a judicious selection with special reference to Materia Medica. We discovered the same thing frequently in our clinics, when we worked with Kishoic Card Repertory, where gradation and evaluation of different remedies have not been punched or indicated. These were omitted partly because of these considerations.

There has been a tendency in the past to consider these difficult concepts as inimical to each other. Boger, as we have already seen, has tried to integrate them.

Hering in his Guiding Symptoms, recorded quite a number of new clinically confirmed symptoms which were not present in the provings of the drugs. The applied Materia Medica is built up on this very basis. Lycopodium's aggravation of 4 to 8 p.m. appeared only in the clinical field and was not noticed in the provings. Fortunately, the earlier pioneers of Homoeopathy, recorded by careful observations this clinically confirmed symptom, and thus, enriched our Materia Medica and Repertory. Unfortunately, the later Homoeopathic physicians have not paid sufficient attention to it, with the result, that upgrading of the Materia Medicas and Repertories has not taken place to the desirable extent Without this activity, provided it is done in a scientific and objective manner, we cannot make our Repertories really useful enough, for meeting the increasing and complex demands of the sick humanity, especially when the sickness itself is developing newer and more complex facets, with the increasing complexity of the civilization.

Even during Hahnemann's times, possibility of such difficulty were seen by men like Boenninghausen, and later by his worthy follower. Dr. Boger, as I have mentioned above. The comprehensive generalisation made it possible for more remedies to have a place of honor in a particular case of sickness.

In actual practice, we sometimes come across quite a number of concomitant symptoms which could be diagnostic of a remedy, but in literature, we do not find them recorded. I am giving below, a few common examples in my practice, where I failed to get the relevant reference in the Materia Medica or in the Repertory.

1. I came across a few female patients who felt quite a desire for salt before menses. Nat-mur etc. had not helped them.
2. Increase of appetite during bouts of sneezing (Hay fever ?)
3. A patient had nausea during urticarial attacks.
4. Anger or irritability while fasting or hunger, from.
5. Urge for urination during pain in rectum.
6. Concurrent itching of palms and soles.
7. Lachrymation while eating or during meals.
8. Inflammation and pain in joints before menses.
9. In the pathological rubric of paralysis agitans in the

Generalities of Kent's Repertory, there are only 14 remedies mentioned. It is quite a common condition and may require a larger number of remedies. We could think of combination etc. of the following rubrics. It is only a suggestion.

(a) Trembling of hands while writing.
(b) Trembling of upper limbs.
(c) Trembling of hands on holding objects.
(d) Trembling, taking hold of, on.
(e) Holding out of hands.
(f) Moving them.
(g) Trembling hands in general.

10. To escape or run after convulsions.
Urge for urination after convulsions.

11. We could extend Boenninghausen's concept of analogy in our need for wider area of selection of a remedy by combining rubrics in certain locations, where signs and symptoms exhibit themselves.

For example. Pain, numbness etc. in the left upper limb and hand could be present in both angina pectoris or cervical spondylosis or spondylitis. Especially for the pathologic rubric of angina pectoris, could we not combine the following rubrics and utilise also the following sensations where relevant.

(a) Numbness (Kent's Repertory page no. 1035)
(b) Pain (K- 1049)
(c) Pain heart extending to left hand (K- 850)
(d) Pain heart extending to back (K- 850)
(e) Pain heart extending to hand (K- 850; Kunjli- 717)
(f) Pain heart extending to neck and shoulder (Kunjli- 717)
(g) Pain heart extending to shoulder (Kunjli- 717)
(h) Pain heart extending to left scapula (Kunjli- 717)
(i) Pain heart extending to left arm (Kunjli- 717)
(j) Pain heart extending to axilla (Kunjli- 717)

For angina, we could also refer to this rubric-

Pain, pressing heart (Kunjli- 725)

Also Chest, constriction heart (Kunjli- 690)

Chest, constriction, grasping sensation (Kunjli- 710)

We have felt the need for combining the same rubrics in certain conditions when we felt the danger of missing the indicated remedy. For example,

(a) Thinking of complaints aggravates and
(b) Occupation ameliorates.

In certain cases, this combination was more fruitful than the single rubric, especially, when we were using them as eliminative symptom or using Kent's artistic method of repertorisation.

These days, the software experts of computerised Repertory have given interesting facilities for doing some of these operations and that does help in the analysis of the similimum. Here I would like to sound a note of warning regarding the place of computer in the practice of Homoeopathic medicine and remedial analysis.

We are confronted with the study of patients, who present themselves with disturbing signs and symptoms. A sign or symptom occurring in any person is not an isolated phenomenon. It may have multiple inter-relationships including causes, associated phenomenon and effects. These may be often apparent or only be a submerged subjective psychological component, sometimes minor, but often of major importance. The responses of the patient to his disorder, his reactions to it and understanding of it are essential, and often deeply revealing parts of the history.

Therefore, the requirement on the part of the physician is-

(a) Understanding and sympathy, kindness and humane consideration.
(b) His intensity of the personal experience in medicine.
(c) Ability in sharing embarrassing confidences and frustrations.
(d) Skill in eliciting stories of the history using 'give and take' philosophy when one is engaged in coming to the most intimate problems.

"Sir James Mackenzie contended that the patient himself is our problem. He is a very cosmos in himself, unlike any other human being that exists. His reactions and response to stimuli, whether of drugs or of disease, are of special interest and importance. Diagnosis must go deeper than the most proximate causation - deeper than those previous conditions which have permitted the disease - deep down into the hidden life - activated, with which curative response is indissolubly bound up." These could have been Hahnemann's words.

Can computers replace the mental processes required in the case analysis and diagnosis ? True diagnosis means deep understanding and can we program such things ?

These subtle and complex aspects of human problems cannot be programmed by computer analysis, Let us, therefore, use computer software for case analysis and repertorisation with great caution, keeping in view its limitations.

Machines can yield highly useful data based upon masses of other data fed into them. Human understanding of human problems is possible only through human thought.

Need for Research in Homoeopathic Repertories

I have already indicated the difficulty of an operator for

the accessibility of certain symptoms and complaints in the existing literature on Repertories, and it may be necessary even to make use of existing rubrics in the Repertory by combining them, especially in certain diagnosed functionally pathological conditions. Apart from it, research workers in the Repertory have to work continuously for indexing of provings of newer drugs, and especially of the confirmed clinical findings of the older drugs in the areas which have not been covered in the existing literature. This activity is very important and I have suggested in some of the professional meetings that we should have an International forum, where we can meet and work together, so that we can take all the sources from all over the world and index them on the commonly agreed basis.

Let us take up, for example, Kent's Repertory- first edition. There are certain rubrics and details which were discarded by the author in the subsequent edition. Could we utilize that material and incorporate it in the newer literature, provided they are dependable and useful ?

For example, he had, as some of the earlier repertorians, placed in one section, alternation of complaints. We could go back again to this pattern and place these alternations in the chapter on Generalities, where they deserve to be placed. Now, we have to hunt through different chapters. For alternation of eruptions with diarrhoea, we may have either to see it in the chapter on Skin or in Rectum, under Diarrhoea.

Similarly,Diarrhoea and Rheumatism.
Diarrhoea and Physical complaints.
Diarrhoea and Heat of head.
Epistaxis and Haemoptysis.
Laryngeal and Uterine complaints.
Mental and Physical symptoms.
Pain in abdomen and Pain in chest.
Palpitation with Pain in lower limbs
and so on.

There are other useful items which could be incorporated. For example, under convulsions, we found in the first edition- Convulsions left side of the body- followed by the sub rubrics

Fright, from- Cuprum.

Motions, from- Graph.

Kent, later, omitted these sub rubrics and put them in the relevant general rubrics and not under the convulsions of the left side of body.

Let us give another example- under faintness (Generalities), he gave in the first edition-

Faintness
forenoon - (certain remedies)
'rising from seat, after'- staph.
'stool, after'- dios.

These two sub rubrics are missing from the later editions. Why? Because he generalized them.

In Faintness from hunger-he gave Crot-c and Sulph but in subsequent editions, he gave Phos and Sulph but not Crot-c.

In the later editions, he gave hardly any attention to aggravation and amelioration due to Moon phases, but in the first edition, he gave a number of remedies.

Moon, new agg.- alum, am-c, bufo, calc, caust, clem, cup, daph, lyc, sabad, sep, sil.

Moon, full agg.- alum, calc, cycl, graph, kali-m, nat-c, nat-m, sabad, sep, sil, spong , sulph, teucr.

Moon, increasing during- arn, clem.

Moon, waning agg.- dulc, thuj

Although Hahnemann and Boenninghausen had observed the influence of Moon Phases on human health and sickness, but it was Dr. C. M. Boger, who made a detailed study and tabulated a chart giving indications of influence of Moon Phases and remedial actions. One may refer to his book, 'Times of the Remedies and Moon Phases'. It may be desirable to reconfirm and extend these researches.

Let us take another example. In the first edition, under Generalities, 'Motions, desire for'- quite a number of remedies have been given. But this rubric is not included in subsequent editions, for which Kent never gave any explanation in the Prefaces or Forewords of the later editions.

Similarly, he has given also other rubrics about motion like 'Motion difficult', 'Motion, false agg.', 'Motion involuntary', 'Motion, sensation of'. These rubrics were taken from Boenninghausen's Therapeutic Pocket Book. Was it his prejudice or were they useless rubrics that he discarded them?

There is another important rubric mentioned in the first edition which had a place in the Generalities, but has been removed to Extremities. It was taken from Boenninghausen, who had registered it as 'Rigidity', as he gave Rigidity in general and Rigidity in Joints. Generalized Rigidity or Stiffness should go to the chapter of Generalities.

In the sub rubrics under Stiffness,

evening, bed, in- sil. is missing.
colic, from- sil. is missing.
descending staircase- rhus-t. is missing.
lying quiet amel.- Gettisburg is missing.
resting, after- rhus-t. is missing.

Also, there was a rubric of 'sensation of stiffness' that also is not given.

Some of the rubrics which had sub rubrics under some definite time modalities were transferred to main general rubric elsewhere.

For example, under 'Weakness,
forenoon,
ascending stairs'- Fago.

underlined sub rubric was merged with
Weakness,
ascending stairs, from.

We Find that Fago is mentioned here. Here he has generalized the modality which was confined only to forenoon.

Many such examples could be cited.

Another rubric taken from Boenninghausen's Therapeutic Pocket Book - 'Yawning agg.', placed under Generalities was also discarded. This could easily be replaced in Kent's Repertory after suitable study. There is also 'Agg. after yawning' and 'Amel. from yawning'.

As indicated earlier, our research activity has, today, to lay a great emphasis on judicious additions to our Repertories, especially of remedies which not only have been proved thoroughly, but also have developed fairly good clinical materials. Take the example of Pyrogen and Calc-fl. Boenninghausen is, of course, very deficient in the listing of both the drugs, but even Kent's Repertory needs additions regarding them. I was surprised to find that there are a lot of rubrics in which both the drugs do not appear in the Kent, in spite of the fact that Materia Medica and clinical provings have emphasized their indications. Somebody has to do this work.

Until only very recent times, Kent's Repertory has gone different editions but they have been only reprints. Recently, Kunjli's work has introduced some additions. Major work was done in Synthetic Repertory. Even Boger's additions were not incorporated. Such a number of important drugs, for example, Kali-m, Nat-p, Calc-fl have not been given due representation.

Certain rubrics have been left incomplete and unsatisfactory. Under Chest, for example, 'Inflammation, lungs, measles, after'- only Kali-c has been mentioned. All of us know from our experience that it is a large rubric. At another place in Kent, under 'Heat', certain vague or outdated terms continue to exist e.g..

'Irritative fever'
'Paroxysmal fever' and
'Pectoral fever'.

In the section on Head, there is no rubric having 'Warts', although, warts have been mentioned in other locations like face, and in clinical experience, we found quite a number of cases having warts on the scalp. In a very recent experience, we found in an old lady, a number of hard warts on the scalp with lot of itching. Sepia 10 M was the only remedy which gave her tangible relief.

In the section of Rectum, page 618 of Kents Repertory, the rubrics 'Flatus, loud, stool, during' contains only four drugs- *aloes,* **Nat-s**, *ph-ac,* and thuj. This is too small a rubric and should contain some remedies like Arg-n, Podo, Calc-p etc.

In the section on Abdomen, the rubric 'Liver, enlarged' (Kent's page 546)- Cardius-marianus is given in the lowest degree. It is not mentioned at all in the enlargement of the left lobe, where it should be given in bold types.

In the Generalities, 'Weakness, eating, after, amel.' has only the remedies Aster, Petr, Sil, and that too, in the lowest degree. This is a most inadequate rubric and should contain a more respectable number of remedies. The section on Generalities has to be augmented and enriched, as that is the most important section, from the point of view of repertorisation. These examples have been taken at random, just to indicate that expert revision of such an important work is long over-due, and it should be done by a team of workers.

Another area where we have to make special addition, is the introduction of Cross References, especially, in the chapter on Mind. Even experienced prescribers need to distinguish different shades of a particular mental symptom.

I am giving below a case from my clinical practice, to show how clinical experience can help us in enriching our Materia Medica and Repertory by unearthing the hidden unknown virtues of some of the even lesser known drugs.

One Mr. R K, aged 27 yrs., approached us on 15th of October 1982 for excessive dandruff and falling of hair, especially during the last three weeks. On inquiring, he disclosed there was lot of work tension during the last few weeks. He complains of headache when he is exposed to the sun for sometime.

In the past history, he had suffered from jaundice, measles, mumps and chickenpox. In the family history he informed that his father suffered from eczema, asthma and diabetes. His mother had hypertension.

He himself is a tense , nervous patient. He weeps when upset emotionally and wants to be alone at that time. He adds extra salt to his food, and is very fond of chilled cold drinks.

Apparently, he appeared to be a case of Nat-m. On 15th of October, he was prescribed Nat-m 200, Nat-m 1M, then Nat-m10M, to be taken on three successive days.

On 19th of November, he reported that his desire for salt has decreased and falling of hair is slightly better. He was kept on sac-lac.

On 29th of November, his hair was still falling, though slightly less, but he was still much worried and anxious, since he was to be married soon. He now developed cramps all over the body. This development forced us to look further into the case, as nature was throwing relevant hints for our next step of action.

We thought of giving Verat-album because of:

(a) Extra salt
(b) Abnormal desire for chilled drinks
(c) Cramps all over the body

He was given Verat 30. Hair falling was further decreased, but did not stop. Later, he was prescribed Verat1M, which stopped fully the abnormal falling of hair and he improved very much in general.

In the Kent's Repertory, we don't find Verat under falling of hair and dandruff. We can certainly add it there. I forgot to mention, he had stopped medication for sometime, and later, there was a relapse of this hair loss, but one dose of Verat 10M restored the normalcy. We could also think of making a note regarding the relationship of Verat to Nat-m i.e. Verat follows Nat-mur, or is complementary to it. This is merely a suggestion, and has to be confirmed in more cases.

There was another incidence of a patient of mine, who had arthritis and muscular rheumatism now and then. His complaints in general were better while eating. He used to have sore pains confined to small spots here and there, but more marked on the right side of body. He was generally better by continued motion, but worse in the morning on beginning to move. He had taken quite a number of remedies, but no definite relief could be obtained. Once he developed pain in the right shoulder, which was better by raising the arm upwards, and worse on letting it hang down, and also better when he played about using his right arm. Sang and Rhus-t gave temporary relief. Two concomitants came to our help. One was twitching of left lower eyelid, and the other was, whenever he sat down for his meals, he ate his food rather hurriedly. He drank water also hurriedly. Zinc, one dose, gave instant relief to the pain in the right shoulder, and in the afternoon, he was not as much fatigued as he usually felt earlier.

Referring to Kent's Repertory, we find that Kent missed to record Zinc in the rubric 'Hurry in general', as well as the rubric 'Hurry in eating and drinking'. I feel that it should be added. In some of the source books. Zinc has been mentioned as having the symptom - Hurried in eating and eating greedily. It may have to be mentioned that some recent workers have added this rubric.

In my clinical experience, I found that Thalaspi bursa pastoris came very handy and useful in cases of haemorrhage in females, due, especially, to fibroids, especially when apparently indicated remedies failed to control the bleeding. It saved a patient's life and my reputation. Another drug which was found to be very useful in such cases was Ficus religiosa. These experiences should stimulate us in making suitable upgrading of our Repertories in general.

Another area, where at times, I have been bogged down, was the Sides of the body. For example, in Kent's Repertory, Ant-t has been listed under side left in the second grade, but in the Hering's Guiding Symptoms, there are more symptoms listed on the right side. It has to be revised. It is also interesting to note that different authors at times changed the indexing of symptoms on sides from one position to another. For example, Boenninghausen, in his earlier writings, listed Apis weakly on the left side, but in later editions, he shifted the emphasis more to the right.

On studying Zinc for example, we found that in the Boenninghausen's Repertory, left sided has greater value than the right, but in the Kent's Repertory, Zinc has been given second grade in the right side, but has not been mentioned in the side left. But on studying the Hering's Guiding Symptoms, we find that there are much more emphasis mentioned in the left side than on the right side. Similarly, Medorrhinum has been mentioned more on the left side than right side in Hering's Guiding Symptoms, but Kent has not listed it at all in any of the sides.

In the clinical literature of Homoeopathic Materia Medica, we come across a lot of references where suppression of one condition like skin eruptions, leads to something much worse. Even in everyday practice, in chronic cases, we tend to suppress certain group of symptoms by a partial similimum, and the result is never ending sickness. It may be desirable to introduce in the Generalities, like, as already suggested- ' alternations of conditions', a paragraph having 'suppression of conditions or symptoms by local applications or crude medications' and certain sickness or illness resulting from such suppressions are also indicated wherever relevant. Suppression of discharges like sweat, menstruation, stools, urine etc. gives rise to disturbed economy. Suppression of skin eruptions may lead to myriad of abnormal functions and structure. All these could be placed under 'Suppression' in the Generalities.

In the earlier chapter, I have already hinted that we may be required to approach different Repertories for working out our cases, depending upon the kind of case we have to deal with. It is often seen that there are cases, where there is paucity of mentals or uncommon generals, and we have to depend upon the particulars that are available. This is often seen in cases of ordinary acute coughs and colds, where we have to depend upon the regional modalities. If there are more of common generals and regional symptoms, then Boenninghausen's approach has to be seriously considered for repertorial analysis and evaluation. It may be mentioned here that numerical totality will pay greater dividends in the working of Boenninghausen or Boger's Boenninghausen's Repertory than with the Kentian Repertory. In the Kentian method, total dependence on numerical summation can be misleading.

In the repertorial exercises, we often come across remedies like Bell, Bry, Sulph, Sep. Nux-v, Puls as the leading remedies. Sepia will emerge much more frequently and prominently than Silicea, and in our actual experience, in many such cases, Silicea happened to be the right remedy. Remedies like Tub, Carc, Syph, Calc-p, Graph, Aur etc. are hardly able to compete with them, although they are deep constitutional remedies. The main reason for this paradox is that some remedies were proved more extensively, and confirmed clinically more often than others. This is evident for a number of pages devoted to these remedies, both in the Allen's Encyclopaedia and Hering's Guiding Symptoms. This is one disability which we have to contend with. We did not make enough efforts, compared to our earlier pioneers in collection and indexing of suitable clinical data. Whether we use any Repertory or Card analysis or computer softwares, this inherent weakness will always tend to vitiate our results, unless we are conscious of this handicap, and try to refer more often to Materia Medica and other storehouses of our experiences.

Very recently, my sister, herself a homoeopathic doctor, suffered frequently from mouth ulcers affecting more of the left side of mouth, tongue and palate. They appeared something like blood boils, bluish dark red papules, and later, bursting and oozing blood. The pain was not that severe, but soreness, and at times, when throat was affected, she had a foreign body sensation and wanted to clear her throat frequently. No thermal modality could be ascertained except that she is very fond of cold chilled drinks, is using lot more salt than others, and cannot relax; desire to move and do things here and there; or go out for a walk; gets depressed often; and likes socialization. There was excessive salivation along with the ulcers. She was hardly totally free from it. We had tried a number of remedies like Phos, Nat-m, Lach, Merc, Nit-ac, Ham etc. but nothing helped her. I decided to give her Carc 200 one dose. The reaction was instantaneous with agg. of symptoms, along with very painful heaviness of the right breast which became sensitive to any touch or clothing. Within a week, all this subsided and for the first time she was free from these mouth sores and remained free for months. Only very recently, after 3-4 months of the last episode, she again developed these sores. Carcinocin 30 was taken without effect. She took a dose of Carc 200 which immediately started an agg. and increased salivation, but it subsided within 3-4 days. She is more relaxed and generally well, although, this time also she had heaviness and soreness of both the breasts for three or four days.

This is a very valuable data and could be utilized as addition to our Materia Medicas, as well Repertories. I may mention that Carc was, most probably, prepared from malignant growth of breast. At present, I have no definite knowledge of origin of Carc as prepared by our pharmacists and laboratories. In this case, the clinical proving of action of Carc on the right breast may be related to this origin.

There is also a great need for preparing an integrated Repertory, as some of the areas covered by Boger in his Repertory, could be brought on without causing any disturbance.

Boger, in his section of General Agg. and Amel., has introduced a rubric 'Agg. when alone', which includes remedies which have various kinds of anxieties, sadness, fear etc. when alone. Kent has not given it at all. He spread it under small different rubrics under Mind. For e.g..-

Sadness when alone
Fear when alone
Anxiety when alone
Weeping when alone.

In my opinion, this broad modality could be kept, may be, under Mind or under Generalities. I am working at an integrated Repertory, which could be much more useful in actual working, especially in computer software.

To help explaining my argument for an integrated

approach in repertorisation, I am reproducing below my article - Remedies affecting the posterior nares. I have added remedies and enlarged the rubrics, introduced a new rubric on Boenninghausen's concept i.e. Remedies affecting the posterior nares.

REMEDIES AFFECTING THE POSTERIOR NARES.

The earlier repertorians had given no attention or space to the Repertory of remedies affecting the posterior nares. Hahnemann, Jahr, and Boenninghausen had not mentioned any remedies for catarrh or catarrhal discharges from the posterior nares. It was Hering, who, in his Guiding Symptoms, described in detail, a number of drugs having catarrhal inflammation of the posterior nares, and gave different kinds of mucous discharges from the posterior nares. Knerr was the first compiler of Repertory to devote a detailed section on it. Gentry, in his Concordance Repertory, also gave different sub-rubrics and mentioned 17 remedies affecting this region.

Lippe mentioned only 1 drug - Cinnabaris for thick, dirty, yellow mucous in lumps from posterior nares.

Kent based his rubrics on Knerr's Repertory, and added some more remedies. It was Hering, who, because of his Germanic thoroughness, had cared to diagnose this condition in the provers, and observed it in the clinical confirmations of drugs.

We still require most painstaking experiments and observations of the effects of the drugs on the post nasal space. It does not require specialists to diagnose this and related conditions. Some drugs are bound to emerge having a more specific influence on the naso-pharyngeal passage. We have to define this influence of such drugs, so that the average practitioners can apply them easily.

Post-nasal catarrhs have been a sore problem with

homoeopaths for a long time. It is more difficult to tackle as compared to sore throats or colds in the chest. Some cases seem to resist even most diligent efforts. This is, unfortunately, a very common condition to be met with, in every day medical practice. We have seen cases suffering from it for years. Such cases do not response except to their constitutional remedies. It would have made our task easier, if homoeopathic prescribers had made careful observations on this aspect of the catarrhal discharges and given us remedies with well defined action on this region. It would have enriched our Repertories.

Recently, I came across a case of a very chronic and inveterate cough which had defied all treatments, homoeopathic and otherwise. It was a dry, irritative type of cough, with practically no modalities. The constitutional symptoms were not prominent. The lungs and sinuses were clear. On examining the throat, I discovered, however, trickling of a thin mucous discharge from posterior nares, with a slight oedema of the uvula. The mucous membrane of the throat seems to be very sensitive. This discharge was the irritant which seemed to excite the cough. Coralium rubrum 30, in repeated doses, helped her considerably. In many cases, I have often observed that the infection from the posterior nares affects the tonsils, and as a result, there are recurrent attacks of tonsillitis and fever.

Anybody who can treat successfully the patient with obstinate catarrhal condition of the posterior nares, is indeed a great prescriber.

Kent has given 3 main rubrics regarding the catarrhal discharges from the posterior nares.

1) Catarrh of the posterior nares.
2) Discharges from posterior nares.
3) Mucous drawn from posterior nares.

Actually, it is not possible to distinguish one from the other. Catarrhal inflammation leads to discharges from the mucous membranes. We should, therefore, have a combined rubric. In my Cards Repertory (Kishore Cards), I have made a separate combined rubric made up of (1) and (2) apart from these as mentioned by Kent. One could have sub-rubrics differentiating different kinds of discharges.

I feel that these rubrics are still far from complete, and need to be augmented with provings as well as clinical verifications. Compared to its prevalence, the disease of posterior nares has received too little attention at our hands. In our case records, we should examine the throats etc. In every case of catarrhal discharges and cough, note down the conditions before and after the treatment. It is this lack of observation, due to which, we have not been able to enrich our literature.

The following rubrics made up our repertoriums of our drugs affecting the posterior nares -

1) Adenoids
2) Catarrah of the posterior nares
3) Crust from posterior nares
4) Diphtheria, posterior nares
5) Discharges from posterior nares
6) Dryness, posterior nares
7) Itching, posterior nares
8) Mucous drawn from posterior nares
9) Obstruction, sensation of, in posterior nares
10) a) Pain, in general, posterior nares
    b) Pain burning -do-
    c) Pain rawness -do-
    d) Pain sore -do-
    e) Pain stitching -do-
    f) Pain tearing -do-
11) Polypus, posterior nares
12) Roughness posterior nares
13) Scraping posterior nares

The following drugs have an affinity of varying degree for the posterior nares. This rubric may be considered as a location of Boenninghausen -

Posterior Nares, Ailments in general-

acon., aesc., agar., agra., all-c., aloe., alum., alumn., alum-sil., am-br., am-c., anac., ant-c., ant-s-aur., ap-g., aral., arg-m., arg-n., ars., ars-i., arnm-tr., asaf., aur., aur-i., aur-m., bals-p., bapt., bar-c., bar-m., bell., berb., bry., bufo, calc., calc-ar., calc-f., calc-i., calc-p., calc-sil., calc-s., camph., canth., **CAPS**., carb-ac., carb-an., carb-v., carl., caust., cench., chin., chr-ac., chlor., cinnb., cist., coc-c., cochl., cop., cor-r., crot-t., dig., dios., echi., elaps., elat., erio., euph., euphr., fago., ferr., **FERR-P**., fl-ac., gal-ac., gels., glyc., gram., graph., helia., **HEP**., hydr., hyper., ichth., ind., iod., irid., iris-v., **KALI-BI**., kali-c., kali-ch., kali-m., kali-p., kali-s., kali-sil., kreos., lac-ac., lac-c., lach., lem-m., lith., lob-c., lob-s., lyc., lyss., mag-c., mag-m., mag-s., maland., malar., manc., mang., med., mentho., meny., merc., merc-c., merc-cy., merc-i-f., merc-i-r., merl., mez., myric., nat-ar., **NAT-C**., **NAT-M**., nat-p., nat-s., nit-ac., nux-m., nux-v., ovi-p., onos., osm., ox-ac., paeon., par., pen., petr., ph-ac., phos., phys., phyt., plb., **PSOR**., puls., quill., ran-b., rhus-t., rumx., sabad., sang., sang-n., sanic., sapin., sel., seneg., **SEP**., sin-n., sol-n., spig., staph., stict., stram., sul-ac., sulph., sumbul., syph., tell., teucr., thlas., ther., thuj., tub., ust., verat., vinc., wye., yucca., zinc., zinc-p., zing.

Adenoids-

agra., bar-c., calc., calc-f., calc-i., calc-p., chr-ac., iod., kali-s., lem-m., lob-s., mez., psor., sang-n., spig., staph., sulph., thuj.

Catarrah of the Posterior Nares-

acon., aesc., alum., alum-sil., alumn., am-br., ant-c., ant-s-aur., arg-n., ars-i., arum-t., aur., aur-i., aur-m., bal-p., bar-c., bar-m., bry., calc., calc-i., calc-s., canth., caust., cinnb., cor-r., echi., elaps., euph., **FERR**., ferr-p., glyc., **HEP**., hydr., iod. **KALI-**

BI., kali-c., kali-chl., kali-i., kali-m., kreos., lem-m., lith-c., lyc., mag-s., manc., mang., med., merc-i-f., merc-i-r., merl., mez., myric., nat-ar., **NAT-C**., **NAT-P**., nat-s., nit-ac., petr., phos., phyt., plb., **PSOR.,** rhus-t., sang., sang-n., sel., **SEP**., sil.,sin-n., spig., staph., stict., syph., teucr., ther. thuj., tub., wye., zinc.

Catarrh and Discharges from Posterior Nares-

This rubric includes-

(1) Catarrh of the posterior nares
(2) Discharge from the posterior nares
(3) Chronic catarrh of the posterior nares; and
(4) Mucous drawn from posterior nares.

acon., aesc., all-c., aloe., alumn.,alum., alum-sil., am-br., am-c., anac., ant-c., ant-s-aur., arg-n.. ars., ars-i.,arum-t., aur., aur-i., aur-m., bals-p., bar-c., bar-m., bell., bell-p., bry., bufo, calc., calc-f., calc-i., calc-s. calc-sil., canth., **CAPS**., carb-ac., carb-an., caust., cench., chin., cinnb., colch., cop., **COR-R.,** dios., echi., elaps., euph., euphr., fago., ferr., **FERR-P**., glyc., gran., **HEP**., hydr., ichth., ind., iod., irid., **KALI-BI.,** kali-c., kali-chl., kali-i., kali-m., kali-si., kreos., lach., lac-ac., lem-m., lith-c., lyc., lyss., mag-s., malar., manc., mang., med., merc., merc-c., merc-i-f., merc-i-r., merl., mez., myric., nat-ar., nat-c-f., **NAT-M**., nat-p., nat-s., nit-ac., nux-v., onos., osm., paeon., penth., petr., ph-ac., phos., phyt., plb., **PSOR.,** rhus-t., rumx., sang., sang-n., sel., **SEP**., sil., sin-n., spig., staph., stict., sulph., syph., tell., teucr., thlas., ther., thuj. tub., wye., zinc., zinc-p., zing.

Chronic Catarrh of the Posterior Nares-

alum., ambr., ant-s-aur., arg-n., ars-i., calc., calc-sil., cinnb., cor-r., fago., glyc., hep., hydr., kali-bi., **KALI-M.,** lem-m., merc-i-r., merc-i-f., nat-ar., nit-ac., penth., phyt., psor., **SANG-N**., **SEP**., sil., sin-n., spig., stict., sulph., teucr., ther., thuj., wye.

Discharges from the Posterior Nares-

all-c., aloe., alum. alumn., arn-br., am-c., anac., ant-c., arg-n., ars., ars-i., arum-t., aur., bar-c., **BELL**., bell-p., bry., bufo., calc., calc-f., calc-s., calc-sil., canth., **CAPS**., carb-ac., carb-an., carb-c., caust., cench., chin., cinnb., colch., cop., **COR-R**., dios., echi., elaps., euph., euphr., ferr., gran., glyc., hep., hydr., iod., irid., **KALI-BI**., kali-c., kali-chl., kali-m., lach., lac-ac., lem-m., malar., mang., med., merc., merc-i-r., mez., nat-ar., **NAT-C**., **NAT-M**., nat-p., nat-s., nit-ac., nux-v., onos., osm., paeon., petr., ph-ac., phos., phyt., plb., **PSOR**., rhus-t., rumx., sang., sang-n., sanic., sel., sep., sin-n., spig., staph., stict., sulph., syph., tell., teucr., thlas., ther., thuj., tub., wye., zinc., zinc-p., zing.

Discharges- Characters

1. ACRID CLEAR MUCOUS-

all-c., ars., ars-i., carb-ac., kali-m., Kreos., lyc., nat-m., sol-n.

2. BLOOOY-

alum-sil., arg-n. (yellow mixed with clots), canth., cench., hep., hydr., kali-bi., lach. (bloody pus), mez., nit-ac., phos., sabad. (bleeding through posterior nares), sang-n., sep. (with yellow green shreds), sulph., tell.

3. BROWN-

kali-bi. (bloody and offensive)

4. CRUSTS, PLUGS. CLINKERS-

alumn., bar-c., calc-ar., cinnb., culx., elaps., hydr., kali-bi., lyc., mang., merc-i., nat-ar., sep., syph.

5. GREEN-

berb., kali-bi., merc., nat-c., phos., puls., sep., thuj.

6. LUMPY-

osm., rumx., teucr.

7. OFFENSIVE-

ant-s-aur., asaf., aur., elaps., graph., kreos., lach., merc., nat-c., nit-ac., sulph., tell., ther., thuj.

8. STRINGY-

am-br., cinnb., coc-c., hydr., kali-bi., sul-ac., yucca.

9. TALLOW LIKE-

cor-r.

10. THICK, TENACIOUS-

alum., am-br., ant-c., calc-sil., carb-an., cench., cor-r., hydr., kali-bi., lem-m., mentho., merc-i-f., nat-c., nat-m., nat-p., nat-s., osm., petr., phos., phyt, sang-n., sapin., sep., sin-n., spig.

11. YELLOW-

alum., ant-s-aur., arg-n., aur., bals-p., berb., bufo, calc., calc-s., caust., cench., cinnb., hep., **HYDR., KALI-BI**., kali-m., kali-s., lyc., meny., merc-i-f., mez., nat-c., nat-m., nat-s., nit-ac., phos., puls., rumx., sang-n., spig., sul-ac., sulph., sumb., ther.

Dryness of Posterior Nares-

acon., aesc., alumn., alum., bell., calc-p., carb-ac., carb-n., carb-v., chin-s., cinnb., cist., coc-c., colch., cor-r., fago., **LYC**., mag-m., maland., merc-c., merl., nat-m., nux-m., onos., petr., phos., plb., rumx., sang., seneg., sep., sil., sin-n., stram., verat., wye., zinc.

Itching in Posterior Nares-

arg-m., kali-p., ran-b., wye.

Membrane-

Dark-

am-br., lach., phyt., yucca.

Red-

arg-n.

Mucous Drawn from Posterior Nares-

alum., alumn., anac., ant-c., arg-n., bry., calc., calc-s., canth., carb-ac., carb-v., caust., cench., chin., cinnb., **COR-R**., elaps., euph., euphr., gran., hep., hydr., ichth., ind., kali-bi., kali-chl., lyss., merc., merc-c., merc-i-f., mez., nat-ar., nat-c., **NAT-M**., nat-p., nit-ac., onos., osm., paeon., ph-ac., phyt., plb., psor., rhus-t., rumx., sin-n., Spig., stict., sulph., syph., tell., teucr., thuj., tub., zinc., zing.

Obstruction, Sensation of, Posterior Nares-

hydr., lac-ac.

Rawness, Scraping and Soreness in Posterior Nares-

acon., aesc., agar., ang., aral., ars., ars-i., arum-t., bapt., carb-v. (on coughing and swallowing), caust., chlor., cist., cop., dig., (morning), ferr-p. (on inspiration), gall-ac., hydr., irid., iris., kali-bi., kali-chl., kali-n., kali-p., kreos., lac-f., lec., mag-c., maland., merc., merc-i-r., mez., nat-ar., **NAT-M.**, nat-s., nit-ac., nux-v., osm., ox-ac., par., penth., phos., ph-ac., quill., sang-n., sep.

Roughness in Posterior Nares-

gall-ac., hyper., staph.

Tumors, Posterior Nares-

osm.

Some of the drugs need clinical confirmation, although they have found a place in some of our standard literature but not found their place in Kent yet.

Fagopyrum for example, has lot of action on the posterior nares: rawness and dryness, formation of dry crusts, granular appearance of the mucous membrane, intolerable itching and burning. This should be used frequently enough.

Aesculus is a neglected remedy. Dr. T.F. Allen pointed that it suits colds which extend downwards from posterior nares: with dryness scraping and burning. At times secreted mucous drops low down and causes choking : patients are weak: with backache, constipation and piles.

Sinapis Nigra may be tried where dryness of the posterior nares is coupled with scanty chunks of tenacious mucous secreted. It requires an effort to dislodge the mucous from posterior nares. The mucous is tasteless and cold, sometimes it causes nausea and even vomiting.

Sensitive to inhaled air is more important in chronic catarrh. This calls for remedies like ars., ars-i., cor-r., fago., ferr-p., hydr., kreos., lith-c., nat-ar., osm., rumx., tub.

Osm. is again a neglected remedy. From its pathogenesis,

it seems to have a very specific action on the mucous membrane of the naso-phyranx. Lumps of mucous are ejected from posterior nares. It is also mentioned as a drug for tumors, in this space.

Although Kent made lot of additions of remedies in different rubrics compared to the earlier authors, but we find that some of the rubrics were not taken up by Kent. It is well known that Kent, to start with, followed Lippe, and took his work as the base to start with. He rationalized many of his rubrics and added remedies, but he did not include others which should have been a useful addition.

For example, Lippe, on page 9 (Indian print), talked about 'solicitude about futurity', which was changed by Kent to 'Anxiety about health'. Lippe had given 'Locality, errors of', but Kent took it away to 'Mistake'. Similarly, 'Dreaming while awake' was kept by Kent as 'Dream, as if in'. There were other symptoms which Lippe had recorded, but they have not found a place in Kent's book.

For example-

1. Anxiety in pregnant women- con.
2. Anxiety at the approach of others- lyc.
3. Anxiety from meditation- ars., calc., camph.
4. Anxiety with pain in abdomen- ars., aur., cham., cup-ac.
5. Anxiety with pain head- acon., alum., bell., bov., calc., carb-v., caust., graph., laur., mag-c., phos., puls., ruta., sulph.

In the last symptom, he changed the remedies and Dr. Kunzli has introduced a few. Kent changed the valuation of remedies in a particular rubric and sometimes changed the remedies also. He must have had some definite reason for doing so. But I think research workers have to go through the original records and provings to confirm them.

I am giving below a few examples. Let us take up the

rubric 'agg. from bread'.

1. Kent has given 31 remedies.

2. In Jahr's Manual, there are 22 remedies. Bar-c is the highest in value (Kent has given second grade)

3. Boenninghausen, in his Anti-psoric Remedies, gave also 6 remedies and Merc is highest.

4. Lippe gave 14 remedies, all in the lowest grade.

5. In my copy of Kent's Repertory, I made the following additions from Boger- Cina., Verat.

Even today, there is a need for having an International forum for reviewing the old literature, as well as covering the newest provings, and set up same standards for doing this work.

For making Kent's Repertory more useful, by adding judicially, rubrics in certain areas, as well as in planning at an Integrated Repertory, I am giving below rubrics in Boenninghausen not to be found in Kent . These were collected by Dr. Elizabeth Wright Hubbard, and published in the journal of the American Institute of Homoeopathy- Aug. 1956.

Rubrics in Boenninghausen not to be found in Kent.
(Elizabeth Wright Hubbard, MD..)

Page No.	Rubric
2.	Disposition generally affected.
18.	Amativeness.
20.	Intellect: activity Intellect: Befogged

23. Drugs which have concomitants of mental symptoms

26. Internal Head: one sided in general

27. External Head: dark hair
External Head: light hair

28. External Head: Beard
External Head: scalp of occiput

29. External Head: hairy siniciput
External Head: scalp of vertex
Internal Head: left side
Internal Head: right side

30. External Head: left side
External Head: right side
Eyes: aqueous humor

32. Eyes: vitreous
Eyes: white of eye (sclerotic)

34. Eyes: inner surface of lids
Eyes: orbits

37. Visions, illusions of form

41. Ears: lobules

42. Ears: left
Ears: right

44. Ears: stopped feeling

45. Nose: back

46. Nose: odors from nose

47. Nose: stopped coryza

49. Nose: accompanying symptoms of nasal discharge

50. (All objective symptoms of Face together)

57. Face: malar bone (antrum)
Face: upper jaw
Face: lower jaw
Face: articulation of jaws

59. Face: left side
Face: right side

61. Teeth: inner gum

77. Diaphragm

79. Epigastrium

80. Loins
Groins (caecum, ileo-caecal region, poupart's ligaments)

81. Pit of stomach
Rings externally
Mons veneris
Abdomen: left side

82. Abdomen: right side

84. Flatulent pain

85. Incarceration of flatus

90. Troubles before stool

91. Troubles during stool
Troubles after stool

92. Ineffectual tenesmus

93. Perineum

100. Troubles before micturition

101. Troubles at beginning of micturition
Troubles during micturition
Troubles at close of micturition
Troubles after micturition

102. Male organs in general: Foreskin

103. Female organs in general
External female organs

108. Menstruation: Gushing

111. Accompanying troubles of Leucorrhoea

114. Accompanying troubles of respiration

116. Cough: Evening with, and morning without, expectoration
Cough: Night with, and day without, expectoration
Cough: Day with, and night without, expectoration

120. Troubles associated with cough
Before and after coughing, and after expectoration
(Agg. page 276 and 281)

123. External Throat and Neck: Nape

124. External Throat and Neck: Thyroid gland
Neck and Nape of Neck: Left side
Neck and Nape of Neck: Right side

125. Sternum and region

126. Heart's action Intermittent
External chest (ribs and muscles)

132. Back of hand

135. Loins (region of hips)
Nates

136. Thigh: posterior part
Thigh: anterior part
Thigh: outer side
Thigh: inner side

138. Tendo achilles
Back of foot (Dorsum)

139. Great toe
Balls of toe

141. Knee, hollow of
Bones of lower extremities in general

143. Asleep feeling, in single parts

144. Benumbing pain

149. Constriction of orifices (sensation of)

153. Crepitation, sensation of

155. Dislocations

157. Dust internal, sensation of

159. Flabby feeling
Forcings

162 Hardened (muscles)

163. Immobility of affected parts

165. Jerking, muscles

167. Motion difficult

168. Mucous secretions increased

181. Splinters, feeling of

194. Vibrations

196. Whiteness (of parts usually red)

200. Glands, ulcers, cancerous

215. Cysts, sebaceous

216. Hair of head falls out: occiput
Hair of head falls out: beard

217. Hair feels pulled

223. Nails generally affected (all nail rubrics together)

239. Wounds: with injuries of bones
Wounds: with injuries of glands

240. Falling asleep late
Sleep prevented by various symptoms
Waking in distress

241. Associated symptoms (see agg. waking- page306)

242. Sleepiness during the day

243. Associated symptoms of sleepiness
Sleepiness caused by various things

246. Symptoms causing sleeplessness

248. Dreams with indifference
Dreams indifferent, to the day's business

250. Dreams waking (daydreaming)

253. Pulse unchanged (with various symptoms)

254. Chilliness in certain parts

255. Chilliness, becomes chilled easily
Chilliness with thirst
Chilliness without thirst

256. Chilliness, symptoms during chill

257. Heat in special parts
Heat in special parts externally

258. Heat, special internally

259. Heat associated symptoms

260. Coldness of special parts

261. Shivering of special parts
Shivering of one side

262. Sweat special parts

263. Sweat without thirst

264. Sweat easy
Sweat odorous, acrid
Sweat odorous of- Camph.

265. Sweat odorous of onions
Sweat odorous of rhubarb
Sweat odorous- sweetish sour
Sweat with associated symptoms
Compound fever in general

268. Before fever
During, fever
After fever.

Aggravation

272. Bending or turning
Bending or turning of affected part
Bent, holding the part
Biting teeth together

273. Blowing nose
Breathing, when not
Breathing, holding breath

273. Bruises
Brushing teeth

274. Chewing, when
Children specially, remedies for
Closing eyes
Closing mouth
Clutching anything

276. Combing hair
Combing hair backwards
Conscious, when half
Dancing, when

277. Drawing off boots
Drawing the limb back
Drinkers, for hard
Drinking, when
Drinking, after

278. Drinking fast

279. Elevation, when on an

281. Expanding abdomen
Expectoration
Expectoration, after
Expiration
Fainting, after
Fatigue

283. Food & Drink, Crumbs
Food & Drink, Garlic, odor of

284. Food & Drink, Oil
Food & Drink, Thought of food, she would like

285. Food & Drink, Water, cold
Food &. Drink, Wine containing lead
Food & Drink, Wine containing sulphur
Gargling
Grasping anything tightly
Heated by the fire

286. Hiccough
Holding together parts.
House, in the
Idleness
Injuries bleeding profusely
Inspiration

287. Inspiration of cold air
Intoxication, after
Jar
Jumping
Labour, manual
Leaning, after
Leaning (against anything)

Leaning, backward
Leaning against a sharp point
Leaning to one side
Licking lips

288. Looking around
Looking straight forward

291. Lying-in women (The puerperal state)

292. Motion after
Motion false
Motion of head
Motion of eyes
Motion of eyelids
Motion of arms

293. Music
Narrating her symptoms
Odor of wood

294. Opening eyes
Opening mouth
Organ, playing the
Persuasion
Piano, playing a
Picking teeth
Pregnancy

295. Putting out the tongue
Raising arms

296. Retching
Retracting abdomen
Riding one leg over the other
Ringing of bell

298. Sewing
Shipboard, on
Shooting
Shrugging shoulders
Singing, after

299. Sitting bent over
Sitting upright

300. Sneezing

301. Splinters
Squatting down
stepping hard
Stooping

302. Stooping, prolonged
Stretching of limbs
Sunburn
Sunrise, after
Sunset, after
Supporting limb

303. Swinging (rocking)

304. Turning around
Turning over in bed

305. Turning head
Turning eyes
Turning neck
Unnatural position
Vertigo, during

306. Violin, playing the
Waking - Being awake at night

307. Walking bent over
Walking on a level
Walking on a narrow bridge
Walking sideways
Walking on a stone pavement
Walking over water

309. Wind, dry
Wind, north

310. Women, for
Writing
Yawning
Yawning, after

Amelioration

311. Bending or turning affected part
Bending backward
Bending inward
Bending sideways
Bending head backwards
Bending holding part bent
Bending head sideways
Biting
Blinking eyes
Blowing nose
Boring in with a finger (ear or nose)
Breath, holding the
Carrying the child in the arms
Chewing

312. Crossing limbs
Dancing
Darkness
Drawing in the affected part
Drinking, after

313. Expiration
Fasting (before breakfast)
Food & Drink, bread

314. Food & Drink, meat
Food & Drink, salt
Gasping
Haemorrhage
Hand, laying, on part
Kneeling
Knitting
Leaning against anything
Leaning against anything hard
Leaning head on anything
Leaning head on one side
loaning head on a table
Licking with a tongue

315. Looking downwards
Looking sideways

316. Lying on hard bed
Lying bent up
Lying horizontally

317. Retracting abdomen
Rising up, from bed
Rising up, from a seat

318. Rising from a seat, after
Shrugging shoulder

319. Sneezing
Stopping hard
Stool, after

320. Stooping
Sucking with tongue
Talking
Tuning at a lathe
Twilight, in the
Tying up the hair

321. Walking bent over
Wiping with a hand
Writing, when
Yawning

I am giving below a few cases for exercise on the art of repertorisation. The readers, especially, the students are expected to work out the cases and then go to the Materia Medica for final confirmation.

REPERTORY TUTORIALS CASE HISTORIES

Case No. 1

Mrs. X - housewife, 44
History of drastic purgatives
Diarrhoea(3) - for 3 days - watery, yellowish, with griping pain(3) in abdomen, agg. before stool; amel. after stool(2)
No response to regular treatment with antibiotics
Clinically - NAD

Case No. 2

Baby boy - 15 days old, returned home from hospital
Soft tender swelling on the scalp since birth in the right parietal region, of the size of a lemon, which has remained the same for 15 days.
Diagnosis -cephalic haematoma
FTND. History of prolonged difficult labor.

Case No. 3

Mr. X
Insanity - tianquilized and sedated in hospital
Refused food
Rudeness
Removed clothings
Passed stool and urine in bed
Gestures - foolish, insensible - catching at imaginary objects in air
Chilly patient

Case No 4

Pious old lady - 70 years
Raving maniac
Restless(3) - agonized tossing about
Ailment resulting from fright (son not returning home at the usual hour, and sensing danger to bis life)

Case No. 5

Miss S.L. - 20 years
Acute depression, (History of 2 previous attacks)
Gazing, staring, face unmoved
Silent, taciturn. Agg. after quarrel with mother
Laughs immoderately
Screams and shouts against mother
Not interested in changing dress
Violent - abusive, lewd talk
Shameless. Behaves in obscene manner- wants to be naked. Eats hurriedly. Thirstless.
Lewd behaviour agg during menses.
sleepless
Suicidal tendencies (threat of drowning)
Erotic insanity.

Case No. 6

Boy 3.5 years
Pyelitis
Fever agg. evening
Scanty painful urination - pain in urethra after urination
Thirst ice cold water
Throat pain amel. cold drinks
Hot (2). Likes sweets

Case No. 7

Mr. X, 21 yrs. Engineer.
Chronic sinusitis, chronic liver affection and dysentery.
Sensitive, emotional, shy.
Modest, diffident
Repressed emotions
Hot patient
Sun headaches.

Case No. 8

Surgeon aged 45 years
Ball- sensation in the forehead
Emptiness in occiput
Outbursts of temper(3), especially at opposite sex.
Suppressed anger and chagrin (Dominating wife).

Case No. 9

Old man, 75 years
impotence (3)
Sexy (3)
Tobacco agg. (3) - smoking and chewing.

Case No. 10

Male, 35 years
Anxiety neurosis with hypochondriasis
Troubles commenced after an unpropitious prediction that his only newborn son will die soon (Ailments from fright and grief.)
Sadness, despair
Unpleasant thoughts torment him
Dwells on past disagreeable occurrences
Indifferent to pleasures
Hot patient (2)
H/o married against wish of his parents
Strained relations with his parents.

Pre-illness personality-

Independent minded
Brooding type- nurses the grudge if insulted or injustice done.

Case No. 11

Lady aged 60 years
Chronic malaria- 20 yrs., with cachexia
chills; 10 am. agg. before fever
not amel. by warmth
Thirst for cold water
Fever 104° F lasting whole day
Fever with hammering headache, extreme weakness and discomfort in chest
Perspiration amel. all complaints.

Case no. 12

Girl- 6 years
Bedwetting (3) agg. night
White spots nails
Chilly
Cold sweats forehead agg. sleep

Case No. 13

Male - 28 years - Married - Engineer
Chronic urethritis, treated with local silver nitrate
Blood KT negative
Discharge culture : B Pyocyaneous
Sensitivity Test : Bacteria resistant to practically all antibiotics.
Discharge : Yellowish-green, thin gelatinous, slimy continuous
Burning pain at the tip of penis agg. during and after urination.
Robust appearance, short, healthy
Thirsty for large amount of cold drinks(3), yet urine scant
Can tolerate icy cold drinks
Desires fan (3)

Case No. 14

Mr. X-41 yrs - Engineer
Headaches agg. reading, with lachrymation and burning in eyes
Agg. 10 am. till evening
Agg. sun in summer
Amel. cold bath, open air
Head heavy, as if pain in eyeballs
Vertigo agg. sun
Hot patient(3), weakness, exhaustion agg. sun
Clinically - NAD. Stout built

Case No. 15

Baby girl - 3 years
General debility, under developed
Scrawny neck, enlarged abdomen
Running nose
Hard knotty stools
Desire salt
Hot patient Sweat scalp agg. sleep

Case No. 16.

Mr. R.H.P. - young man - 23 years
Subject to very severe congestive headaches
A large, fleshy, full- blooded person
Headache- forehead and temples, accompanied with throbbing
Head fees as if it would burst
Agg. stooping forward, noise, usually agg. 3 p.m..
Intolerance of light, must close his eyes
Cannot lie down
Vertigo and sometimes vomiting of bile
Face becomes red with throbbing of carotids.

Case No. 17

Mr. A.R.K. - 34 years
Ate freely of fruits before retiring. During the night was attacked with cutting pain in the bowels followed by vomiting and profuse, watery stools.

Presenting symptoms-

Before stool - severe cutting pain in the bowels
During stool - nausea, vomiting and great weakness with pinching colic
Pallid countenance with cold sweat on the forehead
After stool great sense of weakness and emptiness in the abdomen
Stools are profuse and watery
Countenance pale, eyes sunken, lips dry and blue, tongue cold
Great thirst for very cold and acid drinks
Nausea from the least motion
Very painful cramps of the legs
The skin is cold and lifeless, remaining in ridge when pinched
The breath is cold, voice hoarse and weak.

Case No. 18

Mr. A.G. - 19 years
Second week of typhoid fever.
Mind is confused, wandering when closing the eyes.
Falls asleep in the middle of a sentence.
Stupor and delirium at night
Head feels as if scattered about the bed, tosses about to get himself together, cannot sleep on this account.
Face is hot, dark red, with heavy besotted expression.
Tongue coated brown in the centre.
Teeth and lips covered with sordes.
Breath very offensive.
Frequent diarrhoeic discharges, thin and dark, of an exceedingly offensive odor.
Flesh seems sore.
Complaints of bed being too hard.
Aching of the lower limb.
Slides down in bed, adynamic.

Case No. 19

Mr. K. - 52 years
Applies for relief of periodical headaches which usually commences in the morning, increased by eating.
Feels better lying down indoors.
Pain is usually located in occiput, very severe, worse from mental work, noise, coffee, stimulants or eating.
Often there is a sense of pressure on top of the head, as if a weight was pressing down into the brain.
Determination of blood to the head with sense of heat and burning in it.
Face red. Head sometimes feel very large.
Headache lessens towards evening.
Appetite good but eating causes distress in epigastrium after 2 or 3 hours of eating.
Sense of feeling of weight in the region.
Bowels constipated. Stools- large, hard and difficult.

Alternate diarrhoea with constipation.
History of piles operated.
Because of headache, has taken a lot of purgatory treatmemt. He often wakes up at 3 am., lies awake for 1 or 2 hours, feeling weak and languid.

Case no. 20

Miss K. - 6 years
Recently had an attack of scarlet fever and went out for playing, before desquamation. The condition, now was as follows-

Urine scanty and dark colored.
Swelling of feet and ankles.
Oedematous condition of the eyelids.
Yellowish, watery diarrhoea, worse in the morning.
Complaints of stinging pains like bee stings that occur in different parts of the body.
Great sensitiveness to touch.
Feels much better in the cold air.
All the symptoms agg. in the warm room.

Case No. 21

A young woman - 22 years
Received a kick in the stomach from a horse 3 months ago.
Vomited a large amount of blood.
Present symptoms are soreness all over the body as if bruised.
Bed on which she lies feels too hard.
Bitter, nasty taste in the mouth, foul, like spoiled eggs.
Repungence for food.
Longing for sour things and alcoholic drinks etc.
Stomach tolerates little or no food.
Eructations tasting like rotten eggs.
Considerable flatus from bowels that smells like rotten eggs.
Bowels constipated, always regular before receiving the injury.
Sluggish state of the mind, indifference.

Case No. 22

Mrs. R.R. - 41 years
Suffering from Bacillary dysentery.
Loose motions, large, at times offensive.
H/O jaundice 2 months ago.
Liver enlarged about 1 finger.
The diarrhoea has been appearing off and on.
The examination of stool reveal bacillary dysentery.
Appetite very poor. Takes lot of neat salt
Very fond of ice-cream and cold drinks.
Passes stool while sitting for urination.
Passes lot of flatus with the stools.
During acute stage she passed stools involuntarily while passing flatus.

Case No. 23

Mr. H.F. - 39 years
Occupation - Banjo maker.
Eruptions on forearms, lumbar region and on the legs below the knees.
Eruptions consists of an undefined red base covered with yellowish white scales.
Itching when the patients becomes warm from exercise or from heat of the bed.
Scratching followed by intense burning.
Many desquamated scales in the bed in the morning.
Rheumatic stiffness of the knees, worse especially on rising from a sitting position.
Belching in the early morning and after meals.
Constipation. Appetite easily satisfied.
Extreme thirst.

Inability to concentrate.
Faulty memory.
Dullness. Mental sluggishness. Difficult comprehension.
All aggravated by mental exertion.

Perspiration offensive, even to the patient
Better in general from moving about.

Case No. 24.

Mrs. T. - 39 years - mother of 5 children.
Very fleshy and of fair complexion.
Has been troubled since a baby with eczema, which disappears at time but always returns sooner or later.
Has tried everything but homoeopathy.
Present condition- Rawness and soreness in flexors of limbs, between fingers, bebind ears etc.
Eruptions of vesicular character exuding a profuse, watery, sticky fluid which forms scabs.
Skin is in an unhealthy condition.
Wounds do not heal well, ulcerate leaving painful scars.
Skin inclined to crack.
Nipples always sore and cracked during lactation.
Nails of hands and feet rough and deformed.
Ends of fingers often crack.
Bowels constipated. Stools large and knotty.

Case No. 25

An adult male, has been sick in bed for 2 days. He is restless.
His chief complaint is an agonizing toothache.
His neck is sore and his ear aches.
He resents being spoken to, and shows his irritability in other ways.
One cheek is red and the other pale.
He sweats freely. He does not sleep well.
No other symptom of value could be obtained, except after hot coffee he is much worse. He frequently drinks cold water, which gives temporarily relief.

In the end, I hope that I have been able to excite the readers' interest in Homoeopathic Repertories in general, and bring to their attention the different ways the different workers made their effort in enriching our literature. My colleague, Late Dr. Sarabhai said that our clinical work must be associated with our Repertories. We have not merely to take out from this vital storehouse, we must also add to it our experiences.